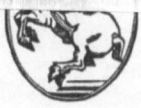

ACTA NEUROCHIRURGICA
SUPPLEMENTUM 23

Stereotactic Treatment of Epilepsy

Symposium under the Sponsorship
of the European Society for Stereotactic
and Functional Neurosurgery, Bratislava 1975

Edited by
F. J. Gillingham, E. R. Hitchcock, P. Nádvorník

SPRINGER-VERLAG
WIEN NEW YORK

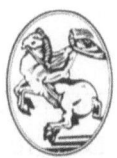

F. John Gillingham

Professor of Neurosurgery, University of Edinburgh,
Western General Hospital and Royal Infirmary, Edinburgh

Edward R. Hitchcock

Consultant Neurosurgeon, University of Edinburgh
Western General Hospital and Royal Infirmary, Edinburgh

Pavel Nádvorník

Professor of Neurosurgery, Comenius University,
Bratislava-Kramáre

With 99 Figures

Library of Congress Cataloging in Publication Data.

Main entry under title:
Stereotactic treatment of epilepsy. (Acta neurochirurgica: supplementum; 23.) Includes bibliographies.
1. Epilepsy-Surgery-Congresses. 2. Stereoencephalotomy-Congresses. 3. Epilepsy-Congresses. I. Gillingham, Francis John. II. Hitchcock, Edward Robert. III. Nádvorník, P., 1923—. IV. European
Society for Stereotactic and Functional Neurosurgery. [DNLM: 1. Epilepsy-Surgery-Congresses.
2. Stereotaxic technics-Congresses. W1 AC8661 no. 23/WL385 S839 1975]. RD594.S74. 617'48.
76-25838.

ISBN-13:978-3-7091-8446-2   e-ISBN-13:978-3-7091-8444-8
DOI: 10.1007/978-3-7091-8444-8

Contents

Acta Neurochirurgica, Suppl. 23, 1—2 (1976)

Department of Surgical Neurology, University of Edinburgh, Scotland

Introduction

F. J. Gillingham

The earliest scientific surgical approaches to the control of the epileptic discharge were aimed at defining the focus of origin and then its ablation by open operative surgery. The contributions of Penfield and his colleagues in Montreal to this field of work are notable for painstaking study and additions to knowledge. The problem has been, however, that the results of focal ablation are not always satisfactory except in temporal lobe epilepsy where the results are conspicuously better. There is also the difficulty of unequivocal definition of the focus of discharge in many instances and even when it is defined and satisfactorily excised the epileptic problem may remain because of established secondary foci which may be inaccessible to ablation by open operation. We then still have the possibility of the existence or not of a primary subcortical focus for the origin of the epileptic discharge: so-called centrencephalic epilepsy, e.g. petit mal. This remains unproven and consequently speculative.

It is not surprising therefore that an entirely new approach to the problem should have been sought, aiming to interrupt the conduction pathways of the epileptic discharge. As one might imagine new ideas are seldom new even in stereotactic surgery. In 1951 Spiegel and Wycis had already obtained promising results in two cases of petit mal epilepsy from lesions placed in the intralaminar nuclei and later they reported success with palliolotomy and pallido-amygdalotomy leading to the more recent work on the effects of amygdalotomy by Reichert (1951), Narabayashi (1958), Chitanondh (1966), Vaernet, Hitchcock and others more recently.

A bonus arising from surgical explorations of the medial structures of the temporal lobe was the immediate re-appraisal of the behaviour disorders and their relief by surgical means as the limbic system was further defined. Thus the field of functional neurosurgery has further broadened controversial though this subject and indeed the results of amygdaloidotomy may be.

It was Jinnai in 1963 who first published his work on the control of intractable epilepsy by interruption of conduction pathways of the epileptic discharge using stereotactic lesions in the field of Forel. This was followed by lesions in the thalamus by Mullen in 1967, and by capsular lesions by Bertrand in 1970 and myself in 1971. In the macroscopic form this was carried out by section of the inter-hemispheric cerebral connections by open operation by Vogel in 1969. This has been an important contribution to knowledge of the basic mechanisms of the propagation of the epileptic discharge and to our understanding of brain function but I would look to stereotactic techniques for the greater development potential. There are, of course, limitations. Bilateral lesions of effective size are difficult to achieve without side effects, particularly in respect of speech (notably dysarthria) and yet are essential if intractable epilepsy is to be con-trolled in severity and frequency. Increased accuracy of target siting and control of the size of lesion are not the whole answer for inevi-tably there are areas where important neuronal circuits are very crowded. But we should not underestimate the contribution of surgery. Increasingly the medical therapy of epilepsy is under scrutiny. Excessive medication for the reasonable control of severe and frequent attacks often reduces the patient to a low level of intel-lectual and physical activity. Also the unpredictable results of medication at acceptable levels, because of variable detoxication by the individual patient, lead to considerable insecurity at times for the patient and his physician. This is particularly so for Phenytoin.

But we should be encouraged in other ways for stereotactic surgery with all its opportunites for recording (during operation and contin-uously on a long term basis) stimulation and biopsy histochemical studies will inevitably advance knowledge not only of epilepsy but also of brain function itself. It has already done so and the notable recent contribution has been the cerebellar stimulation studies of Cooper, although the long term therapeutic benefits have yet to be defined.

Author's address: Prof. F. J. Gillingham, Department of Surgical Neurology, The Royal Infirmary, Lauriston Place, Edinburgh EH 3 9YW, Scotland.

Acta Neurochirurgica, Suppl. 23, 3—8 (1976)

Istituto di Neurochirurgia dell'Università Cattolica, Roma, Italy

"Chronic" Electrodes in SEEG Exploration of Partial Epilepsies *

C. Carapella, G. Colicchio, A. Gentilomo, G. F. Rossi,
and M. Scerrati

With 2 Figures

The rationale of surgical treatment of partial epilepsy is based on a series of different criteria. One of them is the information given by the study of electrocerebral signals on the development of the epileptic process and, in particular, on the topographic location of the lesional-functional epileptogenic complex (see Rossi et al. 1974, for an extensive review on the subject). Actually, there are patients in whom such a location can be defined only on the basis of the analysis of brain electrical activity which therefore becomes a factor of paramount importance for a reliable surgical indication. The use of depth electrodes—or stereoelectroencephalography (Bancaud et al. 1965)—is of substantial help in this connection. The experience accumulated in the last twenty years has brought a large convergence of opinion on the general principles, or tactical considerations, which are the basis of an stereoelectroencephalographic exploration of an epileptic patient regarded as a possible candidate for surgical treatment (Bancaud et al. 1965 and 1973; Talairach et al. 1974; Crandall 1973; Walter 1973; Rossi 1973; Rossi et al. 1974). However, in our opinion, a particular point deserves further discussion, namely the importance of the duration of the stereoelectroencephalographic exploration in order to obtain sufficient and reliable information. Our personal experience indicates that, in most cases, such a goal can be reached only, or can be greatly facilitated by utilizing prolonged and repeated recording, requiring "chronically" implanted intracerebral electrodes. The following findings illustrate our views.

---

* Research supported by the Consiglio Nazionale delle Ricerche.

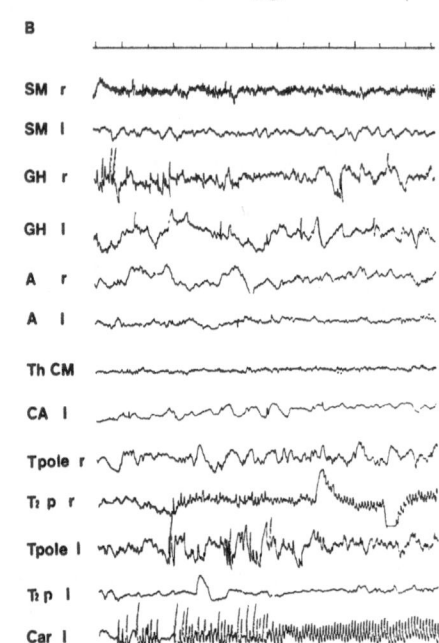

Fig. 1. SEEG recordings. Variations of the ictal epileptic activity on different days. A: first day after electrode implantation. B: after three days. In this and in Fig. 2: *l* left; *r* right; *SM* supplementary motor area; *Th CM* centromedian thalamic nucleus; *Car* temporo-parieto-occipital region; *T pole* temporal pole; *CA* Ammon's horn; *A* amygdala; *GH* hyppocampal gyrus; *T₂* temporal neocortex; *a* anterior; *m* medium; *p* posterior

Material and Method

The findings to be reported have been obtained during 19 chronic stereo-electroencephalographic explorations performed on 17 patients. All patients (7 males, 10 femals; aged between 12 and 49 years) had suffered for several years from frequent epileptic seizures of partial origin. Pharmacological treatment was not sufficient to control the seizures.

The intracerebral multi-electrodes have been built in our laboratory and were introduced into preselected brain sites with the use of the Talairach stereotaxic instrument, following a technique reported elsewhere (Colicchio *et al.* 1973 a).

The recording of the patient's electrocerebral activity usually started on the day of electrode placement. Pin electrodes inserted into the scalp permitted the simultaneous recording of conventional EEG. During the recording, the patient was kept in bed or in an arm-chair. The electrocerebral signals were recorded by one 16 channel and one 10 channel electroencephalographs (OTE-Galileo) and

stored on magnetic tape (14 and 7 channel Philips Analog) for automatic elaboration. Continuous TV monitoring was carried on to record the clinical aspects
of the seizures and to permit their careful correlation with the electrographic
patterns.

The duration of the exploration in the patients considered has been 10 to
30 days. All patients were examined every day, in different physiological conditions (including nocturnal sleep) and under different amount of pharmacological
antiepileptic treatment. No septic complications have occurred so far.

Results

1. Variations of the Ictal Epileptic Activity on Different Days

Ictal discharges, sometimes accompanied by ictal clinical manifestations, can be recorded from different brain structures on different
days.

An example of this is illustrated in Fig. 1, reporting samples
of the stereoelectroencephalogram of a patient with partial seizures of
complex symptomatology which were regarded as being of temporal
origin. Part A of the figure illustrates the recording on the first day
after implantation of depth electrodes; part B illustrates the record
obtained after 3 days. In A, an ictal discharge arises from the neocortex of the right temporal pole; this was the only seizure occuring
on this day. In B, an ictal discharge originates in the left temporo-
parieto-occipital region and then involves the controlateral temporal
neocortex. Other seizures occurred and were recorded on the 6th,
7th and 9th days of exploration. It was confirmed that they could
arise from the right as well as the left temporal lobe.

2. Variations of the Interictal Epileptic Activity in Different Physiological Conditions

The interictal epileptic activity shows large quantitative variations in relation to the physiological state of the patient. These variations become particularly evident during sleep. Fig. 2, A, illustrates
the amount and distribution of the interictal epileptic discharges of
one of our patients regarded as a temporal epileptic during relaxed
wakefulness; antiepileptic medication had been reduced for several
days; numerous epileptic potentials are recorded from most of the
cerebral structures explored; they appear to prevail in the
right temporal lobe. Fig. 2, C, illustrates the recording on
the same day during the REM phase of sleep: the interictal epileptic
activity is on the whole strickingly reduced. However, consistent epileptic discharges are still recorded from the temporal neocortex of the right temporal lobe.

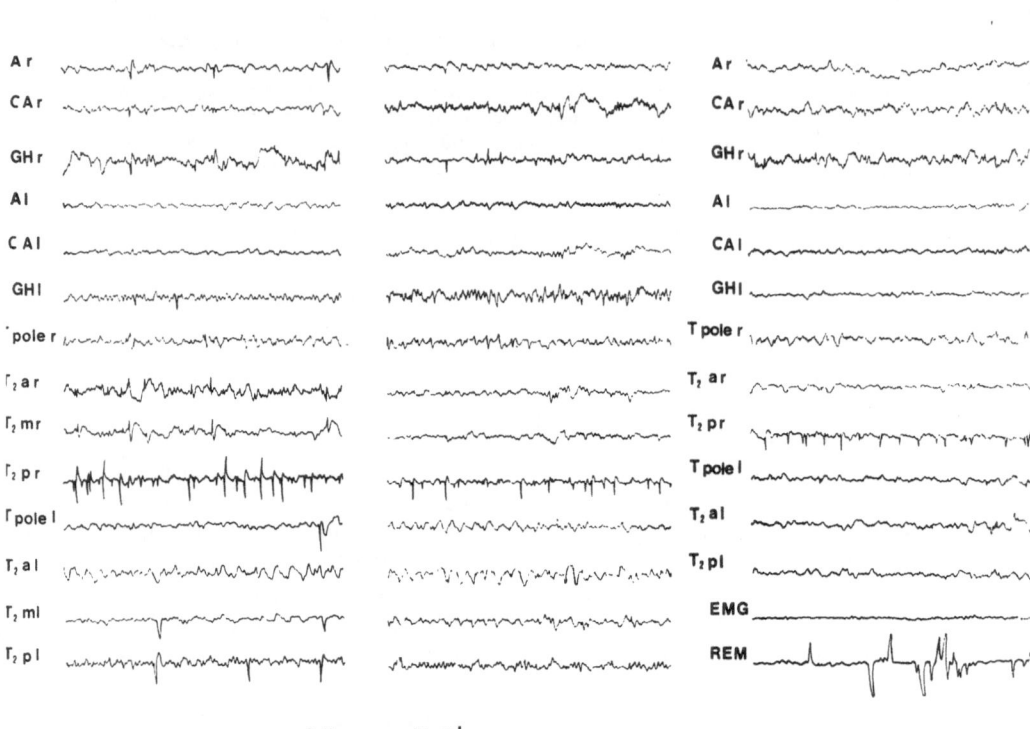

A.N.   50μV ⌐
                   1 sec

Fig. 2. SEEG recordings. Variations of the interictal epileptic activity in different physiological conditions and in relation to the pharmacological treatment. A: relaxed wakefulness; reduced antiepileptic medication; B: relaxed wakefulness; complete antiepileptic medication; C: stage *REM* of sleep; reduced antiepileptic medication. *EMG* electromiogram from submental muscles; *REM* rapid eye movements

3. Variations of the Interictal Epileptic Activity in Relation to the Pharmacological Antiepileptic Treatment

The epileptic activity obviously shows quantitative variations in relation to the use of antiepileptic drugs. The consistent overall decrease of the interictal epileptic potentials due to the latter results from the comparison of parts A and B of Fig. 2. However, as shown in part B not all the epileptic activity recorded appears equally affected by the pharmacological treatment: abundant convulsive potentials persist in the right temporal lobe, and particularly in the right temporal neocortex.

Discussion

From the examples reported above, which were taken from our material of "chronic" stereoelectroencephalographic explorations, we note that:

1. The epileptic activity can show considerable variations in amount and topographical distribution. This appears true for both the ictal and interictal activities. These variations can to a certain extent be related to the change of the physiological conditions of the patient, or to certain manipulations, as for instance the antiepileptic pharmacological treatment. In most cases, however, they occur without any apparent relation to factors which could be recognized. The protracted recording, over a period of several days, can demonstrate this variability of the dynamic of the epileptic process.

2. Not all the recorded epileptic activity is equally subject to the variations mentioned above. There are patients in whom the epileptic potentials recorded from certain structures appear to maintain a steady level of discharge through the whole time of the study and independently of the physiological state of the subject or of the pharmacological antiepileptic treatment. This becomes particularly evident when one carefully analyzes the behaviour of the interictal epileptic potentials (Colicchio et al. 1973 b), which on this basis may acquire a particular diagnostic value (Rossi 1973; Rossi et al. 1974).

3. The stereoelectroencephalographic study limited to the relatively short time allowed by an "acute" exploration may not permit the recognition of the phenomena illustrated and commented upon in 1 and 2 above. Its limitations appear particularly marked when one has to deal with a patient suspected of suffering from a so-called multifocal form of epilepsy.

To conclude, we think that the use of "chronic" intracerebral electrodes is quite useful in verifying the consistency of the electrocerebral phenomena observed. Their use, therefore, increases the value of stereoelectroencephalography as a mean for judging the physiopathological significance and diagnostic value of the recorded epileptic abnormalities.

Summary

The advantages of the stereoelectroencephalographic study of epileptic patients prior to surgical treatment through "chronically" implanted multielectrodes are illustrated and discussed. The reliability of the information provided by the cerebral electrical activity is strengthened by recording the patient on different days, in different physiological conditions and under different pharmacological treatment. The consistency of some of the electrical abnormalities recorded gives them a strong diagnostic value.

References

Bancaud, J., Talairach, J., Bonis, A., Schaub, C., Szikla, G., Morel, P., Bordas-Ferrer, M. (1965), La stéréo-électroencéphalographie dans l'épilepsie, pp. 321. Paris: Masson.

Bancaud, J., Talairach, J., Geier, S., Scarabin, J. M. (1973), EEG et SEEG dans les tumeurs cérébrales et l'épilepsie, pp. 351. Paris: Edifor.

Colicchio, G., Gentilomo, A., Pola, P., Scerrati, M. (1973), Utilità della esplorazione stereoelettroencefalografica „cronica" nella epilessia. Riv. Neurol. *43*, 320—327.

— — Rossi, G. F., Troiani, D. (1973), Analisi dei segnali elettrocerebrali epilettici intercritici registrati mediante elettrodi impiantati „cronicamente" nell'uomo. Riv. Neurol. *43*, 314—320.

Crandall, P. H. (1973), Developments in direct recordings from epileptogenic regions in the surgical treatment of partial epilepsies. In: Epilepsy. Its phenomena in man, 391 pp. (Brazier, M. A. B., ed.), pp. 288—310. New York: Academic Press.

Rossi, G. F. (1973), Problems of analysis and interpretation of electrocerebral signals in epilepsy. A neurosurgeon's view. In: Epilepsy. Its phenomena in man, 391 pp. (Brazier, M. A. B., ed.), pp. 259—285. New York: Academic Press.

— Gentilomo, A., Colicchio, G. (1974), Le problème de la recherche de la topographie d'origine de l'épilepsie. Schweiz. Arch. Neurol. Neurochir. Psychiat. *115*, 229—270.

Talairach, J., Bancaud, J., Szikla, G., Bonis, A., Geier, S., Vedrenne, C. (1974), Approche nouvelle de la neurochirurgie de l'épilepsie. Méthodologie stéréotaxique et résultats thérapeutiques. Neurochirurgie *20*, Suppl. 1, pp. 243.

Walter, R. D. (1973), Tactical considerations leading to surgical treatment of limbic epilepsy. In: Epilepsy. Its phenomena in man, pp. 391 (Brazier, M. A. B., ed.), pp. 99—119. New York: Academic Press.

Authors' address: C. Carapella, M.D., G. Colicchio, M.D., A. Gentilomo, M.D., G. F. Rossi, M.D., M. Scerrati, M.D., Istituto di Neurochirurgia dell'Università Cattolica, Roma, Italy.

Acta Neurochirurgica, Suppl. 23, 9—14 (1976)

Centre for Cerebral Neurophysiology of National Council of Researches;
Institute of Neurophysiopathology of the University, Genoa, Italy

The Role of Focal and Extrafocal Structures in the Triggering of Epileptic Spikes: An Experimental Study

F. Ferrillo, R. Amore, M. Palestini*, and G. Rosadini

With 2 Figures

Epileptic discharges from a cortical focus tend to involve other cerebral areas particularly surrounding neuropil, homotopic contralateral cortex and subcortical centres. They can also induce the development of independent epileptic foci in distant areas of the brain. In these studies the topographic distribution of extrafocal discharges and the chronology of their appearance as independent phenomena have been mainly used (Wilder 1972). On the other side, problems related to morphology and temporal relationships among discharges simultaneously recorded in different structures have been almost neglected (Tharp 1971; Mares 1973).

Preliminary data from our group obtained by a computer averaging technique (Rosadini *et al.* 1974) have shown that the caudate nucleus is the first structure to be involved in the propagation of epileptic spikes from a neocortical focus and that the same structure is also able to elicit time-locked discharges on the focus (Ferrillo *et al.* 1973; Palestini *et al.* 1974).

The present research is designed to investigate the interactions between caudate nucleus and the primary neocortical focus during the development of a cobalt-induced experimental epilepsy in the cat.

Material and Methods

10 adult cats weighing 2.5–3 kg have been used. Under ether anaesthesia trephine openings were made in the skull, the trachea exposed and incised and a tracheal cannula introduced; animals immobilized by intraperitoneally injected

---

* Centro de Psiquiatria Experimental, Universidad de Chile, Santiago de Chile.

D. Tubo-curarine, were maintained in the holder of a stereotactic apparatus and artificially ventilated; wounds and pressure points were anaesthetized with procaine. Cortical electrodes were applied to sensorimotor cortex and depth electrodes inserted in the head of the homolateral caudate nucleus in all experiments. Several structures of both hemispheres including extrafocal cortices, the postero-lateral nucleus of the thalamus, centrum median and the mesencephalic reticular nucleus were alternatively tested. Reference leads against an indifferent electrode on the neck muscles were also used.

The epileptogenic focus was obtained injecting a small amount (10 mg) of cobalt powder in the sensorimotor cortex. The EEG from the various structures was recorded both on paper (OTE Galileo apparatus) and on magnetic tape (Philips ANA-LOG 14), starting one hour before the injection of cobalt and continuing for 12 hours. At the end of the experimental session cats were deeply anaesthetized with nembutal and sacrificed perfusing their brains with 10% formalin saline solution. The site and size of the focus and electrode positions were checked histologically.

The averaging of epileptic potentials (AEP) was carried out off-line by a PDP 12 computer using the technique mentioned above (Rosadini *et al.* 1974).

Results

All animals developed a fairly homogeneous epileptic pattern. The standard pattern of EEG obtained was characterized by periods of desynchronization and short episodes of synchronization, remained substantially unaltered during the first hour from the cobalt injection. During the second hour focal spikes appeared which successively propagated first to the homolateral caudate nucleus (third hour) and later to the other explored structures. Short seizures occurred at first circumscribed to focal area (fifth hour); later they become progressively longer and involved the other structures till their generalization (tenth hour).

The averaging process performed using the focal spikes as trigger permits the following observations:

1. In the early stages of development of the focus epileptic discharges are strictly circumscribed to the focal area; the AEP shows diphasic potentials (negative-positive) in focal leads; no activity time-locked to focal discharges is evident in the caudate nucleus (Fig. 1. T = 50′).

2. Successively, when the conventional EEG does not show any propagated activity, the AEP allows the detection of well featured spike-like potentials in the caudate nucleus; those potentials appear to be time-locked to the focal ones, of opposite polarity and lagging behind them (Fig. 1. T = 110′).

3. In more advanced stages the conventional EEG shows well recognizable spikes both in the focus and in the caudate nucleus. The

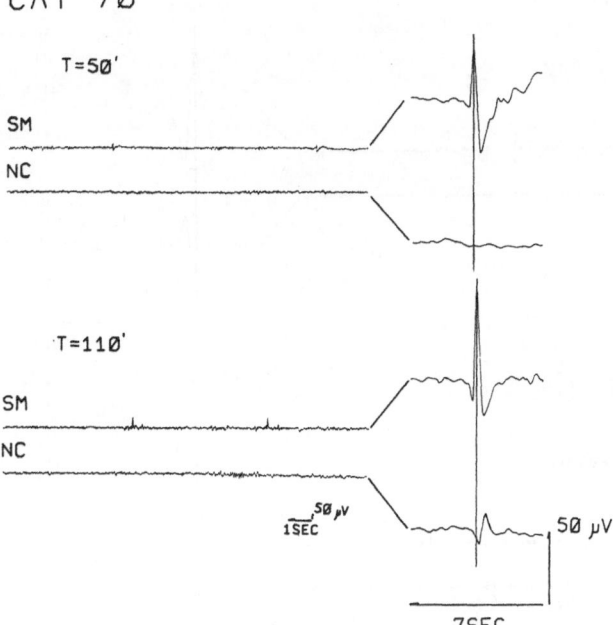

Fig. 1. Early stages of cortical focus. On the left EEG from sensorimotor cortex (*SM*) and caudate nucleus (*NC*). On the right averaged spikes (25 samples) show the absence of spikes in caudate nucleus at T = 50′ and their presence at T = 110′ (T = minute after cobalt)

AEP suggest to distinguish two main groups of local spikes differing both in morphology and in their temporal relations with the caudate potentials. More precisely, diphasic, focal leading spikes belong to the first group; monophasic potentials, which are longer in duration and lag behind caudate spikes, characterize the second group. Spikes belonging to the two groups are mixed in the same epoch of recording (Fig. 2. Cat 72).

4. The AEP performed on spikes that in our experimental model can be easily regarded as starters of seizures shows an analogous behaviour. In this instance too, two types of focal spikes coexist: the diphasic ones leading caudate potentials, the monophasic ones lagging behind them (Fig. 2. Cat 55).

5. In all other explored structures spikes time-locked to the focal ones are detectable in later stages of the experiment; they appear always delayed as regards the focal and caudate activities.

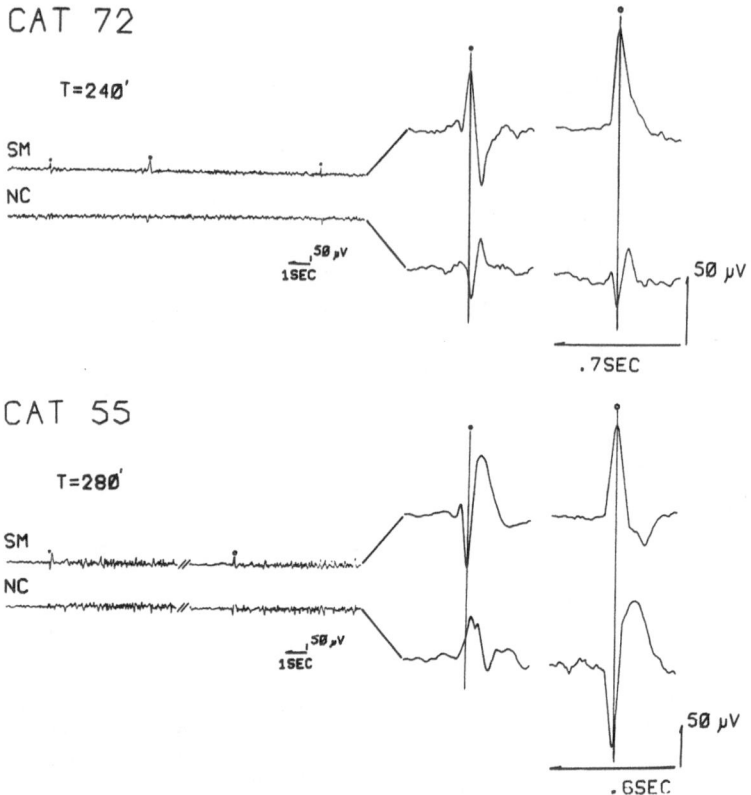

Fig. 2. Two different groups of focal spikes are shown both interictal (Cat 72) and starting ictal episodes (Cat 55); spikes marked by asterisk are diphasic and leading caudate potentials; spikes marked by circle are monophasic and preceded by caudate potentials

Discussion

The reported data lead to the following observations:

A. Potentials time-locked to focal spikes are detectable in the head of the caudate nucleus also in the earlier stages of the development of the focus. Their low voltage and delay suggest the nature of abnormal evoked potentials elicited by projections of the focal spikes (Jasper 1972).

B. Also caudate potentials corresponding to the diphasic, focal leading spikes, can reasonably be regarded as propagated epileptic activities; their high voltage could be the expression of the increased excitability of the caudate nucleus which usually accompanies the development of an epileptic focus in the sensorimotor cortex (Encabo and Buser 1964). When focal spikes are monophasic and follow the caudate ones with a latency consistent with polysinaptic caudo-cortical paths (Kemp and Powel 1972) we can consider caudate spiking as a secondary autonomous epileptic activity able in its turn to elicit propagated activity in the focus. Analogous considerations could be made concerning EEG potentials regarded as starters of ictal episodes.

C. The different temporal relations between the cortex and caudate nucleus are characterized by different morphologies of the focal spikes. It is worth remembering that Wilder and Schmidt (1965), studying Alumina-cream induced chronic neocortical foci in the monkey, noticed two different morphologies of focal spikes depending on the presence or absence of caudate spikes. They assumed that caudate spikes were always propagated from the cortex and deduced that the corresponding morphological changes of cortical spikes were due to the stimulation of a greater number of neurons or to a change in intracortical geometry of the discharging focus to activate projections paths. Our data suggest that the different morphologies could be the expression of different patterns of discharge of the same neural aggregate according to the starting of the spike which can be primary focal or elicited by autonomous activity of caudate nucleus.

The capability of the caudate nucleus to generate secondary autonomous epileptic activity has been stressed by many authors in chronic experiments (Wilder 1972); this is generally ascribed to a continuous and prolonged synaptic bombardment. Our finding concerning the development of secondary autonomous epileptic activity in a relatively short time lead us to stress these close functional relations between the two structures. Spikes recorded from the caudate nucleus following the focal ones could be the expression of phasic corticifuge influences acting on the caudate nucleus and enhanced by the epileptization of the cortex (Encabo and Buser 1964). A similar mechanism, able to act in a corticipetal direction could be postulated concerning caudate leading spikes.

Summary

Experiments carried out in cats with a neocortical cobalt induced epileptic focus demonstrated that focal averaged spikes, obtained by a personal computer technique, can alternately lead the caudate ones or be led by them. Defined morphological alterations of the spikes characterize the two situations.

References

1. Encabo, H., Buser, P. (1964), Influence des aires primaires neocorticales sur les reponses sensorielles visuelles et acoustiques de la tête du noyau caudé. Electroenceph. clin. Neurophysiol. *17*, 144.
2. Ferrillo, F., Amore, R., Cavazza, B., Rosadini, G. (1974), An experimental research on time relationships among focal and secondary epileptic spikes. Boll. Soc. Ital. Biol. Sper. *50*, 1936—1940.
3. Jasper, H. H. (1969), Mechanisms of propagation: Extracellular studies. In: Basic mechanisms of the epilepsies (Jasper, H. H., Ward, A. A., Pope, A., eds.). Boston: Little, Brown & Co.
4. Kemp, J. M., Powel, I. P. S. (1971), The structure of the caudate nucleus of the cat. Philosophical Trans. Roy. Soc. (London) *262*, 383.
5. Mares, P. (1973), Bioelectrical activity of an epileptogenic focus in cat neocortex. Brain Res. *56*, 203.
6. Palestini, M., Amore, R., Ferrillo, F., Rosadini, G. (1975), Interazioni cortico-caudate durante l'evoluzione dell'epilessia da focolai sperimentali neocorticali. Riv. Neurol. *45*, 180.
7. Rosadini, G., Cavazza, B., Ferrillo, F., Siccardi, A. (1974), Simultaneous averaging of epileptic discharges in 14 channels: a computer technique. Electroenceph. clin. Neurophysiol. *36*, 541.
8. Tharp, B. R. (1971), The penicillin focus: a study of field characteristics using cross-correlation analysis. Electroenceph. clin. Neurophysiol. *31*, 45.
9. Wilder, B. J. (1972), Projection phenomena and secondary epileptogenesis-Mirror Foci. In: Experimental models of epilepsy (Purpura, D. P., Penry, J. K., Tower, D. B., Woodbury, D. W., Walter, R. D., eds.). New York: Raven Press.
10. Wilder, B. J., Schmidt, R. P. (1965), Propagation of epileptic discharge from chronic neocortical foci in monkey. Epilepsia *6*, 297.

Authors' address: F. Ferrillo, M.D., R. Amore, M.D., M. Palestini, M.D., G. Rosadini, M.D., Centre for Cerebral Neurophysiology, of National Council of Researches, Institute of Neurophysiopathology of the University, Genoa, Italy.

Acta Neurochirurgica, Suppl. 23, 15—20 (1976)

Neurosurgical Department of Clinic of Neurology and Psychiatry,
University of Medicine, Debrecen, Hungary

The Value of Electrostimulation in Epileptic Focus Localization

R. Gombi, Gy. Velok, and J. Hullay

With 2 Figures

Introduction

Electrical stimulation (ES) for epileptogenic zone localization can be performed in two ways, either on surgically exposed brain, mostly on the cortical surface, or intracerebrally with implanted electrodes. This study is based on the data obtained with intracerebral ES.

Patients with intractable epilepsy which by nature of their electro-clinical seizure pattern and/or lack of appropriate response to anticonvulsant medication are considered candidates for surgical treatment. It is depth recording that may provide important electrophysiological information, confirm the data of routine investigations or clear up confusing findings and prevent an inappropriate surgical intervention. The best way for precise determination of the epileptogenic zone is the electro-clinical observation of spontaneous seizures in the course of stereo-EEG and the information is completed by using peripheral and central stimulation. But the lack of spontaneous clinical seizure during stereo-EEG makes it necessary to provoke attacks mainly by stimulating different cortical and subcortical areas electrically and record and analyse the electroclinical manifestations as well as the propagation of seizure activity. Stereo-EEG is used mostly in a selected group of patients, where severe epileptic manifestations are combined with complex pathology. In such cases precise evaluation of various clinical and electrographic responses elicited by ES is important, or even critical, from the point of view of focus localization and further treatment.

Material

For the last 8 years 41 acute stereo-EEG explorations have been performed in 31 epileptic patients. Most of them had epileptic seizures of several kinds as secondarily generalized convulsions, generalized seizures without convulsions, partial seizures with elementary or complex symptomatology and myoclonus. Before stereo-EEG intervention the electro-clinical symptomatology (initial symptom, mode of propagation etc.) of the seizures were analysed in detail. 26 patients underwent stereo-EEG explorations according to the Talairach-Bancaud method. In the other 5 non-specific surgical intervention was carried out by the Riechert apparatus. ES was used in both kinds of intervention. During stimulation the patients were alert and cooperative.

Stimuli were applied with a Tönnies stimulator which was connected to a cathode ray oscilloscope. Stimulus parameters were as follows: rectangular single and repetitive shocks with duration of 3 and 5 msec and voltage of 0.5 to 10 Volt controlled on the oscilloscope. Duration of the stimulus was 2–5 seconds. Bipolar stimulation was performed in most of the cases. The distance between two poles of electrodes was 4 mm. Monopolar stimulation was also used in some cases, but the bipolar one proved to be more convenient. Whilst trying to standardize stimulation in a given structure, the different sensitivity of brain structures to ES was taken into consideration. The stimulus threshold of electrical and clinical responses was always determined.

The clinical and electrical (recorded only in EEG) responses in different brain areas can be devided into 5 groups:

1. *No electrical and clinical reactions.* The lack of response may be the consequence of various technical and cerebral causes *e.g.* inadequate stimulus frequency or voltage, high stimulus threshold, low functional level of stimulated neuronal population in the actual functional state of the nervous system etc. The lack of response is not uncommon in certain regions of the cortex and the basal ganglia.

2. *Local electrical response with or without clinical signs.* The EEG changes are usually manifested in rhythmic after-discharge, but occasionally they show slowing of activity or, on the contrary, the appeerence of an arousal reaction. When repeating the ES within

---

Fig. 1. Electrical stimulation (2 V, 50 Hz, 5 seconds) of right frontal convexital cortex evokes a seizure with severe abduction and tonic extension of the right arm and leg and with gradually increasing flexion of left extremities. The legs and trunk are turning to right

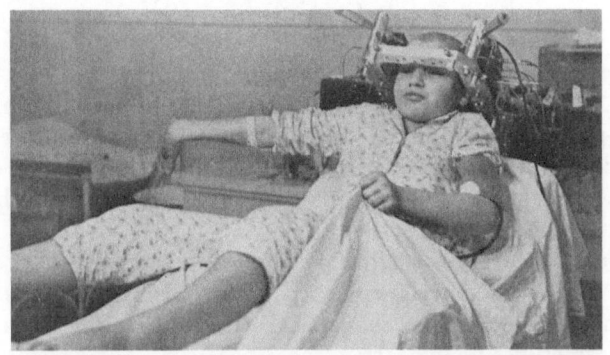

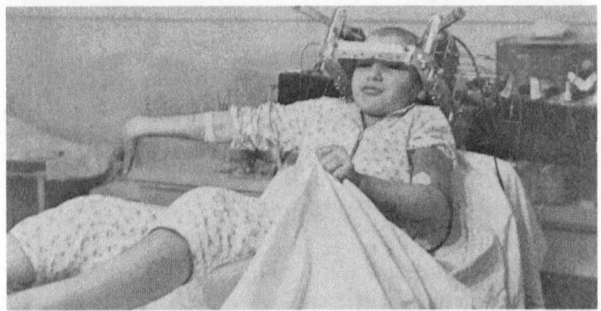

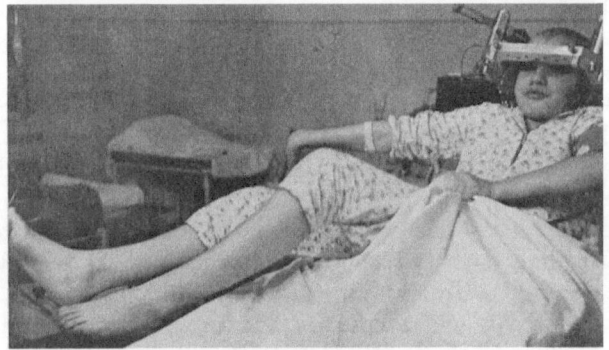

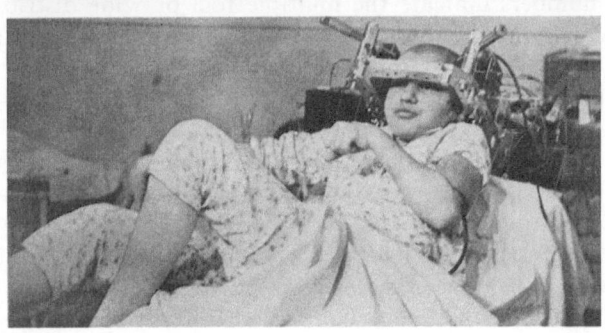

Fig. 1

a short period or increasing the stimulus frequency and voltage, the responses are either increased and prolonged, or may diminish and even disappear. The clinical manifestations were characteristic of the function of the stimulated structure, but it may be an element of habitual seizure, too. This type of response is visible both in the cortical and subcortical structures.

3. *Clinical response without electrical signs.* These clinical responses are usually well-separated from seizure elements. They appear mostly in certain subcortical (thalamic and subthalamic) areas but sometimes in the cortex, too.

4. *Spreading but not generalizing electrical response accompanied by clinical signs.* This clinical response may be either of a "physiological" pattern or elements or fragments of a seizure. If they were identical with the initial symptoms of the usual type of seizure, they often developed into a typical clinical seizures when repeating the ES or after increasing its voltage. If the elements of the seizure pattern were similar to or even identical with one of the late signs of the usual attack, the repetition and increase of ES did not usually evoke the complete electro-clinical seizure pattern. This group of responses can be elicited in many cortical areas in the epileptic brain.

5. *Typical electro-clinical seizure manifestations.* The complete clinical seizure or complex seizure episode with spreading or generalized EEG paroxysm appear during ES or within short latency following the ES. Sometimes either the clinical or the electrical signs develop with longer latency. Fragments of an elicited clinical seizure can be seen in Fig. 1. In Fig. 2. the topography of ES inducing the habitual clinical seizures is demonstrated. They schematically show the medial, interhemispheric surface and the convexity of the brain (according to Talairach's atlas). The numbers from 1 to 26 indicate the patients whose epileptic seizure could be evoked by ES. Identical numbers indicate the multiple foci or wide distribution of epileptogenic zones in the same patients. In some cases certain sites of these areas were thermocoagulated in order to interrupt the seizure mechanism.

In our material 9 patients had circumscribed foci or discharges localized in one lobe focus. This type a localization is generally suitable for surgical intervention, which may be carried out after the stereo-EEG exploration. Bilateral symmetrical foci have been observed in 3 patients, multiple asymmetric ones in 13 and the epileptogenic focus has remained unknown in 6. In 4 of these 6 patients stereo-EEG had not been performed only thermocoagulation of non-specific structures. In patients with multiplex or undeter-

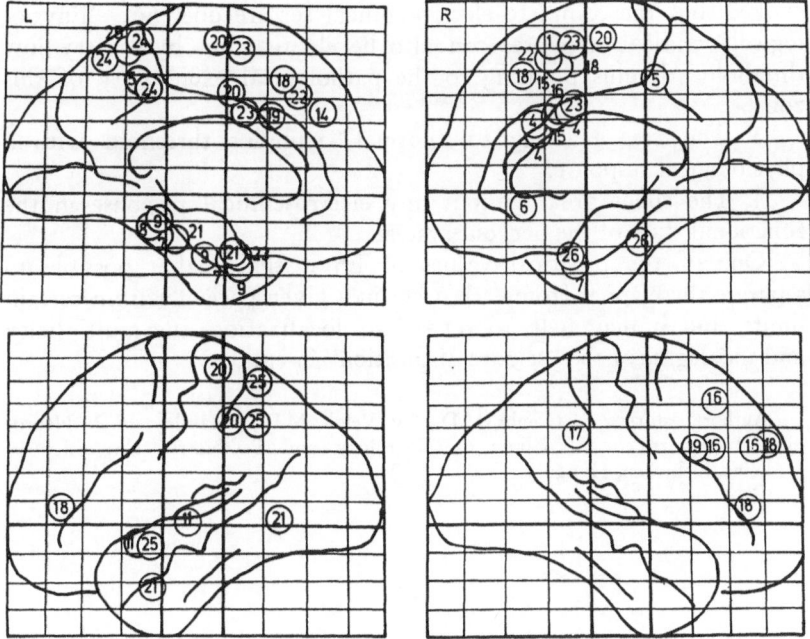

Fig. 2. Topography of ES inducing the usual seizures. See the text

mined foci thermolesions were carried out in non-specific areas of the brain, *i.e.* mainly in thalamus and subthalamus. Observation on the effects of thermocoagulation will be presented in another paper (by Hullay and collab.).

Summary and Conclusions

The ES is a non-physiological stimulus of the brain. However it represents an important and indispensable part of stereo-EEG investigation since it is an easily adjustable method, capable of inducing typical electro-clinical seizures. From the clinical and electrical responses elicited by ES and from the data of the stimulation treshold, we are in agreement with other authors, we feel we can also distinguish several different reacting zones in the epileptic brain:

1. The epileptogenic zone from which the complete or almost complete electro-clinical seizure is reproducible immediately by ES or with short latency. These pathological responses show the severe dysfunction of the given structures.

2. The irritative zones from which seizure elements can be

evoked, but the complete electro-clinical seizure does not. "Physiological" clinical responses can also be elicited, but by a very low threshold stimulus pointing to the pathological excitability of this zone.

3. The area reacting to "normal" stimulus threshold with a physiological response.

4. The silent area without any electro-clinical response in the functional state of the nervous system.

One of the practical values of ES is that makes possible to separate these zones from each other in a given patient within certain limits, and it may help to reveal the localization, the multiplicity and the degree of the "seizure disposition" in epilepsy.

Authors' address: R. Gombi, M.D., Gy. Velok, M.D., J. Hullay, M.D., Neurosurgical Department of Clinic of Neurology and Psychiatry, University of Medicine, Debrecen, Hungary.

Acta Neurochirurgica, Suppl. 23, 21—25 (1976)

Research Laboratory of Clinical Stereotaxis of Neurosurgical Department,
Comenius University, Bratislava, ČSSR

Graphic Representation of the Epileptic Focus

P. Nádvorník, M. Šramka, and G. Fritz

With 2 Figures

The concept of the epileptic focus as a single trigger of the epileptic discharge which then spreads to the environment is still subject to discussion. The evidence about brain damage provoking focal epilepsy, *e. g.* under clinical conditions following head injury [5] or experimentally after application of some chemical compound on the brain [3] appears to be exceptional particularly when the study of electrical brain acitivity is repeated with the recording made not only with scalp leads but within deep brain structures as well. The analysis of epileptic manifestations in both EEG and SEEG records may well affect the wiews of the epileptic focus.

In the course of 87 streotactic operations for epilepsy the brain's electrical activity was always investigated from the surface as well as from deep structures. Chronic multilead deep electrodes were introduced through three standard trajectories to enable comparison of the recordings. Since the introduction of deep electrodes has not been so far carried out in a uniform way, we considered this procedure to be the most important one.

Through a frontal approach, designated coronal, with the first trajectory one can reach along the gyrus hippocampi, the uncus, nucleus amygdalae, commissura anterior, and putamen or pallidum respectively. Along the second trajectory one can reach Forel's field H_2 or by shifting the electrode the subthalamic region as well as the anterior reticulum of the thalamus and head of the caudate nucleus situated over them. Along the third trajectory it is possible to reach the posterior hypothalamus or even red nucleus and, over it, the nucleus centrum medianum of the thalamus. By moving the electrode towards the surface, the medial hemispheric area, particularly areas [24, 32] and also [6, 8, 9] respectively according to the inclination of the electrode. To obtain records for precise analysis the electrodes should be introduced through the three trajectories simultaneously and into both hemispheres.

From the posterior occipital approach, which may well be designated lambdoid, the electrodes are introduced longitudinally into the hippocampal and transtentorially into the nucleus dentatus [6, 7].

After X-ray control of the electrode positions electrical activity is registered from deep structures separately and in various combinations with the scalp recordings.

In some structures it is the rule to find typical epileptic activity showing different intensity. From minimal changes the disturbance of the electric activity often spreads over to remote structures. Pathological wave discharges are sometimes accompanied by clinical attacks.

The changes observed during the series of recordings, *i.e.* not only in the ictal but in the interictal periods as well, are then evaluated and the results of this evaluation are recorded into a scheme (Fig. 1). In this scheme the degree of pathological activity at different brain sites is expressed by numerical values, subjective comparative weighing, and the association of sides are shown by connecting lines. Thus, the scheme is changed into an orientated and evaluated graph showing weights and bonds of structures participating in epileptic discharge.

The standard method of examination before surgery was carried out in 20 patients suffering from generalized epilepsy. The graph showing functional dependency was the basis for selecting structures suitable for surgical treatment of epilepsy.

The systematic study of graphs in generalized epilepsy makes it, possible however, to consider the epileptic focus as well. By the analysis of the graphs the following were determined:

1. The pathological activities in amygdala-hippocampus complexes of both sides are independent of each other. The pathological manifestations are of irregular character with a slower rhythm on the anatomically affected side.

2. The pathological activity in the anterior thalamic reticulum on the thalamus-caudate border recorded from the two sides are dependent on each other, manifested by synchronization spreading periodically to cortical brain areas or conditioning possibly periodical discharges in the amygdala-hippocampus complex (Fig. 2).

3. The pathological activity in the posterior hypothalamus is connected with that of the non-specific thalamic system as well as with medial area of the frontal lobes.

4. The epileptic activity is prevalent, as a rule, in the anterior reticulum of the thalamus amygdala-hippocampus complex, in the

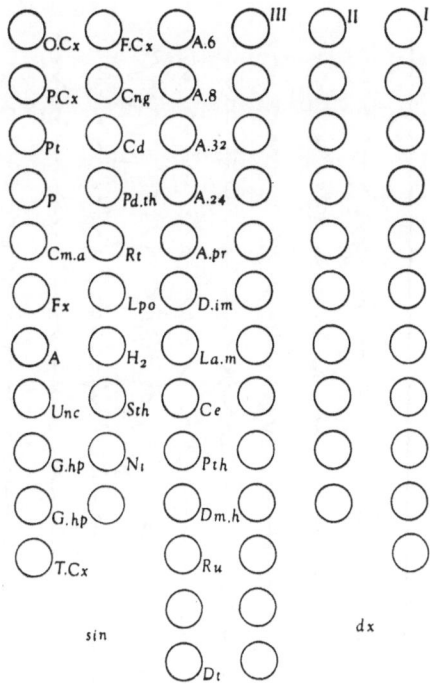

Fig. 1. Scheme of the investigated brain structures. *I, II, III* are trajectories on the right or left side respectively

I. *OCx* occipital cortex, *PCx* parietal cortex, *Pt* putamen, *P* pallidum, *Cm.a* commissura anterior, *Fx* fornix, *A* amygdala, *Unc* uncus gyri hippocampi, *G.hp* gyrus hippocampi, *T.Cx* temporal cortex

II. *FCx* frontal cortex, *Cng* cingulum, *Cd* caudatum, *Pd.th* pedunculus thalami, *Rt* reticulum thalami, *Lpo* nc. lateropolaris, H_2 Forell's field H_2, *Sth* nc. subthalamicus, *Ni* nc. niger

III. *A 6, 8, 32, 24* area 6, 8, 32, 24, *A.pr* nc. anterior princeps, *D.im* nc. dorsomedialis thalami, *La.m* lamina medialis thalami, *Ce* centrum medianum, *Pth* prothalamus, *Dm.h* nc. dorsomedialis hypthalami, *Ru* nc. ruber, *Dt* nc. dentatus

posterior hypothalamus and medial area of the hemispheres as well. The anatomical connections between these structures are most likely to the responsible for their functional dependency. According to our experience as well to the results of surgical treatment, the graph of functional relations reflects the clinical form of epilepsy and may well be considered to be a mode of epileptic focus representation. According to this graph, the focus may be understood as a functional cooperation of those brain structures showing epileptic activity.

The concept of the epileptic focus as the graph of functional groupings is different when compared tho that of the three concentric

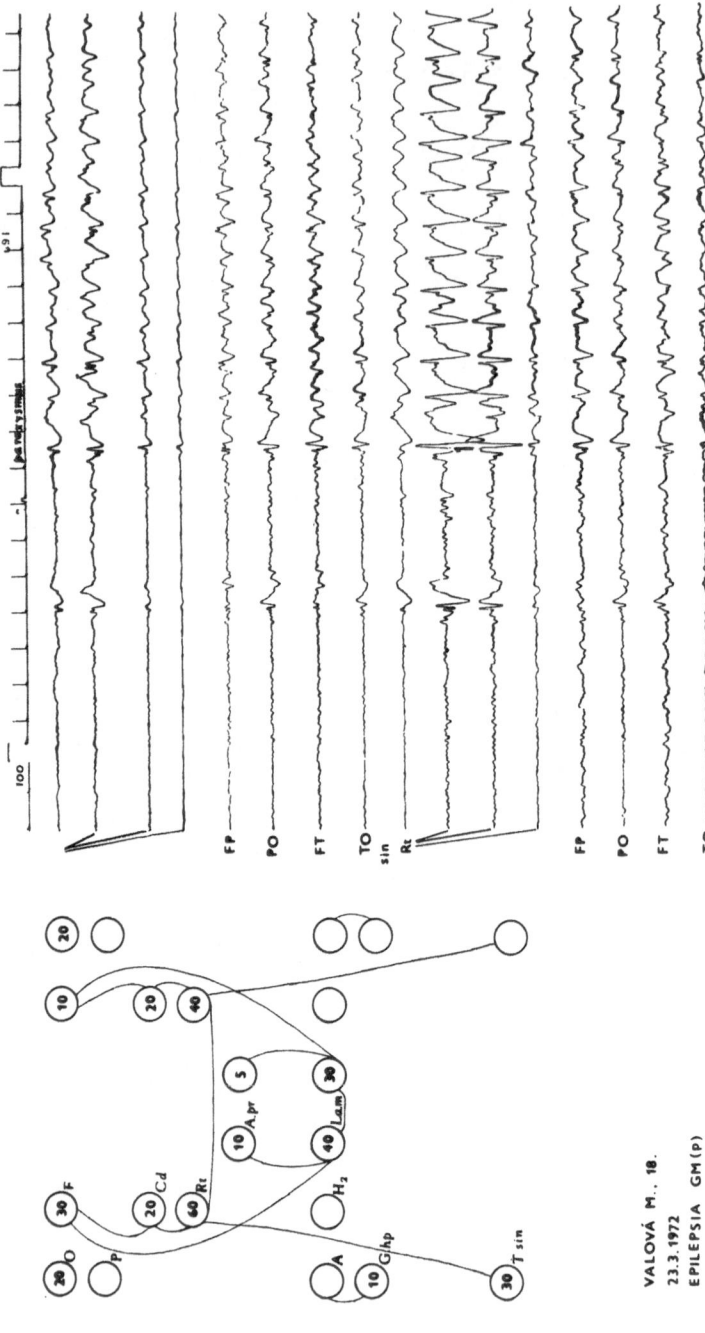

Fig. 2. Graph of functional conjunctions and a specimen of combined EEG and SEEG record

circles on the cortex, where Penfield [4] distinguished the lesion focus, the irritative zone and epileptogenic area respectively. Later Jasper presumed that the lesion [2] as the source of pathological activity occurs excentrically and deep in the brain, probably in the brain stem. With respect to their own experience with SEEG [8] Talairach and Bancoud proceeded to separate the irritative zone from the epileptogenie area which proves to be a convenient source of epileptic attack and they endeavoured to find the epileptogenic area in the cortex.

By the investigation of epileptic patients with electrodes introduced in the standard way into brain deep structures as well as on the scalp we established the concept which treats epileptic foci as functional dependencies expressed by the graph.

Summary

On the basis of systematic examinations of electrical activity of brain deep structures in 87 epileptic patients, an experiment was carried out to replace the concept of the epileptic focus by the graph of functional grouping of structures with epileptic activity. In order to make the graph as realistic as possible, the multi-lead electrodes have to be introduced into the brain systematically and under standard conditions. In this case, the results obtained are comparable. At the same time, the graph proves to be the basis of indications for stereotactic treatment.

References

1. Jasper, H. H. (1958), The ten twenty electrode system of the International Federation. Electroenceph. clin. Neurophysiol. *10*, 371—375.
2. — (1962), Changing concepts of focal epilepsy in Černáček, Cigánek round table conference on the surgical treatment of the epilepsies and its neurophysiological aspects, pp. 175—181, SAV, Bratislava.
3. Kopeloff, L. M. (1960), Experimental epilepsy in the mouse. Proc. Soc. exp. biol. Med. *104*, 500—504.
4. Penfield, W., Erickson, T. (1941), Epilepsy and cerebral localisation. Springfield, Ill.: Thomas.
5. — Jasper, H. (1959), Epilepsy and the functional anatomy of the human brain. London: Churchill.
6. Nádvorník, P., Šramka, M. (1973), Stereotaksičeskaja dentatotomia. Voprosy nejrochir. *57*, 1, 19—23.
7. — — (1974), Anatomical considerations for the stereotactic longitudinal hippocampectomy. Confin. neurol. *36*, 177—181.
8. Talairach, J., Bancoud, J. (1966), Lesion, "irritative" zone and epileptogenic focus. Confin. neurol. *27*, 91—94.

Authors' address: P. Nádvorník, M.D., M. Šramka, M.D., G. Fritz, M.D., Research Laboratory of Clinical Stereotaxis of Neurosurgical Department, Comenius University, Bratislava, ČSSR.

Acta Neurochirurgica, Suppl. 23, 27—31 (1976)

A. L. Polenov Neurosurgical Institute, Leningrad, USSR

Stereoelectrosubcorticography in Epilepsy, the Focus and Epileptogenic System

T. S. Stepanova and K. V. Grachev

With 2 Figures

The progress of knowledge in the field of epilepsy is closly associated with the development of stereoneurosurgery providing unique opportunities for delicate operations on deep brain structures under careful neurophysiological control. In the Neurosurgical Institute of Leningrad 400 stereotactic procedure have been carried out since 1960, of which more than 100 were for temporal and generalized epilepsies. Two kinds of stereotactic performances have been used, viz. the method of implanted long-term multicontact electrodes and one-stage stereotaxis. Stereoelectrosubcorticography, when compared with EEG and electrocorticography and neuronal activity, enabled us to obtain an idea on the functional organization of epileptogenic foci for the cortical, subcortical and extensive multifocal brain lesion.

Electrophysiological characteristics and deep epileptogenic foci differentiation have been determined permitting high locality and spatial isolation of the foci in both the thalamic and pallidal structures, as well as the obscurity of the epileptogenic zone in limbic temporal formations. Cortical foci of convulsive activity were observed extensive as well. These differences prove to be based on morpho-functional particularities of organization of neuronal elements of the aforementioned formations, conditioning either intensification (hippocampus, neocortex) or reduction (thalamus) of the role played by the ephaptic factor in epileptogenesis. Assuming a single "epileptic" neurone not to cause epileptic paroxysms, we carried out, on a model of diencephalic foci, a complex of both microphysiological and histological investigations to determine the minimum dimensions of the cellular population, already functioning as an epileptic focus (K. V. Grachev and T. S. Stepanova, 1971). The analysis made showed that the formation of such a trigger focus producing paroxysmal bioelectrical and clinical phenomena required a "critical" volume of neurone population which, particularly in the human thalamus, amounts to 10^3–10^5 of cells at focus diameter 500 to 3,000 μ. These results are the basis of highly local destruction of brain tissue (anode electrolysis) in stereotactic operations on subcortical formations.

Our long-term investigations of the mechanisms of propagation and interruption of convulsive discharge led to the theory that the escalation of epileptization proceeded via pathological epileptogenic system formation (T. S. Stepanova and K. V. Grachev, 1971) including the following stages: "epileptic" neurone—epileptogenic focus—epileptogenic system—epileptic brain. The analysis of correlations between focus and perifocal structures made it possible to make a thorough study of the possibilities of space-chosing discharge generalization in deep brain regions with intact neocortex. Such patterns were obtained for multineuronal limbic structures, as well as subcortical formations having direct corticopetal and, particularly, thalamocortical projections. These data suggest that the pathological discharge might reverberate for long periods through the range of deep structures within the system of horizontally organized neuronal chains and that the pattern investigated may seem to be the electrophysiological correlate of convulsion-free paroxysm. We showed the role played by provoking factors, such as darkness adaptation, sleep, sleep deprivation, hyperventilation, drugs and the like, contributing to the transfer of epileptic discharge to vertically organized paths resulting in a convulsive attack, and the importance of competing inhibitory brain systems in the limitation and interruption of paroxysmal phenomena. Special investigations made by means of electrostimulation and polarization showed that within the range of pathological systems the foci occurred in complex subordinated, often reciprocal relations; clinically it is difficult to decide which of the foci has to be switched off first. We obtained electrograms showing both the differentiation and heterogeneity of focal constructions in temporal epilepsy indicating the polymorphism of clinical phenomena characteristic of the given disease. In bitemporal epilepsy, particularly complex and dynamic correlations accompanied by precise inter-hemispheral control relations, characteristic for hierarchic systems were found. These facts, as well as the phenomenon of "migration dominance" suggest the unlikelihood of the so-called independent foci in the brain.

The effort to detect the laws governing the interruption of convulsive discharges made it possible to establish the direct participation of basal ganglia not only in generalization mechanisms but also in those of epileptic paroxysms interruptions. It was shown that

therapeutic electrostimulation of n. caudatus brings about, at some
points, interruption of electrographic and behavioural attack components, suggesting both suppression of the epileptogenic and domina-
tion of competing inhibitory systems (effect of the type "brain re-
training"). According to out data, the distant effects on cell level of
epileptogenic focus (Fig. 1) may serve a criterion for determination
such points.

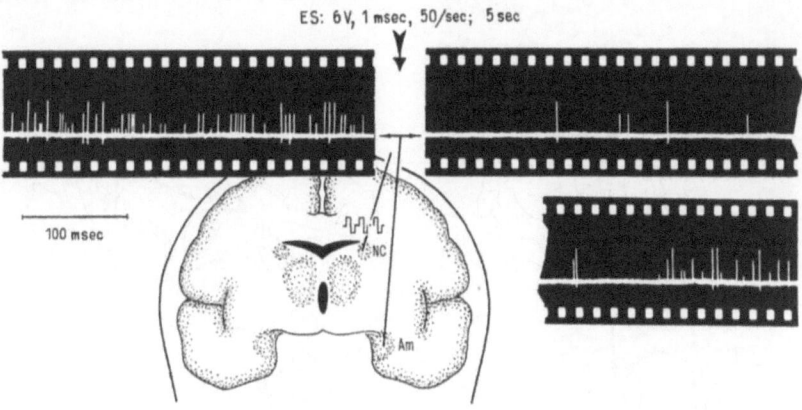

Fig. 1. Neuro-physiological test for intracerebral localization of therapeutic electrostimulation application. Nucleus caudatus stimulation (*NC*) provokes distant
effect: temporary suppression of impulse activity of neuronal pull (extracellular
registration) in nucleus amygdaloideum (*Am*). Lower neuronogram—direct continua-
tion of the upper neurogram

The results were taken as the basis for establishing a conceptual
electrophysiological model of organization of electric brain activity
in epilepsy. On the scheme (Fig. 2), both the horizontally organized
systems of discharge reverberation embracing thalamic, striopallidal,
limbic and mediobasal frontal formations and the vertically organized systems including the cortex into circulation chain, are shown.
Within the interictal period and, particularly, under the influence of anticonvulsants, these systems may disintegrate into
a number of systems, whose time-space organization and structure change in conjunction with afferentation level. We imagine
that in convulsion-free attacks ("psychic equivalents") a long-term
discharge reverberation on cyclical chains of both the diencephalic
and limbic structures, *i.e.*, formations participating in behavioural reactions and motivation integration, appear to be of primary importance. The so-called emotional circle of Pape and basolateral circle

of Livingston-Escobar may well appear to be the structural basis of this pathological system. The convulsive component of the attack may well be associated with discharge transfer on pyramidal and extrapyramidal paths. In bitemporal epilepsy, the pathological system involves the reverberation chain of commissural and subcortical paths and accompanied by the formation of complex facilitating and inhibiting interhemispherical influences. The observations made in the course of night sleep as well as those

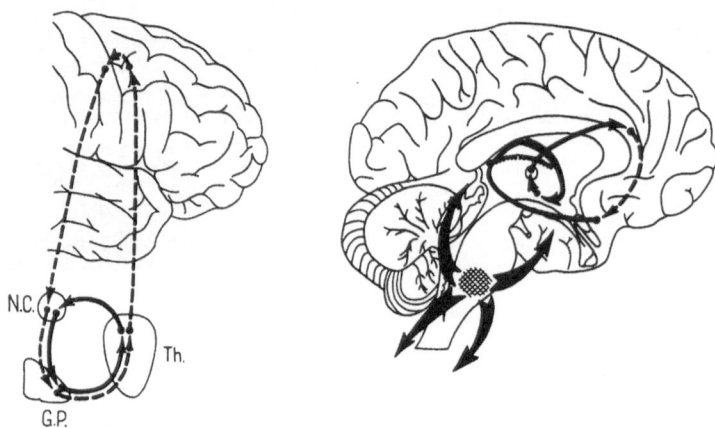

Fig. 2. Model scheme of system organization of electric activity of brain in epilepsy. Explanation to be found within the text

of pharmacological effects suggest that the level of epileptic system excitation is modified partly by control relations of the foci, partly by competing inhibitory systems of the whole brain and particularly, by the inhibitory Buchwald system and caudopontine system with trigger in the zone of the caudal reticulopontine nucleus. We believe that the propagation of the pathological process in these systems is the basis of generalized forms of epilepsy with grand mal attacks when the sharp decrease of inhibitory influences suggest a vast and resistant exciting reverberation simultaneously in a large brain representation. In petit mal, data were obtained of the participation of strio-amygdalorubral pathological system in the mechanism both of the electrographical and clinical phenomena (T. S. Stepanova and K. V. Grachev, 1972).

Thus, the data obtained show that in epilepsy clinics it is no longer possible to be confined to general investigations and findings of pathological focus but necessary to detect the functional organization of an epileptic system with maximum precision of subordinated correlations within its range, and the dominant focus as the trigger switching on the whole system. The material presented showes the large differentiation of focal constructions in the patients investigated. This is why every patient needs individual assessment as well as a strict differentiated approach in the streotactic technique. Depending on the electrographical characteristics and the functional structure of the epileptogenic system and according to indications either destructions of appropriate deep formations or the electrostimulations in the points with the above mentioned criteria may be used.

Summary

According to the conceptual electrophysiological model of epilepsy worked out by the authors earlier (1968–1971) the development of the disease has the following stages: "epileptic" neurone epileptogenic focus epileptogenic system epileptic brain. The mechanisms of the II and III stages are analysed in the given paper. The critical volume of the neuronal population capable of functioning as a triggering focus is shown to be 10^3–10^5 cells (Microsystem). On the II stage the control is achieved by the lateral inhibition. Further on epileptogenic macrosystems and subsystems of discharge reverberation (vertical and horizontal) are formed with complex hierarchy on a reciprocal principle. A morpho-functional organization of pathological systems in petit mal, grand mal, uni- and bitemporal epilepsy was found during ictal and interictal periods. Inhibitory systems (low pontine and caudate) and reciprocal inhibition during the III stage were found to act as controls.

References

1. Gračev, K. V., Stepanova, T. S. (1971), Nekotoryje dannyje k ocenke minimal'noj veličiny epileptogennogo očaga v zritel'nom bugre čeloveka. Vopr. nejrochirurgii *35*, 3, 18—23.
2. Stepanova, T. S., Gračev, K. V. (1968), Nekotoryje osobennosti električeskoj aktivnosti glubokich struktur mozga pri epilepsii. Z. nevropatol. psichiatr. *68*, 2, 1593—1599.
3. — — (1971), Elektrofiziologičeskije ocenki epileptogennych očagov v kortikal'nych i subkortikal'nych strukturach pri chirurgičeskom lečenii bol'nych epilepsiej. V sb.: Chirurgičeskoje lečenije epilepsii. Trudy 1 sesojuzn. sjezda nejrochirurgov, 3. Moskva, 138—141.
4. — — (1972), Elektrofiziologičeskije charakteristiki korkovych, diencefal'nych i limbičeskich struktur mozga čeloveka pri epilepsii v processe nočnogo sna. V sb.: Son i jego narušenija. Moskva, 225—228.

Authors' address: T. S. Stepanova, M.D., and K. V. Grachev, Ph.D., A. L. Polenov Neurosurgical Institute, Leningrad, USSR.

Acta Neurochirurgica, Suppl. 23, 33—34 (1976)

Department of Neurology (Head: Prof. Dr. sc. med. R. M. Schmidt)
Clinic of Psychiatry and Neurology, Martin-Luther-University,
Halle/Saale, German Democratic Republic (Dir.: Prof. Dr. sc. med. H. Rennert)

An Analysis of Routine-EEG-Findings with a View to Surgical Treatment of Epilepsy

E. Grimm

EEG-investigations of epileptic patients in our laboratory usual over ten years have shown that about 50% have typical temporal-lobe-epilepsy and form the greatest group in the so-called symptomatic epilepsy. Most of them (about $^2/_3$) had general pathological bio-electric activity. One or more foci with different functional correlation were found in 70% of our cases. Typical epileptic activity with spikes, spike-waves or high-amplitude sharp-waves was recorded very rarely on the scalp, particularly during the intervall. The most common localisation of epileptic foci was in the sensomotoric area and in the temporal lobe. Sometimes two or more foci occurred with corresponding bioelectric activity, althrough generally the foci were independent.

If a focus could be demonstrated at the onset of the epilepsy the focus usually persists more constantly than one with a later onset.

In about 5% of our cases a temporal focus changed to the other side with less activity in the primary lobe, without surgical excision. In a later examination in 3 cases we recorded a return of the pronunced pathological activity to the original focus.

In all patients with clinical signs of psychomotor epilepsy sleep-EEG was recorded for provocation. These investigations showed 30% more foci than EEG's in the normal alert state. By using other provocative methods such as injections of barbiturates other drugs and flicker-light the original focus was recognizable in cases of bi-lateral pathological acitivity in the temporal lobes, for instance spikes in various forms.

Patients with focal epilepsy should be examined generally by contrast-encephalography, cerebral angiography and radioisotope-scanning for exclusion of tumours before surgical interventions are indicated. In the absence of pathological bioelectrical activity on the scalp in uncontrolled cases of focal, especially psychomotor epilepsy, multifocal depth-electrodes (5–7 evaluation points or wire-bundles bifocal should be used for explorations in the median part of the temporal lobe, in the amygdaloid complex, in the hippocampal formation and in the caudate nucleus to differentiate deep foci and pathological neurophysiological pathways. In hippocampal stimulations especially we recorded a spreading of epileptic activity into the nonspecific epileptic system confirming the observations of Nadvornik and others. Mostly this activity corresponds with grand mal seizures.

In our opinion cases of uncontrolled focal, especially temporo-focal and multifocal epilepsy and special cases of nonfocal epilepsy should have operation in a period before secondary generalization, establishment of independent secondary epileptic foci and associated behavioural disorders.

Author's address: Dr. E. Grimm, Department of Neurology, Clinic of Psychiatry and Neurology, Martin-Luther-University, DDR-402 Halle/Saale, German Democratic Republic.

Acta Neurochirurgica, Suppl. 23, 35—43 (1976

Neuroscience, Broughton Hospital, Morganton, North Carolina, U.S.A.

The Seizure Active Site Demonstrated by Chronically Implanted Electrodes

Y. K. Kim

With 4 Figures

Introduction

In the past two decades open or stereotaxic surgery has actively been applied to seizure disorders. In some cases the results of surgery were encouraging but in others they were disappointing. It seemed to us that the primary reason for these widely divergent effects of surgery was the usual approach of selecting only one target structure without considering the nature of the specific seizure type or that multiple foci were present.

When we started implanting electrodes in subcortical areas we considered three possible ways to stop or reduce the occurrence of seizures. These were: 1. to find and destroy the seizure active site(s), 2. to interrupt the pathways by which the seizure activity was propagated, and 3. to counteract electrically active areas of the brain (the so-called excitatory system) if they could be detected.

In the course of our studies we also investigated the effect of several anticonvulsants on the depth EEG and by means of a neuropsychological battery of tests administrated before and after surgery, evaluated alterations of cerebral functions.

Method and Results

A. Depth EEG

Six bundles of six contact electrodes were chronically implanted in and around the amygdala, hippocampus and anterior part of the thalamus. Eight scalp electrodes were added to correlate depth and surface activities (see Fig. 1). To avoid the activity discharges of surgically traumatized cells, recording was begun three to seven days after implantation. Spontaneous activity was recorded

3*

during waking and sleeping states and under intravenous anticonvulsants. Recordings were also obtained during the stimulation of each structure mentioned above.

In eleven out of twenty four hemispheres the basolateral and periamygdaloid structures were most abnormal in terms of high deltas, single spikes or groups of spikes and waves (see Fig. 2). How-

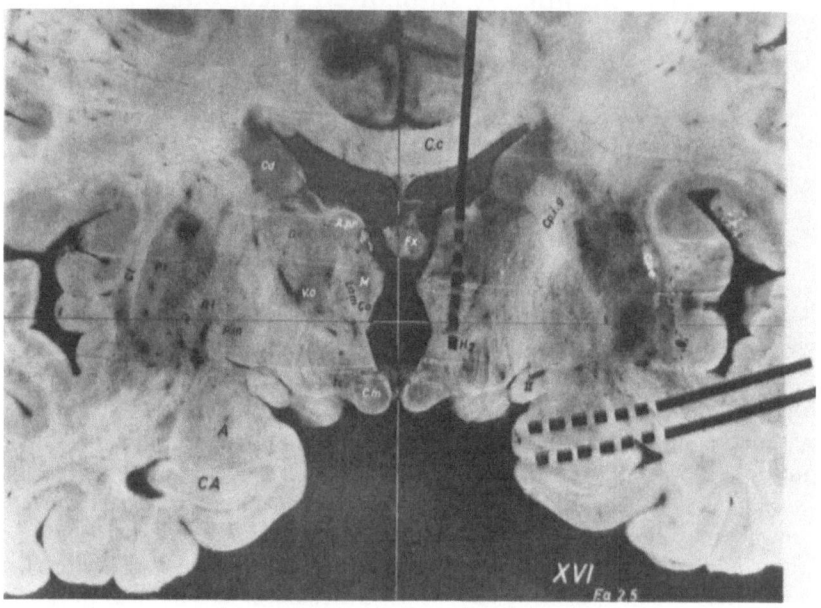

Fig. 1. The location and pathways of the implanted electrodes are shown on the Atlas of Bailey/Schaltenbrand. One bundle of electrode consists of 6 contact electrodes and they are implanted in both hemispheres

ever polyspikes of maximal intensity were seen most frequently in the hippocampus (see Fig. 3). In all cases of temporal lobe epilepsy the anterior thalamus and the subthalamus were essentially silent except for secondary responses to primary foci located elsewhere.

The lateral predominance of foci was more clearly demonstrated by depth than by scalp EEG. For example, those cases which on the basis of scalp EEG were considered to have independent bilateral foci were indicated by depth EEG to have unilateral foci with only secondary responses seen contralaterally. In other instances scalp EEG indicated unilateral predominance whereas depth recordings showed the presence of bilateral foci. Comparisons of scalp and depth EEG recordings were made for the sixteen patients presented in Table 1.

The relation of depth EEG abnormalities to clinical manifestations is shown in Table 2. It may be seen that abnormalities localized in the amygdala were frequently associated with generalized motor

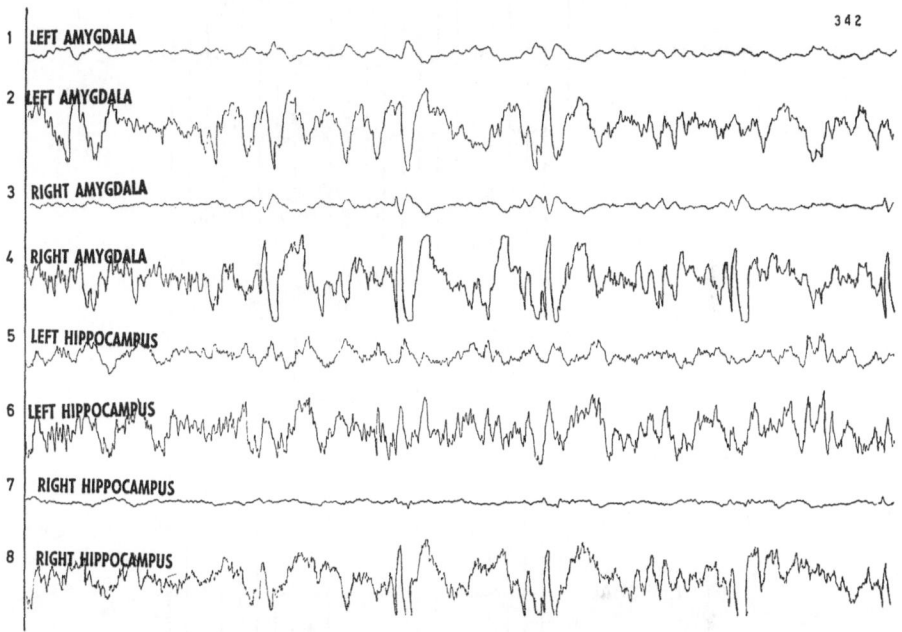

Fig. 2. On this depth EEG the lateral amygdala and the periamygdaloid area are most abnormal. The channel *1, 3, 5,* and *7* is from the medial part and *2, 4, 6,* and *8* is from the lateral part of the named structures

seizures whereas patients with abnormalities confined to the hippocampus tended to manifest automatisms. When a diffuse temporal abnormality was detected, psychiatric symptoms were predominant.

B. Target Selection

Selection of the operative target(s) was based on data obtained from depth recordings. Target selection was easy when seizure foci could be clearly determined but in instances of diffuse abnormality the selection process became difficult. In these cases, several possible

Y. K. Kim:

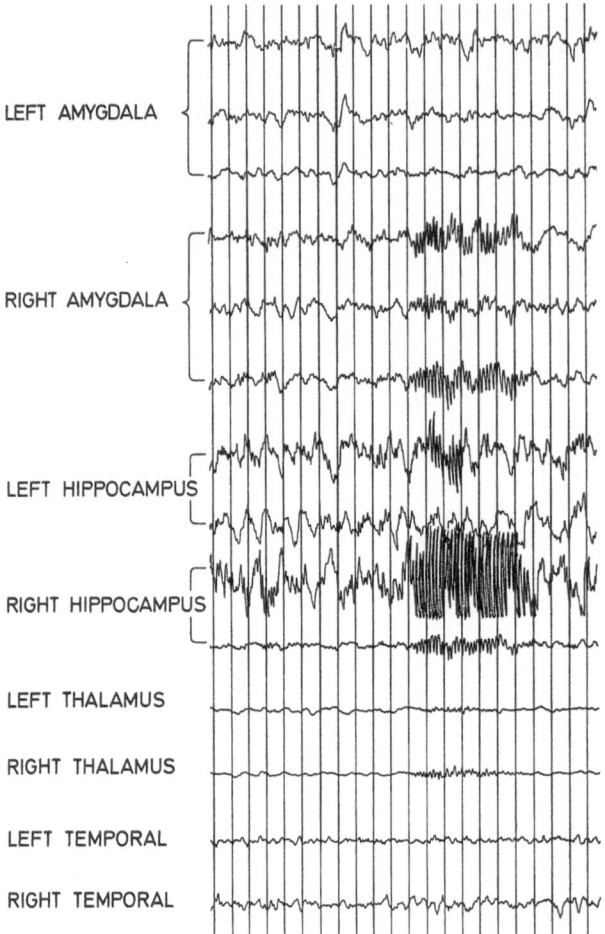

LEFT AMYGDALA

RIGHT AMYGDALA

LEFT HIPPOCAMPUS

RIGHT HIPPOCAMPUS

LEFT THALAMUS

RIGHT THALAMUS

LEFT TEMPORAL

RIGHT TEMPORAL

Fig. 3. Frequent polyspikes are discharged from the hippocampus. (Case of J. B.)
Note the way of propagation of the polyspike discharges

targets were taken into consideration to either interrupt the propagation route or to suppress the excitatory system.

As may be seen in Fig. 3, case J. B. manifested frequent polyspike activity only from the right hippocampus. This was coagulated with excellent results. In contrast another patient appeared to have seizure activities similar to J. B. but originating from the left hippocampus (Fig. 4 a). However after recording for several days a seizure originating in the right hippocampus was detected on one occasion (Fig. 4 b). The hippocampus with polyspikes and greater frequency

Table 1. *Seizure Active Site on Scalp and Depth EEG (16 EEG)*

Scalp \ Depth	Unilateral	Bilateral	Multiple
Unilateral	8 6	1	1
Bilateral	5 1	2	2
Diffuse	3 —	—	3

Table 2. *Most Prominent Symptoms and Seizure Active Site in the Subcortical Structures (21 Major Symptoms)*

Abnormal EEG in	Generalized motor seizure	Automatism	Aggressive behavior	Scizophrenic behaviour
Amygdala	6	3	—	—
Hippocampus	2	2	1	—
Diffuse temporal	1	1	3	2

Table 3. *Postoperative Results on Seizure and the Target Structures*

	Surgery	Excellent	Moderate	Slight/none
Amygdalotomy basolateral periamygdala	8	3	3	2
Hippocampotomy anterior	3	2	1	—
Multiple targets amygdala hippocampus ant. thalamus	5	2	2	1

of abnormality was selected for surgery but in this case the operative results were only moderately successful. Therefore the depth EEG should be studied over a long period of time in order to detect all possible foci and great care should be exercised in target selection.

C. Operative Results

Post-operative results obtained with various interventions are shown in Table 3. While these results are not fully satisfactory, the extent of clinical improvement seemed to be maximized by determination of the target structures through depth EEG.

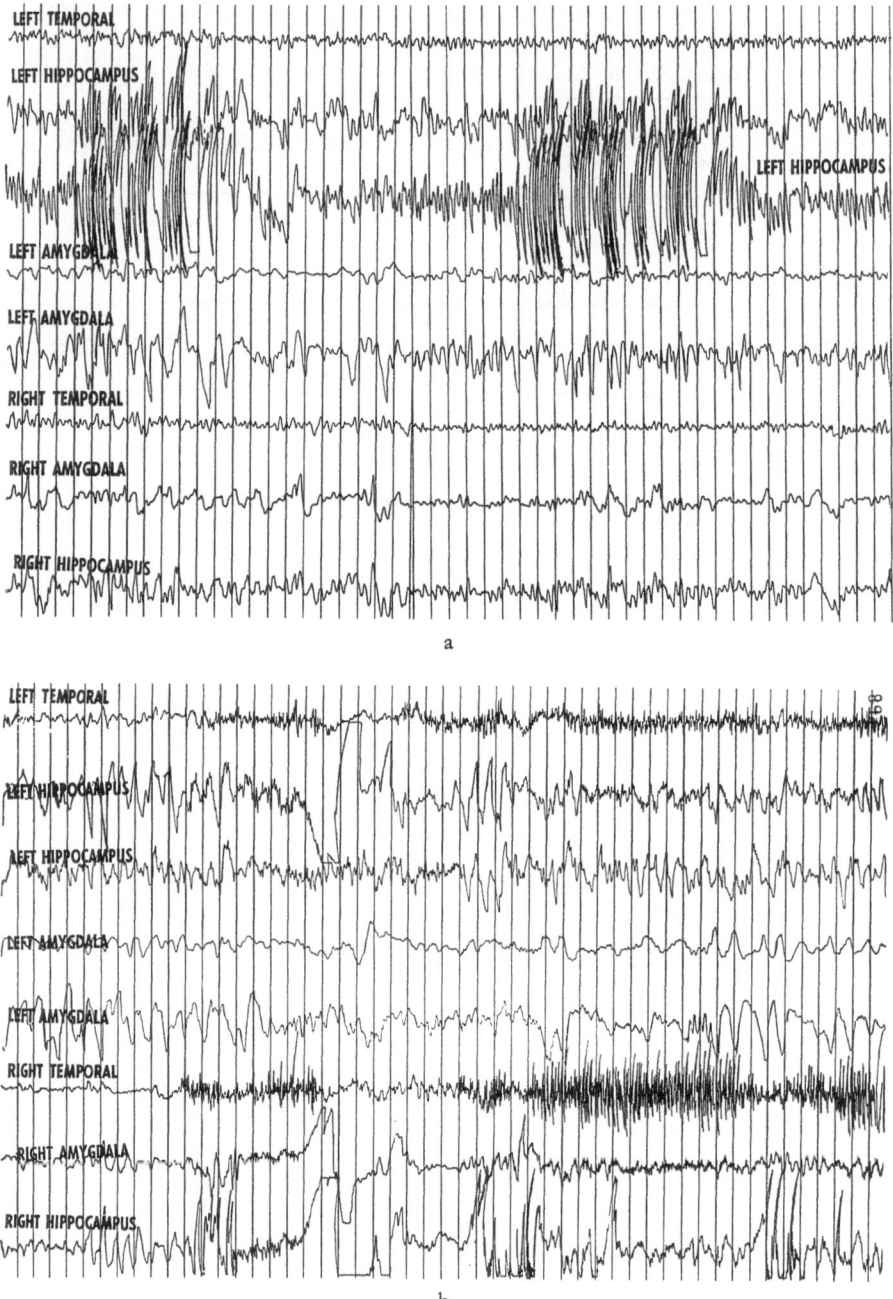

Fig. 4. This patient had constant polyspike discharges from the left hippocampus throughout the recording over 4 days of period (a), however on one occasion of clinical seizure the right hippocampus showed seizure discharges (b). Immediately before the clinical seizure the EEG activities were suddenly suppressed for a second in frequency and amplitude

Table 4. *Summary of Neuropsychological Data*
Patient: G. W. Age: 46. Hand preference: right hand.
Lesion site: left amygdala and right hippocampus

Test	Preoperative data	Postoperative data
Wais-VIQ	87	74
Wais-PIQ	100	97
Wais-FIQ	92	83
Wechsler memory (logical memory subtest)	Immediate: 5.0 Delayed: 1.5	3.0 1.0
Facial recognition test (nonverbal memory)	11 of 12 correct	7 of 12 correct
Digit span	Forward: 5 Backward: 3	6 4
Matching-to-sample	No delay: 100% correct 10 sec delay: 50% 20 sec delay: 33.3%	91.7% 58.3% 41.7%
Verbal learning	Reached criterion: 4 trials	Unable to reach criterion with 18 trials: trials 12, 14, and 17 were correct
	Free Recall	
	Immediate: perfect 2 hours: 1 cue	
Formboard	Right hand: 8 min 36 sec; 0 errors left hand: 8 min 20 sec; 0 errors	3 min 48 sec; 0 errors 3 min 3 sec; 0 errors
Reaction time	0.554 sec	0.612 sec
Trail making	Part A: 50 sec Part B: 142 sec	62 sec 192 sec
Tapping test	Right hand: 52.25 Left hand: 46.0	58.5 47.5

Table 5. *Summary of Neuropsychological Data*

Patient: P. W. Age: 17. Hand preference: right hand.
Lesion site: left amygdala and left hippocampus

Test	Preoperative data	Postoperative data
Wais-VIQ	100	97
Wais-PIQ	78	83
Wais-FIQ	90	91
Wechsler memory (Logical memory subtest)	Immediate: 10.0 Delayed: 8.0	4.5 5.0
Facial recognition test (nonverbal recall)	7 of 12 correct	11 of 12 correct
Digit span	Forward: 4 Backward: 3	5 6
Matching-to-sample	No delay: 100% correct 10 sec delay: 50% 20 sec delay: 50%	100% 50% 66.7%
Verbal learning	Reached criterion: 4 trials	4 trials
	Free recall	
	Immediate: perfect 1 hour: 1 cue 4 hours: 1 cue 24 hours: 1 cue 96 hours: perfect	Perfect Perfect 3 cues 3 cues 4 cues; 1 failure
Formboard	Right hand: 15 minutes, 7 errors Left hand: 15 minutes, 7 errors	15 minutes, 3 errors 15 minutes, 3 errors
Reaction time	0.758 sec	0.87 sec
Trail making	Part A: 103 sec Part B: 484 sec	71 sec 287 sec
Tapping test	Right hand: 21.0 Left hand: 19.0	35.8 28.0

D. Drug Evaluation

The effectiveness of three drugs, Valium, Dilantin and Pheno-barbital was assessed. Of the three, Valium was most effective in altering seizure activities seen in the depth EEG with Dilantin next in effectiveness. Phenobarbital appeared to have no significant in-fluence on the depth EEG.

E. Neuropsychological Results

Comparisons of pre- and post-operative performances on a nine-teen component neuropsychological battery of tests, indicated that four out of six patients with unilateral lesions obtained higher scores post-operatively on most tests. The patient with bilateral lesions had decreased scores on eleven of the nineteen battery components while achieving higher scores on eight. Two extreme cases are presented in Table 4.

The details of anticonvulsant evaluation and cerebral function test will be reported elsewhere.

References

1. Bancaud, J., Talairach, J. et al. (1966), La corne d'Ammon et le noyau amygdalien: Effets cliniques et électriques de leur stimulation chez l'homme. Revue Neurol., Paris, 115, 3, 329—352.
2. Crandall, P. H., Walter, R. D. et al. (1963), Clinical applications of studies on stereotaxically implanted electrodes in temporal lobe epilepsy. J. Neurosurg. 20, 827—840.
3. Gastaut, H., Broughton, R. (1972), Epileptic seizures. Springfield, Ill.: Ch. C Thomas.
4. Kim, Y. K., Umbach, W. (1973), Combined stereotactic lesions for treatment of behaviour disorders and severe pain, surgical approaches in psychiatry, edited by Laitinen, L. V., and Livingston, K. E. Lancaster, England: Medical and Technical Publishing Co., Ltd.

Author's address: Y. K. Kim, M.D., Department of Neurosurgery Neuro-science, Broughton Hospital, Morganton, NC 28655, U.S.A.

Acta Neurochirurgica, Suppl. 23, 45—50 (1976)
© by Springer-Verlag 1976

Neurosurgical Clinic, University of Milan, Italy

Multifocal Epilepsy: Surgical Treatment after Stereo-EEG Study

F. Marossero, G. P. Cabrini, G. Ettorre, G. Miserocchi, and L. Ravagnati

With 4 Figures

The term "multifocal epilepsy" has not been clearly defined. "Multifocal epilepsy" includes all cases of partial epilepsy with multiple independent electrical foci, either unilateral or bilateral (Marossero *et al.* 1975).

The presence, however, of multiple electrical foci does not necessarily imply the presence of multiple epileptogenic lesions. In other words, multifocal epilepsy does not always mean multilesional epilepsy. Both experimental and anatomo-clinical studies on epilepsy have showed without any doubt that a single anatomical lesion may cause multiple electrical foci, either unilateral or bilateral. On the other hand, the possibility cannot be ruled out that multiple electrical foci may be due to multiple epileptogenic lesions.

Identification of epileptogenic lesions is still mainly based on the study of cerebral electrical activities. The anatomical lesion, presumed to be the cause of electroclinical seizures, is very often not found in either pre-operative diagnostic examinations or during operation. The epileptogenic lesion may at times only be evident after microscopic or ultramicroscopic examinations of the surgical specimen. It therefore follows that, at times, an epileptogenic lesion can only be proven "a posteriori".

Evaluation of electrical signals in order to locate the site of the epileptogenic lesions is still being discussed.

We believe that, a general rule by which to judge the aforesaid does not presently exist.

In our experience, great localizing value can be attributed to interictal, paroxysmal abnormalities when they are arhythmic, stationary and persistent and when they are present in a background of abnormally slow, irregular, activity.

Electroclinical seizures, when they start in the same area affected by interictal abnormalities, are the surest evidence of focal epileptogenic lesion.

Particular importance must be given to the reactivity of electrical signals to different levels of consciousness, to convulsant or depressant drugs, and also to electroclinical responses to repetitive electrical stimulations. Study of the temporo-spatial course of electrical ictal phenomena enables us to recognize structures and pathways affected during the seizure itself. Personal experience, which is a factor of greatest importance, and the careful evaluation of all the above mentioned data brings us to the diagnosis of "epileptogenic surgical lesion".

By this term we therefore mean a cortical area which on the basis of all clinical, radiological, EEG and SEEG data, can be considered the sole or principal cause of seizures, excision of which area supposedly will offer best results without causing permanent neurological or psychic impairment to the patient.

Identification of epileptic surgical lesion or lesions in patients affected by partial seizures with multiple independent electrical foci, may be extremely difficult, and at times even impossible.

SEEG study, in our opinion, is mandatory in order to face the problem of diagnosis and subsequent advisability for surgery in multifocal epilepsy. SEEG must be carried out with chronically implanted electrodes (15–20 days). This technique allows a long term evaluation of interictal abnormalities under different conditions.

As has been already mentioned, it is also possible to record spontaneous electrical seizures and evaluate their course in different cerebral structures.

The following case is typical of situations that we came across in the more than one hundred cases of non-tumoral epileptics studied by us with SEEG (Pagni *et al.* 1966, Marossero *et al.* 1971, Cabrini *et al.* 1974).

Scacc. G., 28 years old man, affected by post-traumatic partial seizures with complex symptomatology.

At the admission in 1973, 10 years after the trauma, neurological examination was normal; only a moderate psychic impairment was present. A pneumoencephalogram showed a pseudo-poroencephalic cyst of the right frontal pole, not communicating with the ventricle.

EEG showed independent paroxysmal activities in right frontal and temporal regions, with marked posterior propagation; a spontaneous seizure was characterized by an ictal discharge affecting the whole right hemisphere with important contralateral involvement. Post-ictal reinforcement in the right fronto-central region was present (Fig. 1).

In summary electroencephalographic and neuroradiological examinations

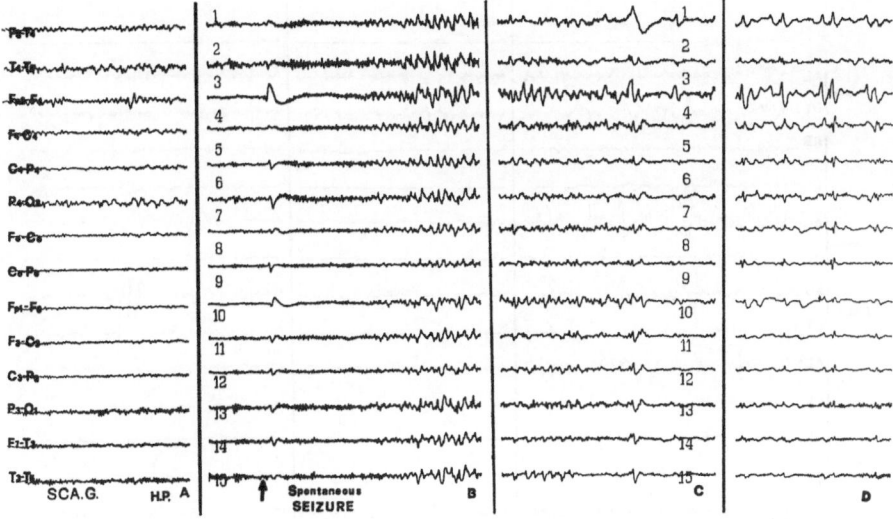

Fig. 1. *Scacc. G.*, 28 years old; post traumatic partial seizures with complex sympto-matology. A. Interictal EEG activity, characterized by independent paroxysmal abnormalities affecting right frontal and temporal areas. B–C. Spontaneous electro-clinical seizure. The ictal discharge starts with a tonic phase followed by spikes and sharp waves affecting the whole right hemisphere, with important contra-lateral involvement. D. Postictal reinforcement in right fronto-central area

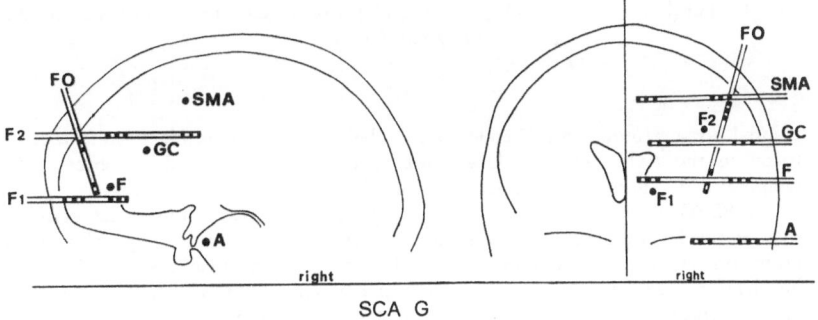

SCA G

Fig. 2. *Intracerebral recording.* Position of seven chronically implanted stainless steel electrodes. Every electrode has two groups of contacts: deep contacts (*A–B*) record from mesial frontal cortex, fronto-orbital cortex and amygdala; super-ficial contacts (*D–E*) record from frontal and temporal convexities. F–O fronto-orbital, F fronto-lateral, G.C. Gyrus Cinguli, S.M.A. Supplementary motor area, F 1, F 2 frontal convexity and frontal mesial surface, A Amygdala and temporal cortex

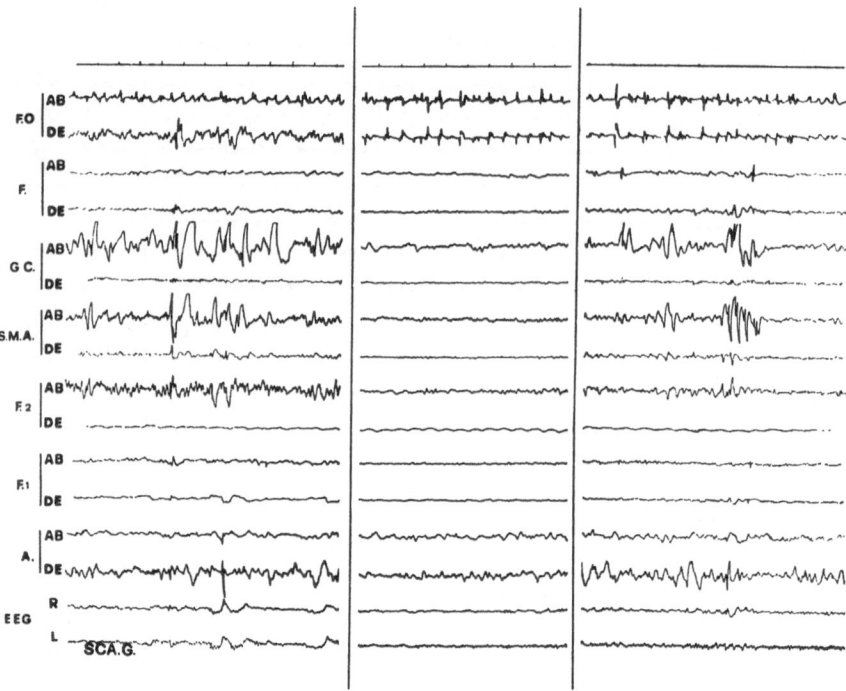

Fig. 3. Different examples of interictal SEEG activity. Paroxysmal activities are affecting independently: fronto-orbital cortex (*F–O, AB*), frontal pole (*F–O, DE,* and *F 2, AB*), Gyrus Cinguli (*G.C., AB*), Supplementary motor area (*S.M.A., AB*), and temporal cortex (*A, DE*). No epileptiform activity is present in the Amygdala (*A, AB*)

pointed to a fronto-central epileptogenic lesion. An independent epileptogenic lesion in the right temporal lobe however could not be ruled out because of temporal EEG abnormalities and because of clinical ictal symptomatology.

A SEEG study was planned (Bancaud 1965). Seven multicontact stainless steel electrodes were implanted in the right fronto-central and temporal regions, using the stereotactic equipment of Talairach (Fig. 2) (Talairach 1957). The interictal recording showed independent paroxysmal abnormalities affecting the mesial surface of the right frontal lobe and fronto orbital cortex; some independent paroxysms were also present on the right anterior temporal cortex (Fig. 3).

Both a spontaneous and an induced electroclinical seizure showed the ictal discharge starting in the mesial surface of the frontal lobe (at the level of gyrus cinguli and supplementary motor area) with secondary involvement of the right temporal cortex (Fig. 4).

In summary SEEG study revealed two independent epileptogenic lesions in the right frontal lobe (mesial surface and fronto-orbital surface). Epileptiform activity on the temporal cortex was probably functional and had no actual clinical significance.

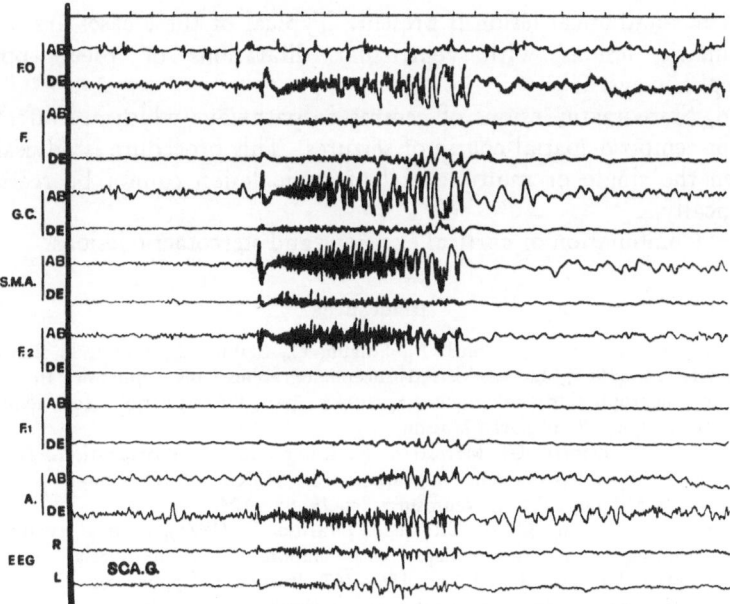

Fig. 4. Spontaneous electro-clinical seizure during SEEG. The ictal discharge is characterized by a tonic phase clearly starting and prominent on Gyrus Cinguli, S.M.A., and F 2 (AB) (mesial surface of frontal lobe). Ictal discharge affects the temporal cortex only secondarily. Paroxysmal fronto-orbital activity remains unchanged during the seizure

On the basis of these data a right frontal lobectomy including supplementary motor area and fronto orbital region was performed. No seizure occurred during one year of follow up. EEG was normal, temporal paroxysms were no longer present.

Conclusion

This case report stresses the importance of SEEG for the diagnosis of epileptogenic lesion or lesions in cases of partial epilepsy with multifocal electrical abnormalities.

After identification of one or more epileptogenic surgical lesions, the following possibilities exist:

a) No surgical treatment in cases of many cortical lesions which extend over one or over both hemispheres, and presenting seizures having different origins and different temporo-spatial courses.

b) Cortical excision when it can be shown that multiple electrical foci are due to a single epileptogenic lesion.

c) Multiple cortical excisions or excision which include multiple adjoining epileptogenic lesions. In most of these cases a large and evident anatomical lesion is present. Typical of these cases are post-traumatic lesions with ventricular dilatations or pseudo-poro-encephalic cysts.

d) Stereotactic lesions of centres or pathways which are affected in the temporo-spatial course of seizures. This procedure is advisable when the single or multiple epileptogenic lesion cannot be reached surgically.

e) Combination of cortical excisions and stereotactic lesions.

References

Bancaud, J., Talairach, J., Bonis, A., Schaub, C., Szikla, G., Morel, P., Bordas-Ferrer, M. (1965), La stéréoélectroencéphalographie dans l'épilepsie. Informations neurophysiopathologiques apportées par l'investigation fonctionnelle stéréotaxique, 321 p. Paris: Masson.

Cabrini, G. P., Ettorre, G., Marossero, F., Miserocchi, G., Ravagnati, L. (1975), Surgery of epilepsy: some indications for SEEG. XXIII Congr. Soc. It. Neuroch. Milano, 1974. J. Neurosurg. Sci. *19*, 95—104.

Marossero, F., Cabrini, G. P., Ettorre, G., Infuso, L. (1971), Critical evaluation of SEEG in psychomotor epilepsy with temporal focus. In: Special topics in stereotaxis (Umbach, W., ed.), pp. 156—167. Stuttgart: Hippokrates.

— — — Miserocchi, G., Ravagnati, L., Indicazioni chirurgiche nelle epilessie multifocali. Simposio sulla epilessia multifocale. Roma, 1975. In press.

Pagni, C. A., Marossero, F., Infuso, L., Ettorre, G., Cabrini, G. P. (1966), La SEEG nella diagnostica delle epilessie non tumorali. Minerva Neurochir. *10*, 145—201.

Talairach, J., David, M., Tournoux, P., Corredor, H., Kvasina, T. (1957), Atlas d'anatomie stéréotaxique, 294 p. Paris: Masson.

Authors' address: Dr. F. Marossero, Dr. G. P. Cabrini, Dr. G. Ettorre, Dr. G. Miserocchi, and Dr. L. Ravagnati, Neurosurgical Clinic, University of Milan, Via F. Sforza, 35, Milano, Italy.

Acta Neurochirurgica, Suppl. 23, 51—57 (1976)

Institute of Neurosurgery, Budapest, Hungary

The Motor Mechanism of Some Types of Epilepsy

S. Tóth, J. Vajda, and P. Zaránd

With 3 Figures

In most cases it is very difficult to find a correlation between cortical or subcortical electrical and clinical electro-myographical activity during epileptic fits. This difficulty arises not only from the mechanism of epilepsy, but from the mechanism of the motor system itself. In our previous studies (Tóth 1972, Tóth, Zaránd, Lázár 1974) we have found that the direct connection between the stimulated site of the central motor system and the answering muscles depends on many conditions. The main conditions are: the intensity, the frequency of the stimulus and the functional state of the motor system, rest activity and the transitional states.

After the stimulus within the motor system there is no only a momentary phasic answer, but a longlasting 200 msec–1 sec or more change in motor activity of reactivity state. This change we can follow with evoked potentials within the motor system, with the evoked motor response at the periphery and especially by means of double stimuli *i.e.* conditioning and test stimuli.

According to these changes the stimulated site influences the other parts of the central motor system, spinal segmental motor activity, the evoked peripheral motor response and evoked activities all feed back to the starting point. So develops a decreasing circulation of the facilitatory and inhibitory effects within the motor system. Epileptic activity is a repetitive irritative process and motor signs have to follow the frequency of this irritative process.

If we stimulate the motor system the motor response at the periphery follows the 100 cps frequency too but it is quite clear that with such a series of events every event will be influenced from the previous one. From our earlier studies we know that stimulation of the motor system with different frequencies will influence, enhance or depress the frequency properties of the motor system (Tóth *et al.* 1974).

4*

To simplify the problem—from the point of view of motor activity—we have chosen as the epileptic model petit mal epilepsy and an epilepsy with very short tonic fits.

In these two types of epilepsy there were two common characteristics. It was much easier to elicit cortical, subcortical and motor

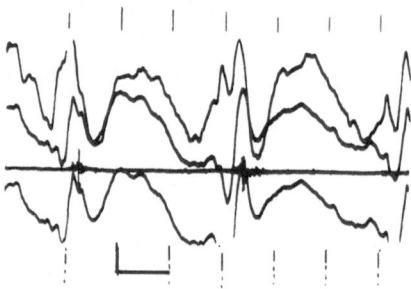

Fig. 1. Petit mal activity in both cingulate areas with motor activity in the left biceps muscle. Calibration: 100 msec, 0.1 mV for the cortical traces and 1 mV for the muscle

epileptic activity at rest. In comparison the resting state enhances some part of the evoked potential and the motor activity enhances the other parts more than during motor activity. To every epileptic wave there belong a motor activity group. As well as that petit mal epileptic activity has a very strict 3–4 cps rhythmic feature and peripheral motor activity appears during the spike phase of the spike and wave complex (Fig. 1).

Fig. 2. Patient with short tonic epileptic fits. Stimulation of different parts of the brain on the right side. Registration of the evoked potential on the same side (dentate nucleus on the left side) and of the motor responses in the left biceps muscle. *On the left:* recording after the first stimulus in rest. *In the middle:* recording after the second or third stimulus at rest. *On the right:* recording during voluntary contraction. With the first stimulus of the motor system, temporal motor cortex and amygdala, it is possible to evoke epileptic spikes and a late short tonic activity. The same is not possible with the second or third stimulus at rest or during voluntary contraction. One can clearly see the spike potential during the period of the short tonic burst or immediately before it. During voluntary contraction the motor rebound activity is in the same period as the short tonic activity at rest and clear after the stimulation of the motor cortex. Naturally after stimulation of the temporal cortex and amygdale there are no motor responses during voluntary contraction. Calibration: 100 msec, 50 microV for the deep electrodes, 500 microV for the muscle. Stimulus: 25–50 V, 0.05 to 0.2 msec. square wave impulses

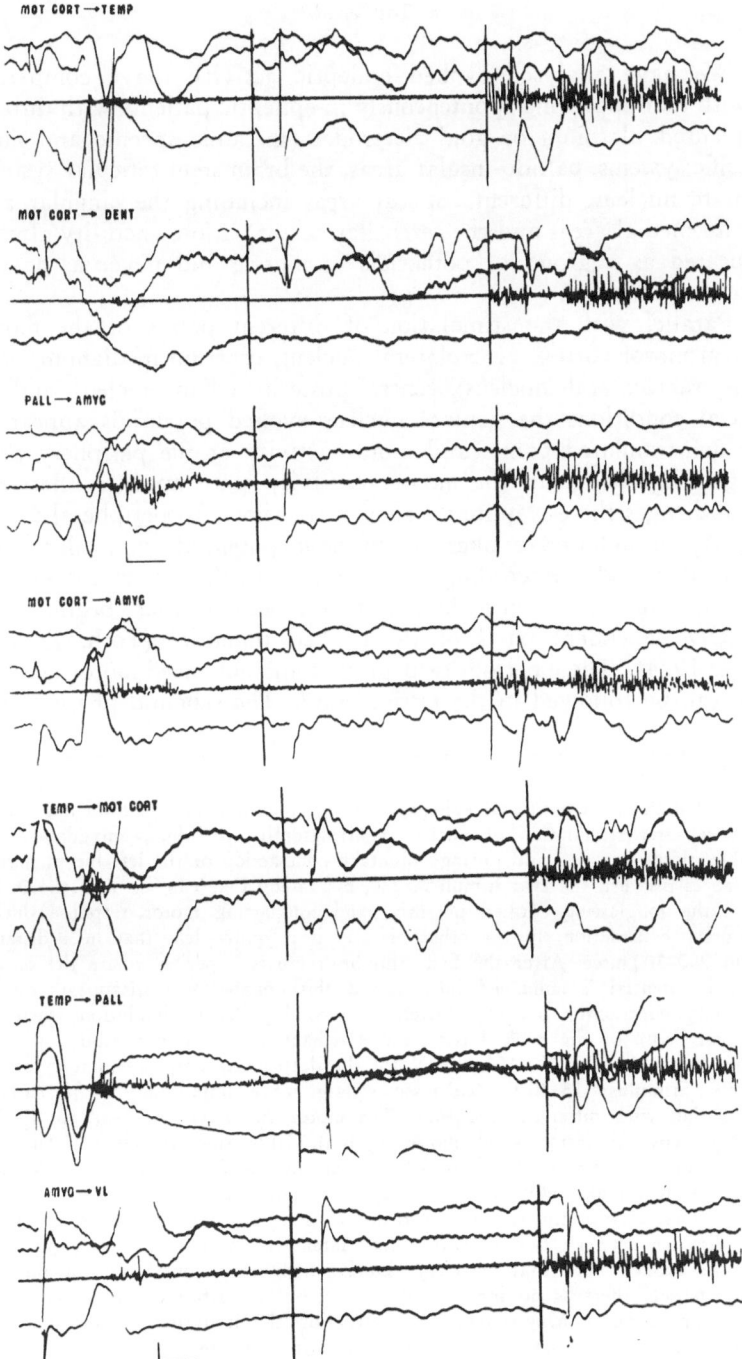

Fig. 2

We have analysed evoked epileptic activity thave comparied it with that appearing spontaneously in epileptic patients with chronic implanted platinum or gold electrodes (thalamic specific and non-specific systems, pallido-insular areas, the brain stem reticular system, dentate nucleus, different cortical areas including the cingular and fronto-medial areas and the cerebellar cortex). Motor activity always appeared as a group of potentials in muscle and never as a synchronous potential.

Parallel with the stimulation of different points of the motor system motor cortex, ventrolateral nucleus, centrum medianum, ventral-posterolateral nucleus, ventral-posteriomedian nucleus and in special conditions the dentate nucleus evoked potentials appear at the nonstimulated points and motor activity at the periphery or a longlasting change in the motor reactivity state appears. Between these changes there is quite a strong correlation. In peripheral motor activity stimulation evokes synchronous potentials and silent and rebound periods. According to this there are changes in the evoked potential an usually with the first motor rebound there begins functionally dependent parts of the evoked potential (Tóth, Zaránd, Lázár 1974). These periods of depressed and enhanced motor activity also can be followed in the resting state. The rebound phase of the

---

Fig. 3. Patient with petit mal epilepsy. *On the left:* Evoked potential and motor response after stimulation of nucleus ventrolateralis, pallidum, amygdala—with double stimuli—in rest and during voluntary contraction of the left biceps muscle (distances between the two stimuli 0, 280, 300 msec). One can see with the 0 distance the longlasting evoked potential and longlasting motor response during voluntary contraction. In the other pictures it is quite clear that in a distance about 280–300 msec. After the first stimulus there is a period where the second evoked potential is enhanced in rest and this enhancement disappears during voluntary contraction but clear after the second pallidal stimulation when the rebound phase of the evoked potential is enhanced with motor rebond at rest. Calibration: 100 msec, 50–100 microV for the deep electrodes, 100 microV for the muscle. Stimulus: 15–40 V, 0,05 msec square wave impulses. *In the middle:* stimulation with different frequency. The motor responses are 3–3,5 cps during 3,5 and 7 cps stimulation (stable motor rhythm). Calibration: 100 msec, 100 microV for the deep electrodes, 1000 microV for the muscle. Stimulus: 40 V, 0.05 msec square wave impulses. *On the right:* repetitive potentials in the motor and cingulate areas, after stimulation of the frontobasal region, with increasing amplitude and distance between two potentials and later with group of muscle potential at rest (evoked petit mal activity). During voluntary contraction of the left biceps muscle there is no increase of the repetitive irritative process after the same stimulation. During voluntary contraction the irritative process does not appear after double stimulation either. Calibration: 100 msec, 100 microV for the deep electrodes, 100 microV for the muscle. Stimulus: 50 V, 0.1 msec. square wave impulses

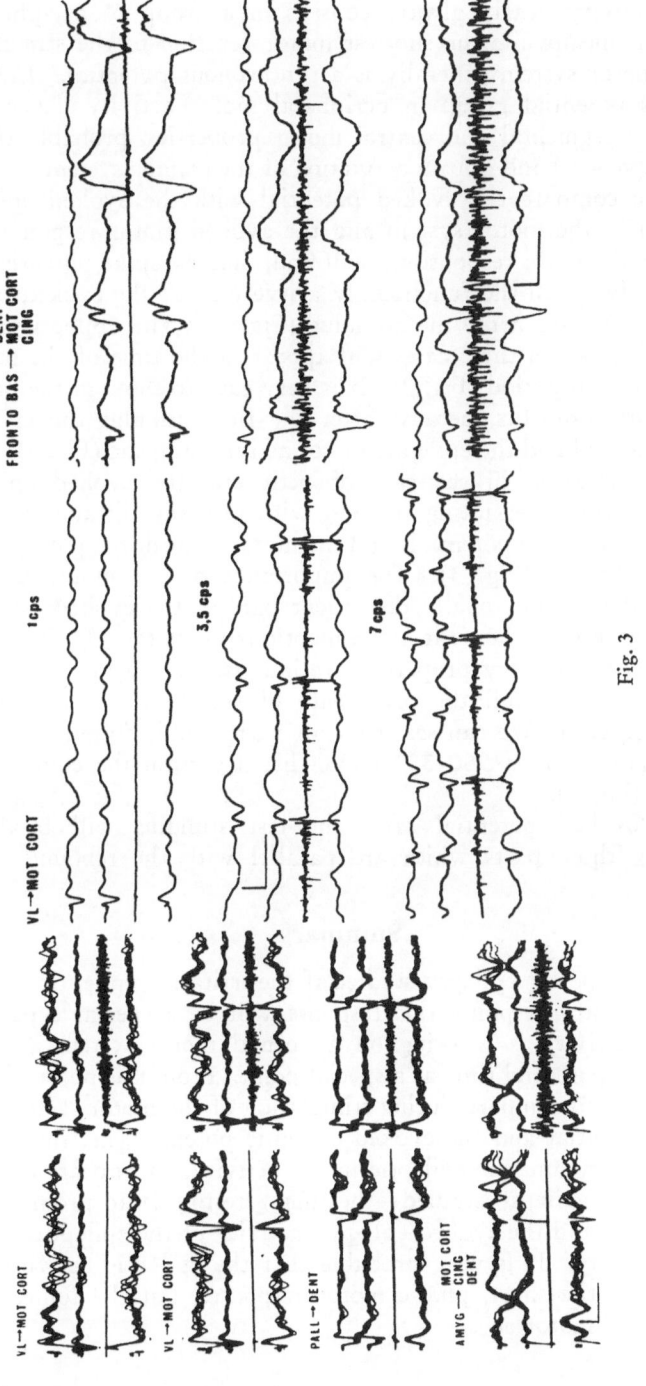

Fig. 3

motor activity nearly always consists in a group of asynchronous potentials meanwhile the shortest motor reaction to the stimulation of the motor system generally is a synchronous potential. The synchronous potential group in peripheral motor activity depends on the spinal segmental and central motor properties, probably on the spinal segmental and central activation of the gamma system.

If we compare the evoked potential with the evoked epileptic potential in the motor system and the avoked motor response with the epileptic motor response we will find, that the spike potential will develop always in the functionally acitve part of the evoked potential 30–500 msec after the stimulus (Fig. 2). The epileptic motor potential group in these cases will appear at the time of the normal motor rebound period (Fig. 2). It is very easy to show in the patient with short tonic fits, because after the first stimulus the epileptic spike potential and the epileptic motor activity appears (Fig. 2).

In comparison in the case of petit mal the evoked epileptic activity needs a recruiting process, with growing distance between the following spike potentials and the motor signs develop only at the 3–4 cps rhythm (Fig. 3). The importance of the motor rebound phase and the functionally dependent part of the evoked potential is quite clear with the petit mal epileptic patients too. In these cases the 3–4 cps frequency properties are important. During stimulation with 1–8 cps stimuli the prevalence of the 3 cps mechanism are obvious (Fig. 3). We can see the same with double stimuli when the test stimulus is in a 260–320 m/sec distance from the conditioning stimulus (Fig. 3).

The evoked potential after the test stimulus will be larger especially those parts which are parallel with the rebound motor activity.

Summary

In the types of epilepsy studied if the irritative epileptic activity evokes a motor response this response will be a special type. The epileptic activity is working on a normal motor system and will affect it in space and time at a special point. From this point of view it is possible to compare-during stimulation of the motor system—the evoked potential and the evoked epileptic potential, i.e. the evoked motor activity and the epileptic motor activity. It appears that—in the types of epilepsy studied—the motor resting state promotes the spontaneous and the evoked epileptic activity or the epileptic evoked motor activity. It is very probable that the epileptic activity does not employ the short, phasic motor responses, but the tonic, automatic, reflex motor ones.

References

Tóth, S. (1972), Effect of electrical stimulation of subcortical sites on speech and consciousness, pp. 40—46. Neurophysiology studied in man. Amsterdam: Excerpta Medica.
— Zaránd, P., Lázár, L., Vajda, J. (1975), Effects of voluntary innervation on the evoked potential of the motor system. Proceedings of the Sixth Symposium of the International Society for Research in Stereoencephalotomy. Tokyo, 1973. Confin. Neurol. 37, 49—55.
— — — (1974), The role of the cortex and subcortical ganglia in the evoked rhythmic motor activity. Acta Neurochir. (Wien), Suppl. 21, 25—33.

Author's address: Dr. S. Tóth, Dr. J. Vajda, and Dr. P. Zaránd, Institute of Neurosurgery, Budapest, Hungary.

Acta Neurochirurgica, Suppl. 23, 59—64 (1976)

Department of Neurology, Research and Teaching Center,
Warsaw Medical Academy, Warsaw, Poland

Clinical and Electrophysiological Effects of Chronic Epileptic Lesion in Split-Brain Cats*

(Preliminary Report)

J. Majkowski, W. Pisarski, B. Bilińska-Nigot, A. Sobieszek, and A. Karliński

With 3 Figures

Summary

The development of the clinical and EEG manifestations of intracortical alumina cream epileptogenic lesion is described in 14 split-brain cats. In 4 animals contralateral and/or ipsilateral, cortical and subcortical secondary epileptic foci were present. The results indicate that integrity of interhemispheric transfer through the corpus callosum and anterior and posterior commissures is not necessary for the transmission of epileptic activity to contralateral hemisphere. Partial epileptic seizures of Jacksonian type were observed in 6 cats. In 1 cat grand mal epileptic seizure developed. The possible mechanisms of secondary epileptic foci and generalized type of seizure are discussed.

Introduction

This report is concerned with the electrophysiological and clinical manifestations of epilepsy in split-brain cats. Observations were made on split-brain animals which had epileptic lesions (alumina cream injections) in the right motor-sensory cortical area (pericruciate cortex). This experimental model was used because it resembles in many ways the development of epilepsy in human patients. This communication is a part of more extensive study including the effect

---

* This investigation was supported by a grant under Polish-American Agreement PL 480, NIMH, No. 05-276-2.

of diphenyl-hydantoin (DPH) on the epileptic lesion and the effects of DPH and/or epileptic lesion and seizures on learning and retention. The detailed results are being prepared for publication.

Material and Methods

Experiments were performed on 14 adult cats which were subjected to surgical separation of the optic chiasm and cerebral commissures. Detailed description of the surgical procedure may be found elsewhere [5]. Each cat had alumina cream (0.1–0.15 ml) injected in the right motor-sensory cortex and subcortical white matter. Alumina cream was prepared according to Faeth *et al.* [2]. Bipolar cortical and subcortical electrodes were next implanted symmetrically in the visual, auditory and motor-sensory cortical areas and in hippocampus for monitoring functional changes occuring in the brain during maturation of the epileptic focus. The EEG was recorded every week or two in each animal. Antiepileptic drug diphenylhydantoin (DPH) was given orally in food in animals with clinical seizures. The localization of the epileptic foci and comissural section was verified histologically.

Results

Several types of EEG patterns could be identified in animals with intracortical alumina cream injection. Focal depression of background activity in the region of the lesion was the first sign observed within the first two weeks after production of epileptic lesion. This depression was characterized by decrease of amplitude and assymetry of EEG rhythms and was considered as a post-traumatic effect. Three to four weeks after injection focal sporadic slow waves in the theta range and of higher amplitude than background activity became distinct. From the 11th week on this type of activity was present in all cats. Spike and sharp waves were the third type of the EEG changes, which usually occured still later than the type 2 (Fig. 1, 2, 3). The proportion of animals with spike and sharp waves was about 55–70%. This type of activity was always present in cats with developed clinical epileptic seizures. Paroxysmal epileptic discharges were the last sign o fthe maturation of the epileptic lesion. They were mainly composed of high voltage spikes or sharp waves accompanied by slow waves in theta or delta range. This type of activity was more pronounced at the time corresponding to occurence of clinical seizures.

In 4 out of 14 cats secondary contralateral and/or ipsilateral focal epileptic discharges developed. They were observed in the left motor-sensory cortex and in the right temporal and left and right visual cortex. They also appeared in the right or in both hippocampi.

Clinical seizures developed in 8 out of 14 cats from about 3 weeks to 5 months after alumina cream injection. Left Jacksonian

C-118

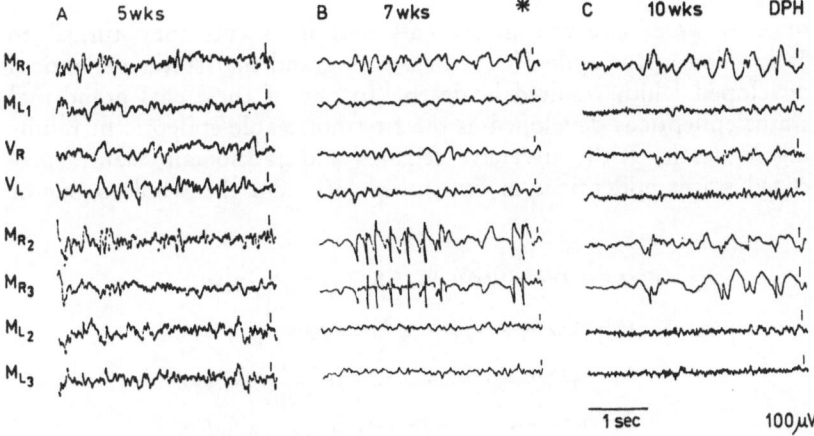

Fig. 1. EEG records in the split brain cat C-118 with epileptic lesion in the right motor-sensory cortex. Focal multiple spikes and spikes and waves in the lesioned area (M_{R1}, M_{R2}, M_{R3}) developed on the 7th week after alumina cream injection (B), while on the fifth week only discrete focal abnormality could be detected (A). * Indicates left Jacksonian seizures which were observed at that period. After diphenylhydantoin (*DPH*) clinical seizures were to some extent controlled and EEG discharges were modified (C). Section of the corpus callosum in this cat was complete but section of the anterior and posterior commissures was partial. Abbreviations: $M_{R1,2,3}$ = indicates derivations from the right motor-sensory cortex, $M_{L1,2,3}$ = the same from the left hemisphere, v_R, v_L = right and left visual cortex

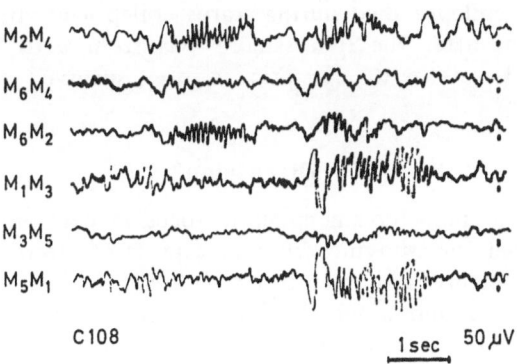

Fig. 2. EEG records from the right (M_2–M_4, M_6–M_4, M_6–M_2) and left (M_1–M_3, M_3–M_5, M_5–M_1) motor-sensory cortical areas in the cat C 108 with complete section of the corpus callosum and posterior commissures and epileptic lesion in the right hemisphere. There is clear assymetry of the electrocortical activity between the two hemispheres with slower rhythms and spindles on the right (lesioned) and sharp wave followed by a spindle in the left (normal) hemisphere

seizures were observed in six cats and in 3 cats they turned to Jacksonian status epilepticus. In 3 cats grand mal status epilepticus developed which resulted in death. In one of these cats grand mal status epilepticus developed as the first noticeable epileptic fit resulting in death. Ritht adversive seizures and Jacksonian seizures preceded status epilepticus in two other cats. On the whole 5 out of

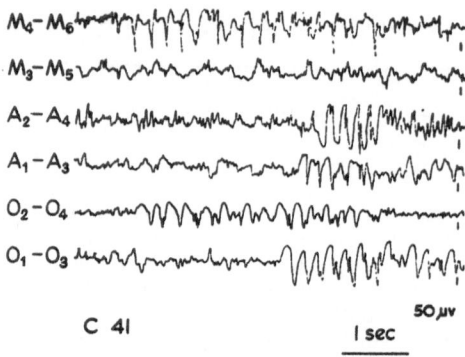

Fig. 3. Multifocal epileptic activity in the cat C 41 about 1 year after alumina cream injection. Clear spike and sharp wave activity can be seen in the primary epileptic focus $(M_4–M_6)$. Abbreviations: $M_3–M_5 =$ left motor-sensory cortex, $A_1–A_3$, $A_2–A_4 =$ left and right auditory cortex respectively, $O_2–O_3$ and $O_2–O_4 =$ left and right visual cortex

8 cats with epilepsy died during status epilepticus. In these 5 cats survival time after the first seizure was from 0 to 8 days. The remaining 3 cats with epileptic seizures survived 62, 157 and 793 days.

Discussion

Chronic alumina cream epileptic focus in cats provides a convenient model for studying different aspects of electrophysiological and clinical seizures in human being. It seems evident that section of the corpus callosum alone does not prevent development of secondary epileptic activity in opposite hemisphere and generalized seizures or status epilepticus.

Commissural section or surgical isolation of the epileptogenic focus was reported to be effective in preventing spreading of seizure discharges and formation of a mirror focus [1, 3, 4, 6]. Our observations support the hypothesis that the interhemispheric commissural pathway is not entirely responsible for the formation of the secondary epileptic discharges on the contralateral hemisphere [7]. Some electro-physiological studies also support this possibility [8]. However, second-ary contralateral epileptic focus may be explained by different mech-anisms. First, usually some commissural pathways are partly intact eg. commissura posterior, anterior or commissura fornicis. It is well known that even a small part of residual pathways in brain may be sufficient for transmission of epileptogenic activity. In our studies usually commissura posterior was intact or partially cut. Also section of the anterior commissura in some animals was not complete. However, in 2 cats all interhemispheric commissures were cut and still, partial epilepsy and secondary generalized grand mal seizures developed. This might be explained by the possibility that epilepto-genic material could be transported by granular cells to other parts of the brain — being responsible for secondary epileptic discharges in homo — and contralateral hemisphere. Such cells were observed in our cats and in one cat in the lateral ventricule. Transcallosal axoplasmic flow of alumina cream agent which could be responsible for mirror focus formation has to be ruled out since in our case corpus callosum was cut. Finally we should take into consideration brain-stem mechanism responsible for propagation of epileptic activ-ity to the opposite hemisphere. However, it seems that in such cases, one of the prerequisites would be the development of a very active epileptic activity involving entire hemisphere and spreading to brain-stem and then centrapetally to other hemisphere. This was observed in cat C 41 (Fig. 3).

It is emphasized that we did not observe mirror focus. The focus of secondary epileptic activity was never dependently discharg-ing from the primary focus (Fig. 2). Thus, formation of a mirror focus would require an intact corpus callosum in contrast to secon-dary epileptic foci for which this main commissural pathways is not essential.

References

1. Bogen, J. E., Fischer, E. D., and Vogel, P. J. (1965), Cerebral commissurotomy. A second case report. J. Amer. med. Ass. 194, 1328—1329.
2. Faeth, W. H., Walker, A. E., and Andy, O. J. (1956), Experimental sub-cortical epilepsy. Arch. Neurol. Psych. 75, 548—562.
3. Gazzaniga, M. S., Bogen, J. E., and Sperry, R. W., (1962), Some functional effects of sectioning the cerebral commissures in man. Proc. nat. Acad. Sci. 48, 1765—1769.
4. Guerrero-Figueroa, R., Barros, A., Heath, R., and Gonzales, G. (1964), Experimental subcortical epileptiform focus. Epilepsia (Amst.) 5, 112—139.
5. Majkowski, J. (1967), Electrophysiological studies of learning in split brain cats. Electroenceph. clin. Neurophysiol. 26, 521—531.

6. Morrell, F. (1965), Secondary epileptogenic lesions. Epilepsia (Amst.) 6, 297—309.
7. Okudzava, V. M., Chipashvili, S. A. (1973), Concerning the role of callosal and extracallosal connection in the interhemispheric distribution of epileptic activity (in Russian). Zhur. Nevropat. Psich. (Korsakov), Moskwa 73, 1679—1684.
8. Wilder, B. J., Schmidt, R. P. (1965), Propagation of epileptic discharge from chronic neocortical foci in monkey. Epilepsia (Amst.) 6, 297—309.

Authors' address: Doc. dr hab. med. J. Majkowski, Department of Neurology, Research and Teaching Center, Warsaw Medical Academy, Grenadierów 51, Warsaw, Poland.

Acta Neurochirurgica, Suppl. 23, 65—70 (1976)

Centre for Cerebral Neurophysiology of National Council of Researches,
Institute of Neurophysiopathology of the University, Genoa, Italy

Determination of the Functional Hierarchy in Multifocal Epilepsy

B. Cavazza, F. Ferrillo, B. Gasparetto, and **G. Rosadini**

With 2 Figures

Our previous research on interictal electrographic epileptic potentials of human scalp recordings, carried out using a simultaneous
multichannel averaging technique (Rosadini *et al.* 1974), showed that:
1. different morphological spike models can be present in various
structures as well as within a given structure in every single patient;
the distribution pattern of their frequency components can be exactly
defined by Fourier analysis in order to characterize objectively the
identified models (Cavazza *et al.* 1974). 2. The presence of different
morphological models could be related to the functional conditions
of the subjects, such as wakefulness and various sleep stages (Cavazza
et al. 1973). 3. The improvement of the signal to noise ratio allowed
the detection of spikes which were not evident at a conventional
inspective analysis of the EEG because masked by background activity (Siccardi *et al.* 1973).

The present research concerns a study of interictal epileptic
potentials recorded from cortical and subcortical structures in patients
suffering from multifocal epilepsy and in cats carrying a neocortical
cobalt induced epileptic focus. The aims were: i) the verification in
recordings directly performed from the human brain of what was
observed in scalp recordings of large neural populations and consequently less precise from a technical point of view and ii) a new
approach to the interpretation of human interictal epileptic potentials
on the basis of observations obtained from simple experimental
models.

Material and Methods

Bipolar recordings of patients were made using multipolar electrodes chronically implanted in different cerebral structures (Rossi 1973); sessions lasted several
hours and were repeated over a period of 2–3 weeks. Monopolar recordings of

cats were made using electrodes chronically implanted in the focus (sensorimotor cortex), in extrafocal cortical areas of both hemispheres and in various subcortical bilateral structures; the Nucleus Caudatus (NC) and Ventralis Posterolateralis thalami (VPL) were always implanted in all animals (Ferrillo *et al.* 1973). In all human and animal recordings, spikes were present in several channels; in the conventional EEG the temporal relations among spikes belonging to different leads could not be defined. Using as trigger spikes of various leads, repeated multichannel simultaneous averagings were carried out at various times during the whole period of the exploration.

Results

Data derived from human recordings.

In recordings characteristic of multifocal epilepsy, the following events can occur:

1. There are spikes, simultaneously present in several structures, which display a defined chronology (Fig. 1 A); consequently the cerebral zones generating them can be considered as belonging to a neural path through which the pathological electrical event propagates.

2. There are spikes which do not show any temporal relation with other structures and are always confined to one lead only; in this case they can be considered as autonomous (Fig. 1, *RAT 2; A–B*). The structure generating them can also belong to the previously mentioned neural path; in the two cases the morphology is different.

3. There are structures which can generate spikes both autonomous and led by more than one structure; in this case too the morphologies differ (Fig. 1, *RH; A–C–D*).

4. Spikes which are not evident in the conventional recordings can be shown by the averaging process used and quite often such spikes precede those which are more evident in other leads.

5. Finally, a constant morphology of the spikes in all leads and a steady chronology among the epileptic potentials of the different channels is seldom observed.

Data derived from animal recordings.

As shown in Fig. 2, during the development of an experimental

---

Fig. 1. On the left EEG recorded in different cortical and subcortical structures of an epileptic patient. (*R* right; *L* left; *A* amygdala; *CA* Ammon's horn; *H* hippocampal gyrus; *AT 2* anterior part of the second temporal convolution; *PT 2* posterior part of the second temporal convolution; *TP* temporal pole). Under *A*, *B*, *C*, and *D* the simultaneous averages of epileptic potentials concerning the same epoch of recording and carried out using as trigger spikes belonging to different structures (arrows). The chronology of the spikes and their morphological alterations in the different temporal patterns are shown

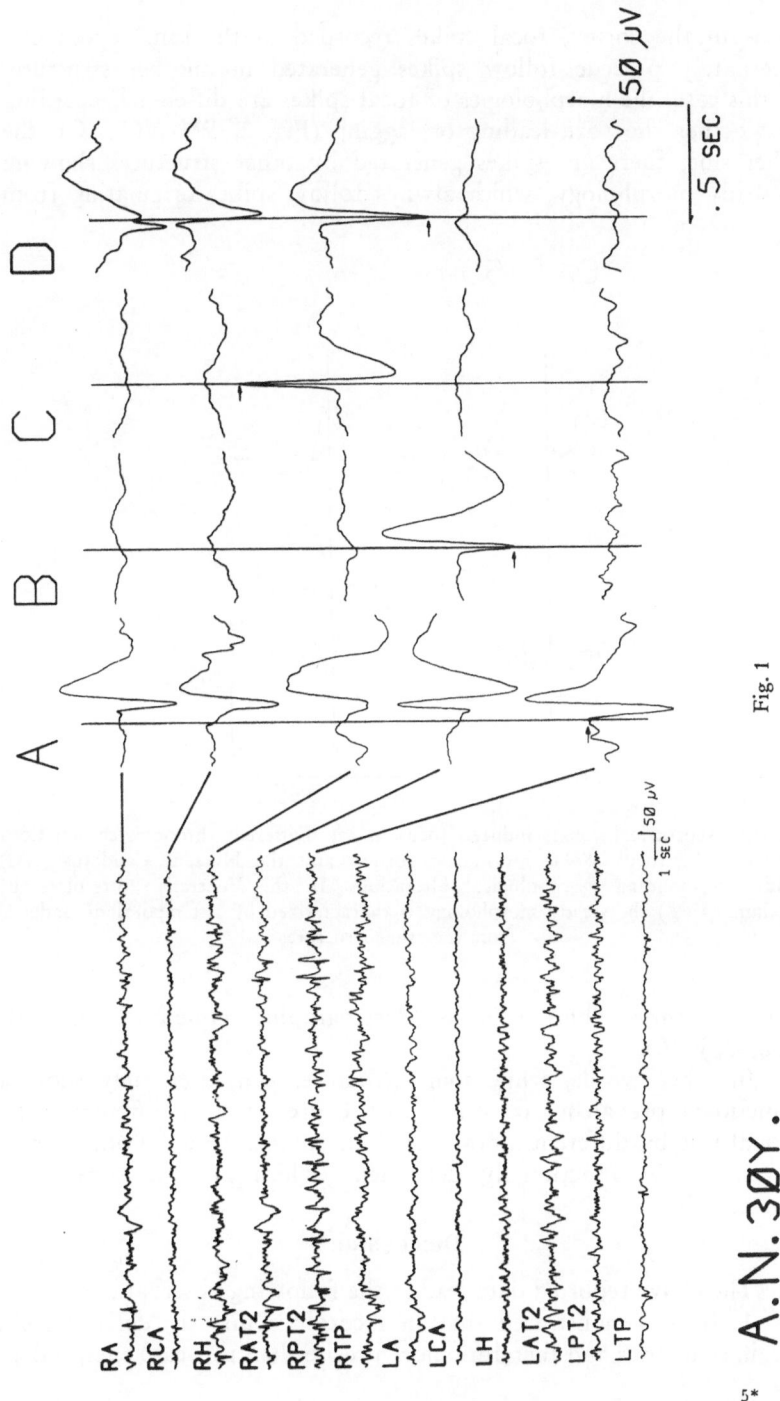

Fig. 1

focus in the cortex, focal spikes recorded in the same epoch can alternately precede follow spikes generated in another structure. In this case, the morphologies of focal spikes are different, according to whether they are leading or lagging (Fig. 2, *SM–NC*). On the other side, there are spikes generated by other structures showing a steady morphology, which always follow spikes originating from

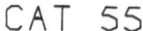

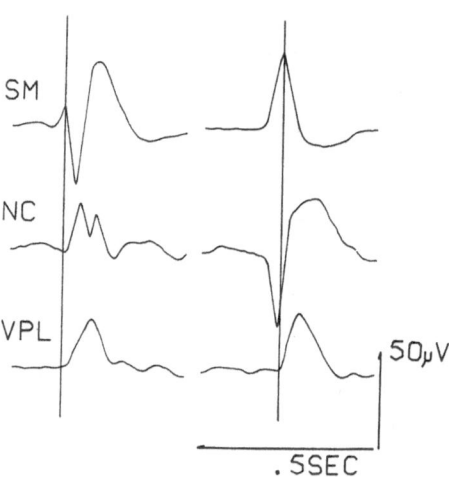

Fig. 2. Neocortical cobalt induced focus in cat. Different chronological relations between the focus (*SM* sensorimotor cortex) and the Nucleus Caudatus (*NC*) and corresponding morphological alterations. In the Ventralis Posterolateralis thalami (*VPL*) the steady morphology is characterized by a temporal dependence from the other structures

the structures able to lead electrographic epileptic potentials (Fig. 2, *VPL*).

In other words, while some structures can alternately show a functional prevalence on others and express such a different functional role by different morphologies of spikes, there are other structures, always functionally dependent, which produce stereotyped spikes only.

Discussion

The above reported data lead to the following observations:

1. It is demonstrated that in recordings directly derived from brain structures and therefore more precise than the scalp ones, epilep-

tic spikes can also be present and detected only by the averaging technique employed, able to separate the examined potential from the background activity which in this case can be considered as a noise.

2. Such spikes can also precede those which are more evident in other structures; this means that in the epileptic brain we can find structures which unexpectedly are precociously involved in the epileptic event.

3. The reported system of data processing gives the exact chronology of spikes belonging to different leads and allows discrimination between structures generating spikes which remain circumscribed and structures involved in the propagation of spikes through the brain. Consequently it supplies important criteria for the definition of the neural paths involved in the dynamics of the epileptic process.

4. A given cerebral zone can be stimulated by an autonomous pathological activity and, in the same epoch, by spikes propagated by one or more than one distant structure. In these different instances the morphology of the spikes generated by the considered structure shows conspicuous alterations. Data derived from animal recordings demonstrated that the morphological changes of the spikes recorded in a certain cerebral zone express the alternation of the functional prevalence of different brain structures. If we transpose such data of experimental pathology to the human situation we can infer that: i) when several chronological sequences among spikes recorded in different channels are detectable, the geometry of the neural systems involved in the dynamic of the considered epilepsy is not uniform an ii) when during a stereoelectroencephalographic exploration of the epileptic brain changes in morphology of the spikes of a given structure occur, the functional relations of this structure with others must be carefully investigated in order to define its role. If and how much such a consideration could be utilized when planning the strategy for a possible neurosurgical treatment of epilepsy is a decision which should be taken only after suitable comparison with other clinical and instrumental parameters.

We believe that this new technological procedure can improve the diagnostic possibilities of the epilepsies of neurosurgical interest and lead to a better utilization of the interictal epileptic EEG activity in the study of the epilepsies from a clinical and experimental point of view.

Acknowledgements

The Authors wish to thank Drs. G. F. Rossi, G. Colicchio, A. Gentilomo, and M. Scerrati for collecting and supplying human recordings.

Summary

An averaging technique of epileptic spikes, carried out on human stereoelectroencephalographic explorations, allowed the detection of morphological alterations of spikes peculiar to a given structure, associated with variations of temporal relations among spikes simultaneously recorded in different structures. On the basis of experimental data it can be supposed that these variations reflect the alternance of the functional prevalence among the different structures involved in the epileptic process.

References

1. Cavazza, B., Rosadini, G., Siccardi, A. (1973), The sleep control of the genesis and transmission of epileptic discharges in man. In: Sleep (Koella, W. P., and Levin, P., eds.), pp. 524—527. Basel: Karger.
2. — Ferrillo, F., Rosadini, G., Sannita, W. (1974), A computer analysis of human interictal epileptic spikes. In: Epilepsy (Harris, P., and Mawdsley, C., eds.), pp. 65—73. Edinburgh: Churchill Livingstone.
3. Ferrillo, F., Amore, R., Cavazza, B., Rosadini, G. (1974), An experimental research on time relationships among focal and secondary epileptic spikes. Boll. Soc. Ital. Biol. Sper. *50*, 1936—1940.
4. Rosadini, G., Cavazza, B., Ferrillo, F., Siccardi, A. (1974), Simultaneous averaging of epileptic discharges in 14 channels: a computer technique. Electroenceph. clin. Neurophysiol. *36*, 541—544.
5. Rossi, G. F. (1973), Problems of analysis and interpretation of electrocerebral signals in human epilepsy. A neurosurgeon's view. In: Epilepsy: its phenomena in man, UCLA Forum in Med. Sci. No. 17, pp. 260—285. New York: Academic Press.
6. Siccardi, A., Cavazza, B., Ferrillo, F., Gasparetto, B., Rosadini, G., Sannita, W. (1973), A computer technique for multichannel analysis of epileptic spikes. In: Die Quantifizierung des Elektroencephalogramms (Schenk, G., ed.) pp. 393—406. Zurigo.

Authors' address: Dr. B. Cavazza, Dr. F. Ferrillo, Dr. B. Gasparetto, and Dr. G. Rosadini, Centre for Cerebral Neurophysiology of National Council of Researches, Institute of Neurophysiopathology of the University, Genoa, Italy.

Acta Neurochirurgica, Suppl. 23, 71—84 (1976)
© by Springer-Verlag 1976

University of Oregon Medical School, Portland, Oregon

Computer Analysis of the Telemetered EEG in the Study of Epilepsy and Schizophrenia*

J. R. Stevens

With 7 Figures

As has long been appreciated, significant abnormalities of electrical activity in the deep structures of the brain are often entirely undetectable in the scalp EEG. Because of medical risks and ethical objections associated with the introduction of intracerebral electrodes in the study of patients with generalized epilepsy, behaviour disorders and psychoses, we have sought to develop non-invasive methods for localization of the subcortical EEG abnormalities in patients with these diagnoses. Two techniques which use episodic disturbances in behaviour to examine EEG power spectra associated with periods of abnormal and normal behaviour have been developed in our laboratory: 1. the sorting of averaged brief epochs of EEG spectra on the basis of normal or pathologically prolonged reaction time; 2. correlation of power spectra from 24 hours telemetered EEG with clinical seizures and during normal and abnormal behaviours in patients with epilepsy and schizophrenia, respectively.

Reaction Time Studies

Grey-Walter (1947) predicted many years ago that computer methods should permit the resolution of distant or asynchronous transients coincident with disturbed attention or perception found in some patients with epilepsy. Brazier (1966) has been a pioneer in the development of techniques for detection and localization of subcortical or remote spike activity in patients with temporal lobe epilepsy and equivocal scalp EEG.

Previous studies in our laboratory demonstrated that spike free

* This research was supported by National Institute of Mental Health grant 18055.

EEG epochs recorded from hypothalamic and septal electrodes in the cat, coincident with spike activity from an amygdala epileptogenic focus, were associated with a rather specific EEG spectrum which we designated a "ramp" function, and which was characterized by

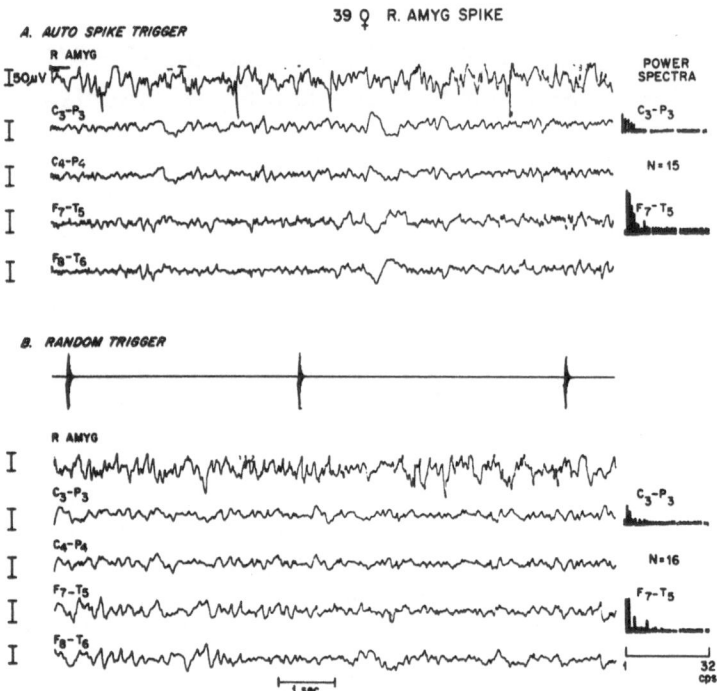

Fig. 1. A) EEG from right amygdala demonstrates spikes which serve as trigger to select simultaneous 1 second samples of EEG from scalp montages. Power spectra from contralateral scalp leads averaged from 28 1-second epochs immediately following the spike are shown on the far right side of the figure adjacent to the channel from which calculation was made. Note smooth "ramp" like configuration of spectra from spike-free scalp leads time-locked to spike. B) Automatic trigger between spikes selects 1-second epochs of scalp EEG from the same patient as in A). Average power spectra for 1-second epochs from same leads during same recording period do not show monotonic decline in power following random trigger in contrast to the EEG samples coincident with the amygdala spike

a smooth monotonic decline in power from lowest to highest frequency (Stevens 1972 a). This spectral pattern could also be demonstrated from spike-free scalp EEG epochs coincident with amygdala spikes in patients with focal epilepsy and chronic implanted electrodes (Fig. 1). We then attempted to develop programmes for detection of subcortical spike activity from spike-free surface EEGs in the absence of intracranial electrodes in patients with epilepsy and schizophrenia by taking advantage of the well known association between spike-wave discharge and delayed reaction time in the epilepsies, and the reported relationship between subcortical spike activity and disturbances of attention and behaviour in schizophrenic subjects.

Having demonstrated that a characteristic "ramp" function was associated with epochs averaged from the spike-free EEG coincident with subcortical spike activity, we reasoned that this characteristic ramp pattern, derived from montages remote from the spike focus, if associated with disturbance in responsivity might serve as a template in searching for subcortical spike foci in the absence of intracranial electrodes or visually detectable abnormalities in the scalp record. To implement such a search we have examined the power spectra of the EEG from four scalp derivations during a reaction time task by sorting and averaging scalp EEG spectra associated with short and long reaction times.

Methods

Following a routine scalp EEG, subjects were seated in a comfortable reclining chair with head rest. A response box was placed near the right hand. Patients were instructed to close their eyes and press the response lever either upward or downward as quickly as possible after hearing each of a list of short words read to them by the technician who sat close by. If the word contained one of the letters G, N, I or K, the subject was instructed to press the response lever downward as quickly as he could do so. If the word did not contain one of the letters, he was to press it upward as quickly as possible. After several practice trials, 40–60 words were presented to each patient, the pace of the task being adjusted to the rapidity of response. Successive words followed the patient's response by 5–10 seconds. The entire test procedure was limited to 15–20 minutes to avoid drowsing, irritability or undue fatigue. A continuous recording of 4 channels of EEG from right and left homologous central-parietal and anterior temporal-posterior temporal montages was made on 7 channel FM tape after amplification by a Grass Model 8 electroencephalograph. A simultaneous record of stimulus and response was recorded by a voice-operated relay that placed a positive or negative pulse on 2 channels of the tape recorder. The positive or negative signal of the patient's response was recorded on the 6th channel. Responses delayed more than 10 seconds were scored as no response trials. An ink record was made of the entire experiment from the output of the tape recorder. The taped data were processed by a program for the PDP 12 computer which detected and displayed the stimulus-response latencies, response direction and indicated whether the response was correct or incorrect. Following digitization at a sampling rate of 256 per second, reaction times were displayed and placement of cursors permitted calling up averaged spectra for 1″ epochs preceding designated reaction times, correct or incorrect response, and non-response trials. Ten patients with epilepsy and 18 normal control subjects were studied.

Results

Comparison of control subjects with epileptic patients demonstrated a wider range of reaction times and higher error rates for individuals with epilepsy. The range of latencies for controls was 0.3 to 4 seconds, with a mean of 0.9 second and a standard deviation (S.D.) of 1.4 seconds. For subjects with epilepsy, reaction times ranged from 0.3 to 10 seconds, with a mean of 1.85 seconds (S.D., 1.6 seconds). The mean error rates were 4.4 percent for control subjects, and 10 percent for patients with epilepsy.

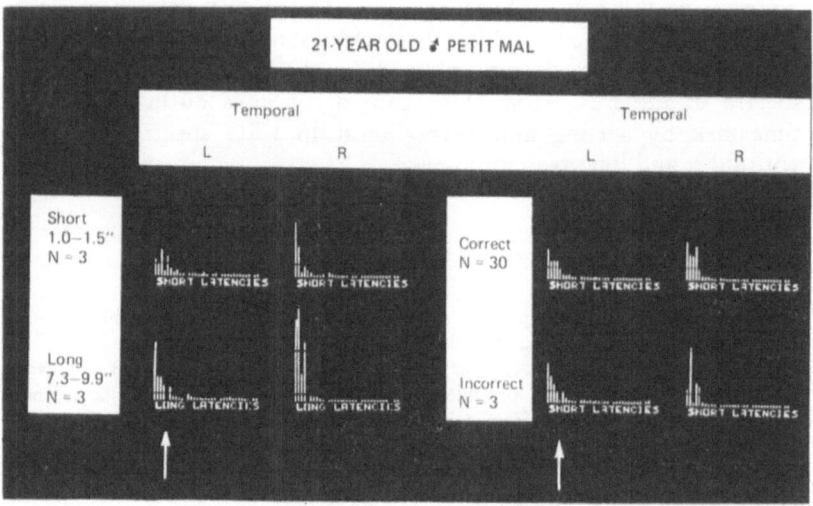

Fig. 2. Power spectra from 21-year-old patient with petit mal epilepsy demonstrates "ramp" pattern in left temporal region coincident with long latency or incorrect response. Patient's routine scalp EEG demonstrates classical 3 cps spike-wave bilaterally, and seizures are typical "absence" attacks. Each bar represents power at 2 cycle band widths from 2–32 c/sec

Shift to lower frequency bands preceded prolonged response latency in half the control subjects and three-quarters of the patients with seizures. No consistent localization was noted although right and left temporal regions were most often affected. Localized slow spectra were highly correlated with the site of the epileptic focus in patients with focal seizures and were identified over one or both temporal regions in all patients with generalized epilepsy.

Using the previously recognized "ramp" pattern as a template, we then searched through the spectral histograms generated by the

FDP 12 from EEG epochs immediately preceding the stimulus. Ramp spectra were identified in the prestimulus intervals from nine of ten subjects with epilepsy from at least one pair of electrodes in the prestimulus interval for prolonged or erroneous responses. The ramp spectra were localized to the scalp region corresponding to the seizure focus in patients with psychomotor epilepsy, and were from left or right temporal montage in patients with generalized seizures (Fig. 2).

This ramp pattern is consistent with the power spectrum from an epoch dominated by a single high-voltage transient, such as the EEG spike. In contrast, only one out of 18 normal control subjects displayed a similar "ramp" configuration.

Applications for Schizophrenia

Several investigators, including Heath (1950), Hanley et al. (1971), Adams (1975) and Sem-Jacobsen (1956) have reported spike activity from subcortical sites in patients diagnosed schizophrenia—most consistently from the medial frontal-basal region including septal nuclei, nucleus accumbens and head of caudate nucleus. We are particularly interested in this evidence of pathological activity in the region of the anterior (limbic) striatum because of recent hypotheses which suggest that the mesolimbic dopamine system, which terminates in anterior striatal structures may be of particular significance in schizophrenia (Andén 1973, Stevens 1973). Because of the restriction in the study of subcortical EEG abnormalities in patients with schizophrenia and other severe behaviour disorders, we and others have attempted to develop computer programmes for detection of putative subcortical spike activity from the scalp EEG of schizophrenic subjects. Saltzberg et al. (1971) reported some success in detecting these "septal spikes" by digital filtering of coincident scalp EEG while Hanley et al. (1972) used stepwise discriminant analysis of power spectra. These methods have the disadvantage of being initially dependent upon recording the spike from the intracranial site in each subject in order to establish criteria for spike recognition in the scalp tracing, although Hanley et al. (1970) demonstrated a statistically significant association between stereotypic activity and rhythmic subcortical fast activity in a single schizophrenic patient. Since identification of the "ramp" spectra from the spike-free surface EEG appeared to be relatively specific to our patients with epilepsy preceding long reaction-time trials, and since this spectral configuration appeared identical to that recorded from remote electrodes during averaged spike initiated trials, we sought to determine whether a similar analysis could detect the presence of subcortical spike

activity in the apparently normal scalp EEG of patients with schizophrenia or other psychiatric disorders.

Episodic disturbances in attention, perception, thought or motor
control in some schizophrenic patients often resemble interruptions
in the stream of consciousness noted in patients with psychomotor
and petit mal epilepsy. In addition, schizophrenic patients share

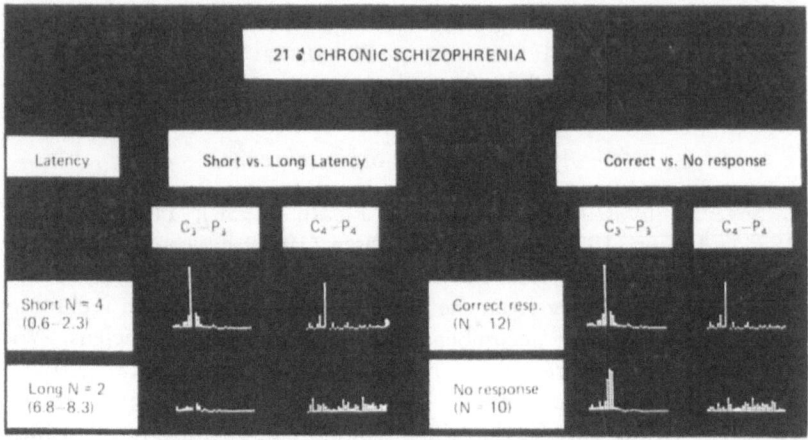

Fig. 3. Flat "noise" pattern from average spectra for left and right central-
parietal regions precedes stimuli followed by long latency or no response trials
in a 21-year-old male with chronic schizophrenic psychosis and marked psychomotor blocking. Note predominant alpha pattern during short latency and correct
response, and loss of central frequency tendency before delayed response or no
response trials. Each bar represents power at 2 cycle band widths from
2–32 c/sec

with epileptics a wide scatter of reaction times to a uniform stimulus-
response task, suggesting fluctuating attention, perception or responsivity. The long latencies so characteristic of schizophrenia (psychomotor blocking, "le barrage") are not however accompanied by
visually detectable changes in the scalp EEG. To maximize the
possibility of recognizing subcortical transients which might correspond to interruptions in perception and behaviour in schizophrenic
patients, we have applied the same reaction time task described above
for subjects with epilepsy and compared averaged spectra derived
from 1 second epochs preceding normal latency responses with those
preceding long reaction times, correct, failed or incorrect response
in 46 patients hospitalized for severe psychiatric disorders.

Seventeen patients hospitalized for chronic schizophrenia, 12 with acute schizophrenia and 17 patients with other severe psychoses were examined with the same reaction time procedure described above for the patients with epilepsy. Three patients with acute schizophrenia and 5 patients with chronic schizophrenia displayed the "ramp" function during long latency or erroneous response trials. Nine of the 17 patients diagnosed chronic schizophrenia but only 2 depressive patients and no normal controls demonstrated a power spectrum characterized by loss of central frequency tendency and a relatively even distribution of power across the frequency spectrum preceding delayed or erroneous response trials (Fig. 3). Although localized to any montage, this pattern was most common over the right temporal region. The flat "noise" pattern did not appear to be related to intrusion of high frequency muscle components as it was frequently unilateral or limited to the central-parietal leads rather than over the temporal regions where muscle potentials are typically more prominent. Review of spectra from our previous study of epileptic, acute psychiatric and normal control groups demonstrated this pattern in only 3 patients—2 with psychoses and 1 with seizure disorder and interictal psychiatric disturbance.

Telemetered EEG Studies

We have previously reported on the use of the 24 hours telemetered EEG for the localization of epileptic foci (Stevens *et al.* 1969, 1972). Since frank ictus is readily recognized on the ordinary scalp EEG, no special programme is required to resolve abnormalities when readily recognizable spike and seizure activity occur. Power spectra analysis of serial samples of EEG does however permit compression of 24 hours of EEG data into a more manageable format and allows rapid evaluation of background activities as well as frank ictus. Epileptic seizures are readily detected by the presence of subharmonics in the power spectrum (Fig. 4). The situation is very different in schizophrenia, in which simple visual inspection of the scalp EEG has not been generally useful. Accordingly, we have applied a programme similar to that used in epileptic subjects for continuous 24-hours monitoring of the telemetered EEG in patients with acute and chronic schizophrenia. Thirty patients have been studied to date by the continuous recording method described for study of epilepsy in several previous publications (Stevens *et al.* 1969, 1971, 1972).

The patients wear a small 3-ounce 4-channel FM transmitter attached to the electrodes on head and are free to move about the hospital ward and carry on their usual daily activities. Antennas

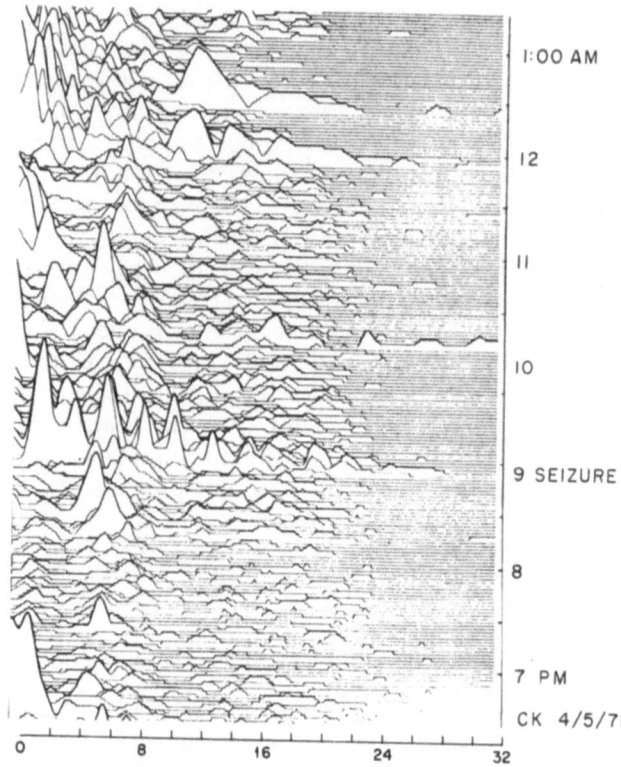

Fig. 4. Frequency spectra from 21-year-old patient with petit mal epilepsy. Time proceeds from the bottom to the top of graph, each line representing 4 seconds of EEG, with 4 consecutive samples taken every 5 minutes. Frequency is plotted on the abscissa from 1½–32 cps; square root of power is plotted on the ordinate. Note predominance of low frequencies and subharmonics during seizures

are placed in the ceiling of the patient's ward and lead to a small 4-channel receiver demodulator unit which delivers the physiologic data to an FM tape recorded monitored by an ink writing polygraph. Homologous central-parietal montages (C 3–P 3; C 4–P 4), electro-oculogram, electromyogram, electrocardiogram, behavioural events and time code are continuously and simultaneously recorded on the 7-channel tape recorder. The data are analyzed off-line by a pro-gramme for the PDP 12 computer which digitizes 4 consecutive 4-second samples of EEG every 5 minutes, performs Fourier analysis, and plots the square root of the power spectra in the compressed spectral array format of Bickford et al. (1971). Additional 16-second

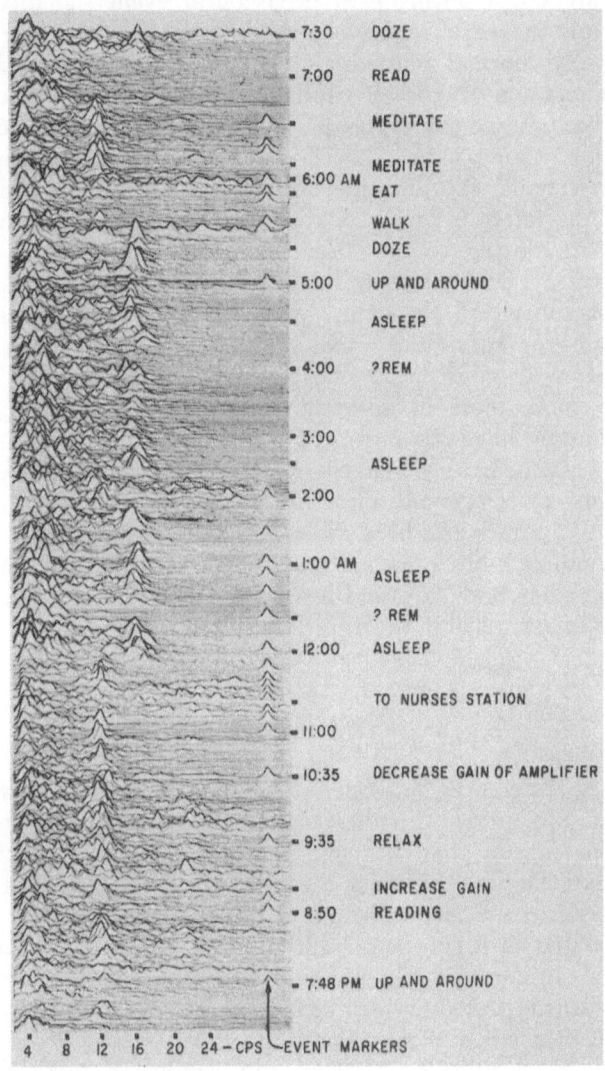

Fig. 5. Spectral array from normal control subject, a 22-year-old woman recorded by telemetry during a 20-hour stay on psychiatric ward, plotted as in Fig. 6. Note predominant alpha when awake, transition to 13 cps activity during slow wave sleep, separated by REM periods. High voltage slow activity at the left side of the graph represents eye movement contamination of the EEG. High voltage signals at 30 cps are event markers which correspond to the behavioural observations noted on the right side of graph. An extra 4-second EEG epoch is plotted coincident with each event mark

samples are taken during each behavioural event signalled by the observer and these are recorded on the final graph.

Typically, normal individuals display power spectra characterized by alpha activity at rest which shows some considerable fluctuation between 9 and 11 cycles per second, shifts to desynchronized activity alternating with 14 cycle per second spindles during sleep, and some irregular fast and slow activity during activity and arousal. Some of the latter is surely related to both movement and muscle artifact. In contrast to the normal control subject demonstrated in Fig. 5, patients with epilepsy have a distinctive pattern dominated by slow activity and clear emergence of subharmonics of slow frequencies during spike and wave discharges (Fig. 4). Patients with schizophrenia demonstrate a variety of unusual patterns none of which resemble those of epilepsy. Spectra from individuals with acute catatonia have demonstrated a flat or "white noise" spectrum (Fig. 6). Hallucinatory behaviour may be accompanied by either desynchrony or hypersynchronous alpha activity (Fig. 7). A psychotic impulsive attack has been associated with a flat frequency spectrum resembling white noise spectra. Drug treatment introduces significant changes in both slow and fast components. Most of our patients have thus been studied in the drug-free state.

Conclusions

Marked differences between power spectra in patients with epilepsy and schizophrenia in the reaction time and 24-hour telemetry evaluations suggest that although there is evidence for subcortical spike activity in both disorders, the pathophysiologies are very different. Intermittently delayed reaction times in patients with epilepsy appear related to subcortical spike activity which is propagated to the cortex. In contrast, a minority of schizophrenic patients display similar spectra preceding delayed response trials or during telemetered EEG, while more than half display focal "white noise" spectra without evidence of cortically conducted spike discharge. These spectra resemble those derived from the surface EEG in patients using amphetamine and hallucinogens (Itil and Fink 1966). Our findings are consistent with those of Hanley et al. (1972) suggesting that although subcortical spike activity is recorded in the paraseptal region of patients with schizophrenia, the behaviour disturbances we have focused upon are not, in contrast to epilepsy, associated with wide propagation of that spike activity. Rather, focal dispersion of background frequencies and in particular, increased fast

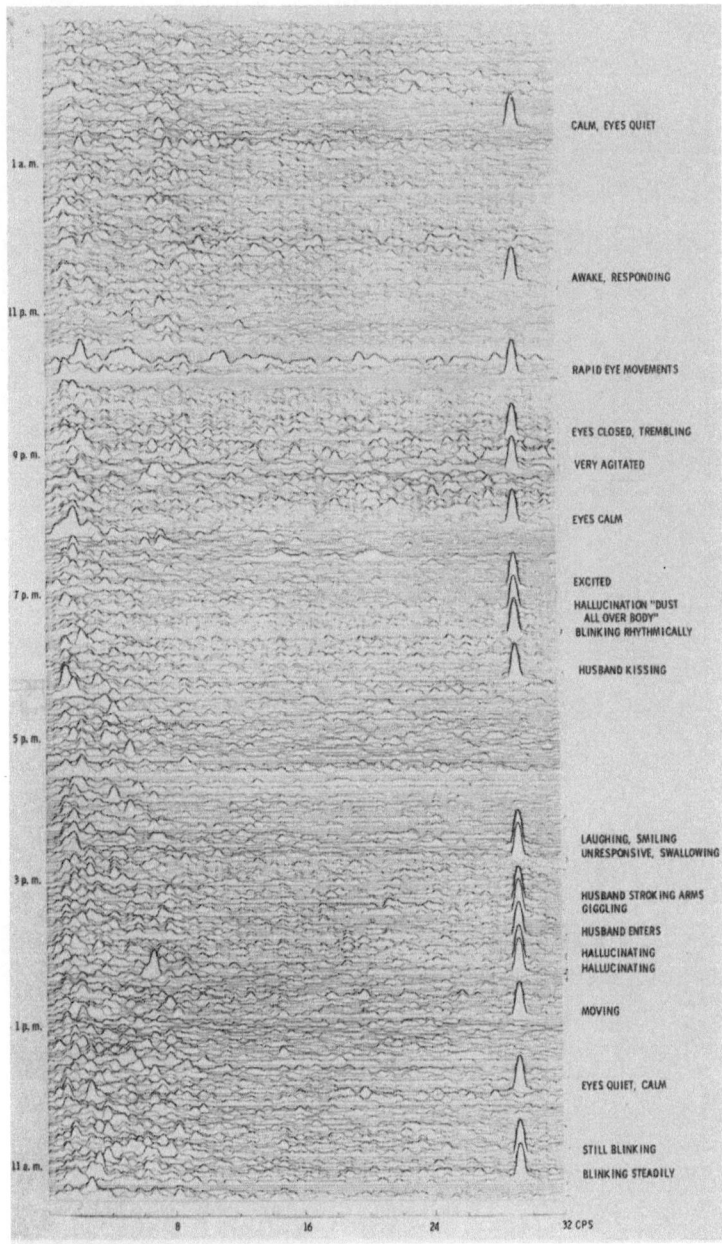

Fig. 6. Compressed spectral array representing 24 hours of consecutive EEG recorded by telemetry from right vertex-occipital derivation of a 22-year-old beauty operator with acute catatonic schizophrenia. Dispersion of amplitude into higher frequencies during excitement may include muscle contamination. Very slow activity represents eye movements. Legend as for Figs. 4 and 5

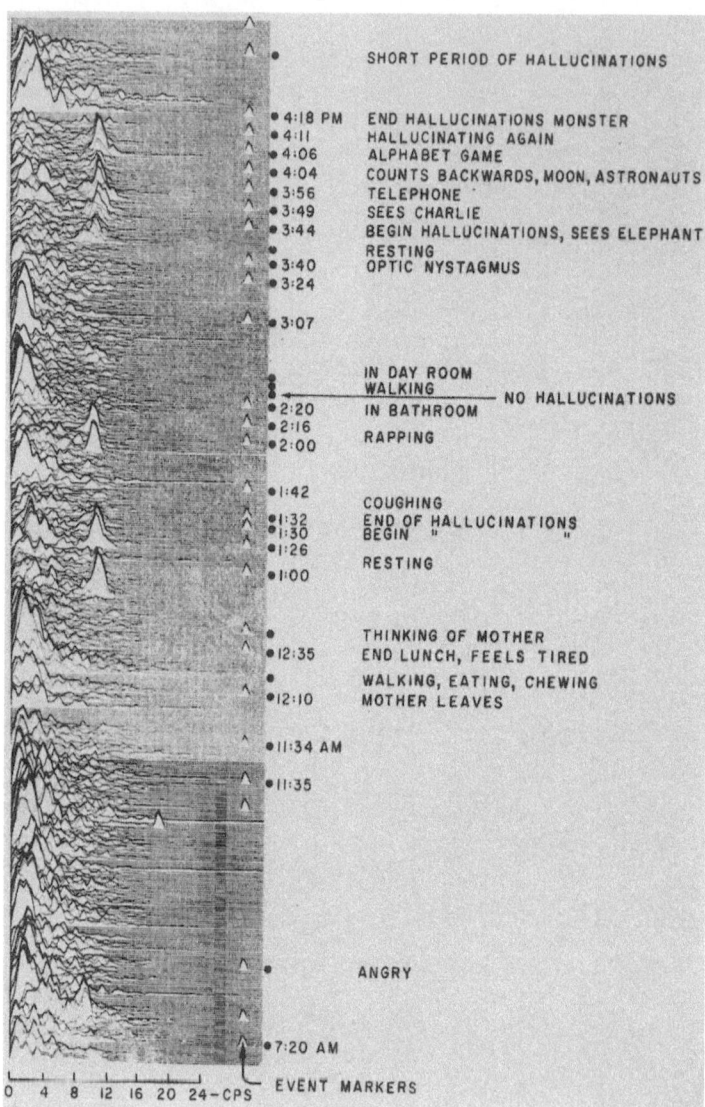

Fig. 7. Power spectra from right central-parietal (C 4–P 4) EEG recorded by radio telemetry from 23-year-old man with chronic paranoid schizophrenia. Time proceeds from below upward. Note onset of monorhythmic 11½ cps activity during hallucinated periods. Slow activity in record represents largely eye movement. Legend as for Figs. 4 and 5

activity emerges during delayed response. Utilization of computer methods combined with careful behavioural analysis suggests that sub-cortical spike activity, which we consider an electrical sign of de-nervation hypersensitivity, when crucially located may be associated with loss of regulation of normal background activity in distant areas. Treatment methods based on stimulation of crucial pacemaker or inhibitory structures may provide more rational treatment than the use of generalized convulsive therapies or destructive lesions.

Summary

Computation of power spectra from averaged brief epochs of spike free scalp EEG coincident with the subcortical spike has rev-ealed a distinctive spectral configuration characterized by smooth monotonic decline in power from lowest to highest frequencies. Nine out of 10 patients with epilepsy display similar patterns preceding long latency responses to a verbal motor reaction time task. Although subcortical spike activity has been recorded from the paraseptal region of patients with schizophrenia by several investigators, half of our patients with schizophrenia displayed a different pattern which resembles a "white noise" spectrum during the delayed reaction time of incorrect response trials. Power spectra derived from 24-hour telemetered scalp EEGs from patients with epilepsy and schizophrenia are also sharply differentiated by similar criteria. These non-invasive methods for analysis of the scalp EEG in relation to careful and controlled behaviour observations may give useful information re-garding subcortical activity when intracranial electrodes cannot be utilized.

References

Adams, J. (1975), Personal communications.
Andén, Carlsson, Haggendal (1972), Dopamine turnover in the corpus striatum and the limbic system after treatment with neuroleptic and anti-acetylcholine drugs. J. Pharm. Pharmac. 24, 905—906.
Bickford, R. G., Fleming, H. F., Billinger, T. (1936), Compression of EEG data. Trans. Amer. neurol. Ass. 96, 118—122.
Brazier, M. (1966), Proceedings of a symposium at Lidice, Czech. In: Comparative and cellular pathophysiology of epilepsy (Servit, V., ed.), 124, 112—125. Amsterdam: Excerpta Medica.
Grey-Walter, W. (1947), Analytical means of discovering the origin and nature of epileptic disturbances. Res. Publ. Ass. nerv. ment. Dis. 26, 237.
Hanley, J., Rickles, W. R., Crandall, P. H., Walter, R. D. (1970), Automatic recognition of EEG correlates of behaviour in a chronic schizophrenic patient with schizophrenia. Electroenceph. clin. Neurophysiol. 28, 90.
— — — — (1972), Automatic recognition of EEG correlates of behavior in a chronic schizophrenic patient. Amer. J. Psychiat. 128, 1524—1528.

Heath, R. G. (principal author) (1954), Studies in schizophrenia. A multidisciplinary approach to mind-brain relationships. Cambridge, Mass.: Harvard University Press.

Itil, T. M., Fink, M. (1966), Behaviour and quantitative EEG changes induced by hallucinogenic drugs. In: Biological and physiological problems of psychology (Vinogradova and Ulyanova, eds.). Moscow.

Saltzberg, B., Lustick, L. S., Heath, R. G. (1971), Detection of focal depth spiking in the scalp of monkeys. Electroenceph. clin. Neurophysiol. 31, 327—333.

Sem-Jacobsen, C. W. (1957), Intra-cerebral electrographic studies in schizophrenic patients. Report of Second International Psychiatric Congress, Zurich, 2, 247—248.

Stevens, J. R., Milstein, V. M., Dodds, S. (1969), Prolonged recordings of EEG by radiotelemetry: An aid to localization and treatment of epilepsy. EEG Clin. Neurophysiol. 27, 544.

— Lonsbury, B. L., Kodama, H., Mills, L. (1971), Ultradian characteristics of spontaneous seizure discharges recorded by radiotelemetry in man. EEG Clin. Neurophysiol. 31, 313—325.

— — Goel, S. L. (1972 a), EEG spectra and reaction time in disorders of higher nervous system. Science 176, 1346—1349.

— — — (1972 b), Seizure occurrence and interspike interval. Arch. Neurol. 26, 409—419.

— (1973), An anatomy of schizophrenia? Arch. Gen. Psychiat. 29, 77—189.

Author's address: J. R. Stevens, M.D., University of Oregon Medical School, Portland, Oregon.

Acta Neurochirurgica, Suppl. 23, 85—91 (1976)

Neurosurgical Department, Comenius University, Bratislava, and
Department of Computers, Electrical Engineering Faculty, Slovak Technical
University, Bratislava, ČSSR

Investigation of Epileptic Structure Properties by Transfer Function

S. Neuschl*, L. Hluchý*, P. Nádvorník, and **M. Šramka**

With 4 Figures

The efforts aimed at the objective analysis of the electrical activity of the brain have recently become increasingly intensive. The development of mathematical methods and computer science have greatly stimulated this research. Since the first experiments with Fourier analysis, many more complex methods have already been put into practice out of which correlation analysis appeared to be the most convenient one. The latter was recommended for detecting similarities and dependencies between signals, and registrations from various brain structures. The method was expected to facilitate determination of the source of epileptic activity as well as an aid in finding ways of its propagation. But the simple application of these methods, such as Fourier analysis or the correlation analysis may, however, lead to formal conclusions which, apart from evoked potentials, do not show any functional dependencies among the brain structures investigated which, in our case, were epileptic structures. If it has to be found, how in EEG signals represent the structural brain organization from the standpoint of both information processes and the transfer dynamics within the brain, more complicated mathematical procedures have to be assumed.

Brain tissues can be regarded as a communication channel, which has distributed parameters, where signals are spreading from one side to the other. In this case the channel may be examined either from the standpoint of information, such as decoding or pattern recognition, or from the standpoint of the dynamics of transfer paths or channels, respectively.

---

* Department of Computers, Electrical Engineering Faculty, Slovak Technical University, Bratislava.

In the present paper we tackle the latter, assuming that

a) the medium is both linear and stationary;

b) the bonds between individual points of structural brain organization may be expressed by concentric parameters and represented by means of a network similar to electrical networks,

c) the theory of statistical dynamics and the linear theory of control may be used.

We are, of course, aware that these conditions are not fully satisfied and therefore, we consider the model suggested as the first and linear approximation of the real brain system. The basic idea is the following: By means of computing methods we are in the position to suggest an oriented graph of a chosen brain structure with indicated signal propagation directions and to try both to calculate and interpret the characteristics among the individual structure points starting from the conception that one of the points emits and the other receives the signal. As an example of this procedure, we chose a four-element structure, by means of which the hypothesis was verified, as outlined in Fig. 1. In an epileptic patient the record of electrical activity signal was taken from lamina medialis thalami, reticulum thalami and hippocamus, respectively. The graph shows the orientation of the individual transfer paths. The recorded signals, i.e. the actual stereoelectroencephalographic record from chosen brain structures were taken as the initiating data. Fig. 2 shows an example.

Except for the traditional record of EEG potentials by the recording device of electroencephalograph (Elema Co) EEG was recorded by the 14-track tape recorder (EMM 140), simultaneously watching EEG on the 8-track slow-time-base oscilloscope (OPD 280). The time interval of the EEG record ranged from 40 sec to 220 sec. Digitization of the suitable EEG sections was made by the computer (GIER). Sampling time of digitization was 8 msec in most cases. This sampling interval fully satisfies the Shannon-Kotelnikov theorem which gives the connection between the upper cut-off frequency and the sampling interval. Let the upper cut-off frequency of the EEG signal be *e.g.* 60 Hz. Then the length of sampling interval is 8.3 msec.

The statistical properties were checked by means of the autocorrelation function as well as tests for stationary and ergodic properties. We found that the statistical conditions could only be satisfied if the record lasts at least 4 seconds. From the decrease of the amplitudes of autocorrelation functions it 50 function points could be used. This corresponds to a duration of 400 msec of the realization. Fig. 3 shows the auto- and cross-correlation functions. The orientation of transfer paths (channels), between two points can

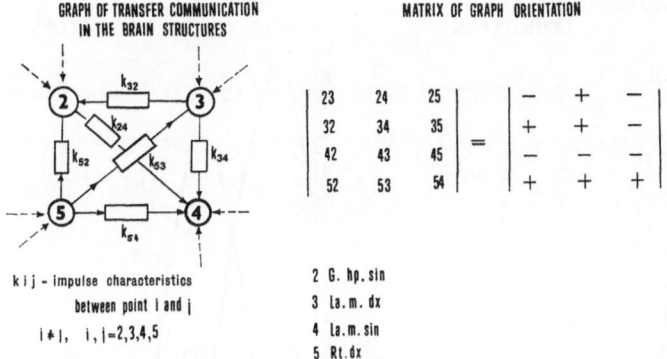

Fig. 1. The graph of transfer paths in the brain structures and the matrix of the graph orientation

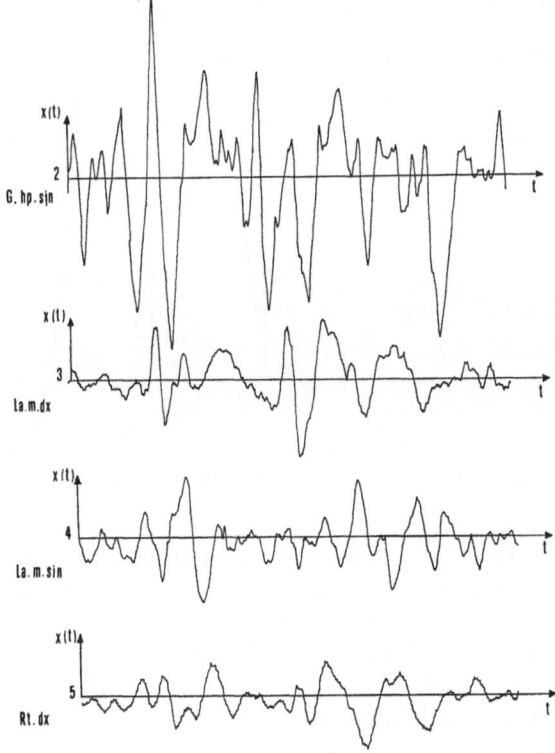

Fig. 2. EEG records from 4 points

S. Neuschl *et al.:*

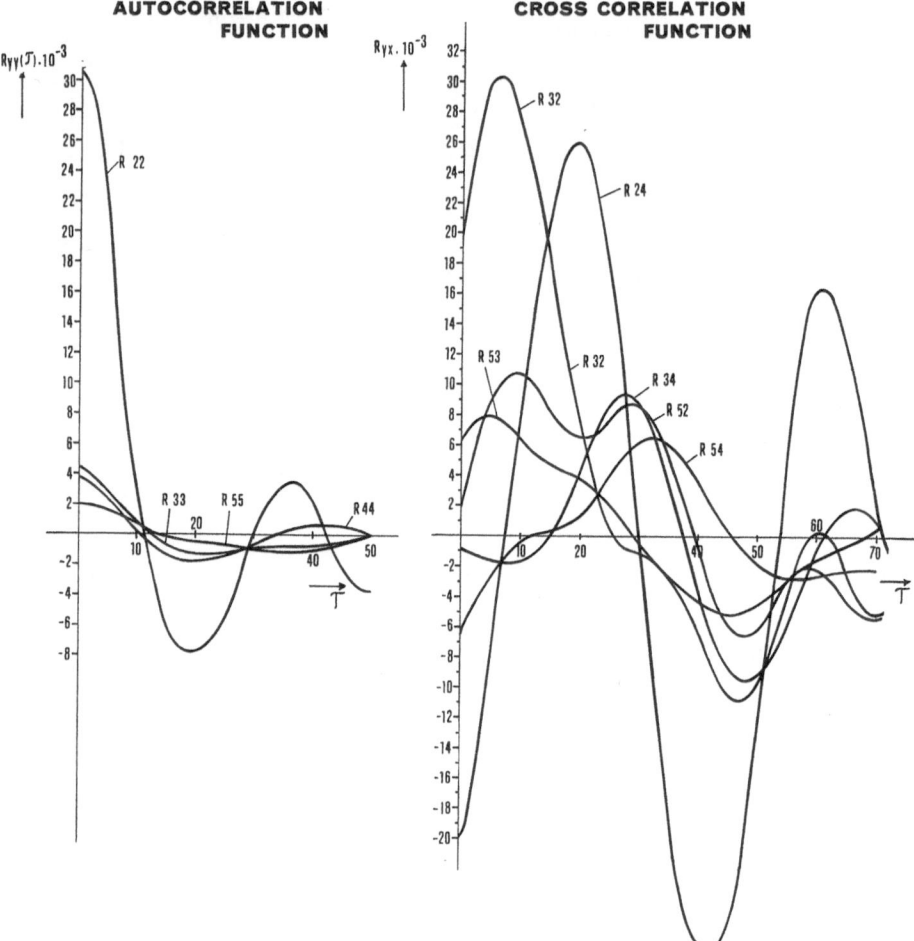

Fig. 3. Auto and cross correlation functions of EEG signals

be defined from the crosscorrelation functions. To investigate
transfer path properties we used impulse characteristics, stated as the
response that would be measured in one point to the impulse emitted
from another point. Theoretically this is the so-called Dirac impulse.
The values of impulse characteristics were obtained from the discrete
form of Wiener-Hopf equation.

$$R_{xy}(r) = \sum_{m=0}^{\infty} k(m) . R_{yy}(r-m)$$

where R_{xy} is the cross-correlation function between points x, y,

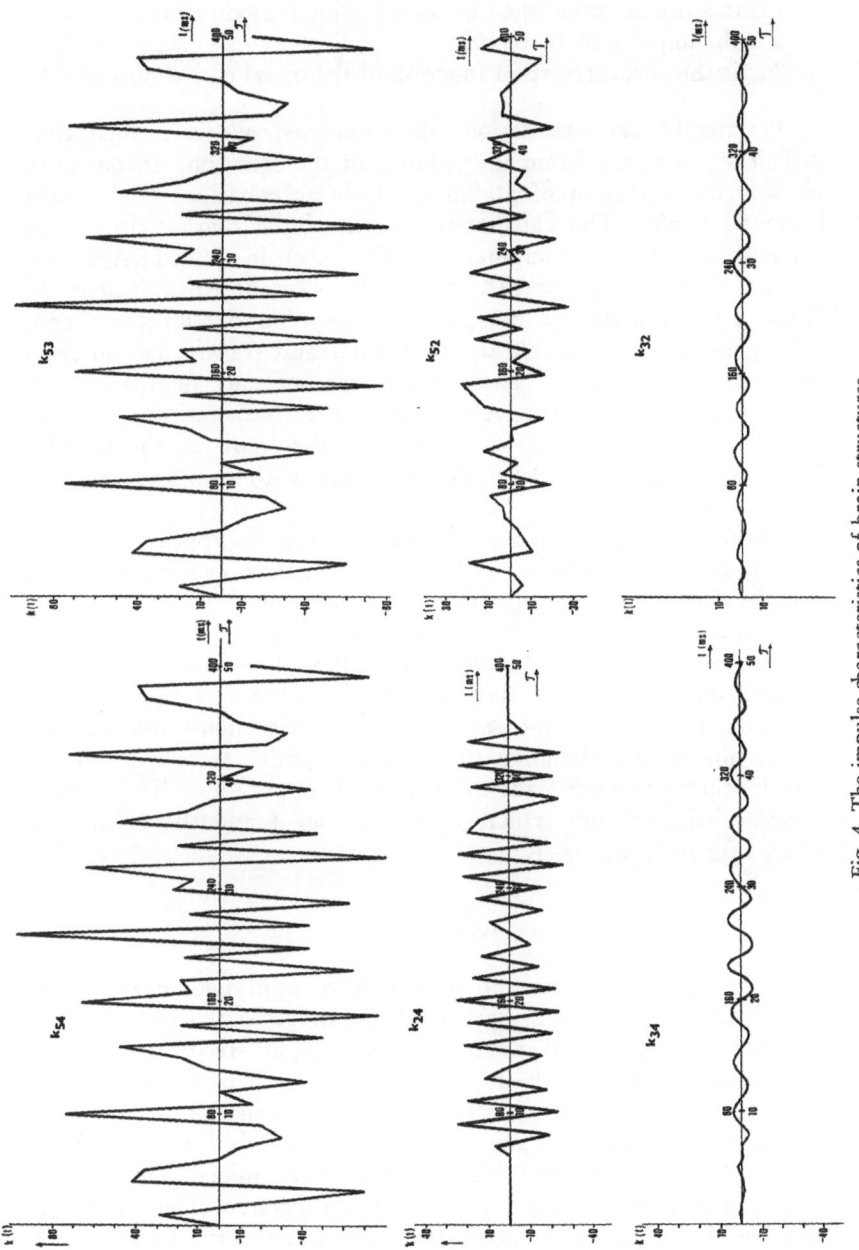

Fig. 4. The impulse characteristics of brain structures

m is the time coordinate of impulse characteristics,
r is the discrete time (the time to sampling period ratio),
k is the impulse characteristic,
R_{yy} is the autocorrelation function of the signal on the output side.

Practically, the calculation was completed within a final time sufficiently long to obtain the validity of the equation. In our case, we solved the system of 50 linear algebraic equations (the matrix being 50 × 50). The calculation of all of the characteristics was carried out on the computer (MINSK 22) in FORTRAN language. From the properties of impulse characteristics it may be deduced which of the transfer paths is susceptible to "vibrations" and, consequently, to non-stable signal transfer and transformation from one point to the other. These results are not only qualitative but even partly quantitative. Also other EEG characteristics, such as transfer characteristics (as a response to the step) or, the transfer functions and the frequency characteristics with complex variables are to be considered.

We believe that the most valuable contribution appears to be the basic graph orientation as well as approximative evaluation of the transfer path. By investigating the conjunction between structures and epileptical activity, the method described allows detection of the source of pathological activity as well as the ways of its spreading and the properties of such structures. In the case described, the reticulum thalami was the output structure with non-stable transfer on the non-specific thalamus system of both sides, from where a relatively quiet pathway leads toward gyrus hippocampi. The impulse characteristics of such structures are in Fig. 4 and the orientation of transfer paths in Fig. 1.

Summary

The paper deals with the possibility of applying linear control theory and the theory of statistical dynamics to the complex and quantitative analysis of electroencephalographic records. The aim is to specify signals in the brain environment, in particular sources, speed and direction of signals, and the determination from results gained of the model of signal transfer. The possibilities of applying Fourier analysis and correlation analysis are examined. The methodical approach of the transient analysis is suggested. Conditions are discussed for approximate application of linear theory. Experimental results, as well as the calculation of transfer parameters of signals are evaluated. The method of magnetic EEG records, the scanning and processing of data on analogue and digital computers are introduced.

The method described of correlation and transient analysis arises from the necessity to detect epileptic structures from an evaluation of SEEG records of the deep brain structure.

References

1. Beneš, J. (1961), Statistická dynamika regulačních obvodů. Praha: SNTL.
2. Brazier, A. B., Barlow, J. S. (1957), Correlation analysis of depth recordings from the basal ganglia. Electroenceph. clin. Neurophysiol. *9*, 171—180.
3. Vojtinskij, E. Ja., Prianišnikov, V. A. (1974), K voprosu o verojatnostnom analize elektroencefalogram. Voprosy psichologii *4*, 99—105.

Authors' addresses: Dr. S. Neuschl and L. Hluchý, Department of Computers, Electrical Engineering Faculty, Slovak Technical University, Vazovova 5, 88019 Bratislava, ČSSR, and Prof. Dr. P. Nádvorník and Dr. M. Šramka, Neurosurgical Department, Comenius University, Limbová 17, 809 46 Bratislava-Kramáre, ČSSR.

Acta Neurochirurgica, Suppl. 23, 93—100 (1976)
© by Springer-Verlag 1976

Institute for Neurobiology, Okayama University Medical School,
Okayama, Japan

Catecholamine Levels in Penicillin-Induced Epileptic Focus of the Cat Cerebral Cortex

K. Kobayashi, T. Shirakabe, H. Kishikawa, and A. Mori

With 8 Figures

Chen *et al.* (1954) first reported that pretreatment with reserpine lowered the threshold of experimental seizures. Since then the relationship between brain monoamines and susceptibility to epileptic seizures has been studied by many investigators by means of electro-convulsion (De Schaepdryver *et al.* 1962, Azzaro *et al.* 1972, Kilian and Frey 1973), pentylenetetrazol (Kobinger 1958, Lessin and Parkes 1959) and audiogenic seizures (Lehmann 1967, Boggan and Seiden 1971, Jobe *et al.* 1973). From the results of this work, it has been suggested that treatment lowering the total brain levels of monoamines generally facilitates epileptic seizures, and vice versa. However, there has been little agreement as to the brain monoamines (dopamine, norepinephrine and serotonin) most intimately involved in the seizure susceptibility.

This work was experimentally performed to clarify the role of catecholamine in the epileptic focus.

Materials and Methods

Twenty-five adult cats, weighing about 3 kg, were used for the first series of experiments. After being lightly anaesthetized by intraperitoneal injection of sodium pentobarbital (50 mg/kg), two cats were placed in a stereotaxic apparatus and the bilateral parietal cortex was exposed by means of skull resection and opening of the dura. The electrocorticogram was recorded with two pairs of cotton electrodes applied on the pia (Fig. 1). In the left side of cortex (middle suprasylvian gyrus), an epileptic focus was produced by intracortical injection of potassium benzyl penicillin G (400 U/10 µl saline solution). On the other hand, sham-operation was done on the right side by injection of the same volume of saline solution without penicillin. At three different stages of propagation of penicillin spikes, bilateral cerebral cortices were excised and frozen rapidly in liquid nitrogen. Catecholamine in brain tissues was adsorbed on alumina, eluted with 0.2 N acetic acid and then trifluoroacetylated. Catecholamine analysis was performed within a few days after sampling by using gas chromatography with electron capture detector in nanogram order.

In the second series of experiments using 15 adult cats, the effect of catecholamines and their precursor l-DOPA on penicillin-induced spike activity was examined. When the epileptic activity had fully developed, a piece of 4 mm square filter paper soaked with 10^{-3}–10^{-5} M catecholamine or l-DOPA was topically applied on the penicillin focus. In some experiments, l-DOPA was slowly injected through the femoral vein. The efficacy of a given drug was evaluated by the change of spike counts per minute throughout the experiment.

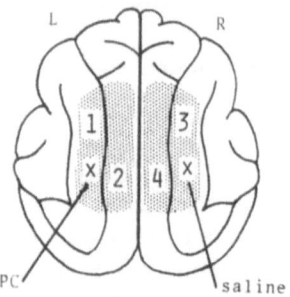

Fig. 1. Dotted areas of cerebral cortex were excised. *PC* and aline: penicillin-treated and sham-operated points. *1–4:* positions of cortical electrodes

Results

1. Catecholamine Levels in Epileptic Focus

Fig. 2 shows the three stages of propagation of penicillin-induced spike activity on the electrocorticogram. In the first stage, dopamine and norepinephrine both decreased in the focus of all 8 cases (Fig. 3). The mean decrement of dopamine and norepinephrine in the focus was the level of 60.9% and 59.0% of the non-focus, respectively.

In the second stage, dopamine and norepinephrine in the focus still remained in low levels than those in the non-focal cortex except for one case as shown in Fig. 4. Both amines in the focus decreased to the level of 63.7% and 52.8% of the non-focus, respectively. In the third stage, on the other hand, no differences existed in each dopamine and norepinephrine levels between the focal and non-focal cortex (Fig. 5).

Catecholamine levels in these three stages were summarized in Fig. 6. The statistical significance of the difference in the catecholamine levels between the focal and non-focal cortex was tested by means of the Mann-Whitney's U test. In the first stage, both dopa-

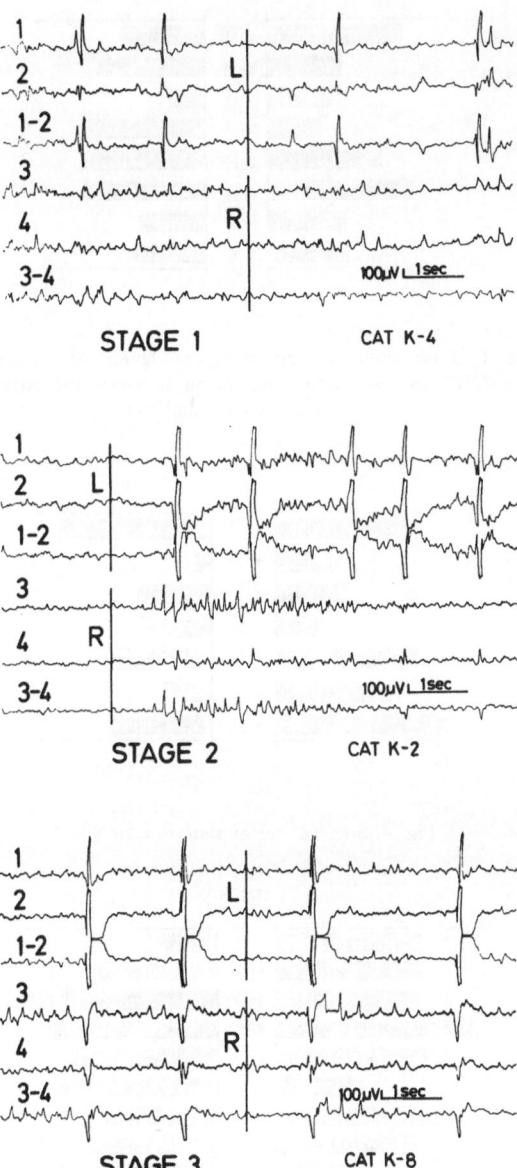

Fig. 2. Three stages of propagation of penicillin spikes. Stage 1: spikes localize in the focus. Stage 2 and 3: spikes slightly and fully propagate to the non-focus

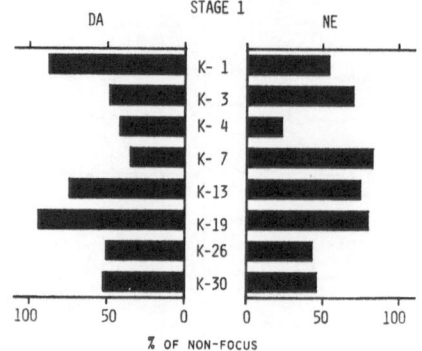

Fig. 3. Stage 1. Each columns represent the levels of dopamine (*DA*) and norepinephrine (*NE*) in percentage comparing between the focal and non-focal cortex. *K* cat number

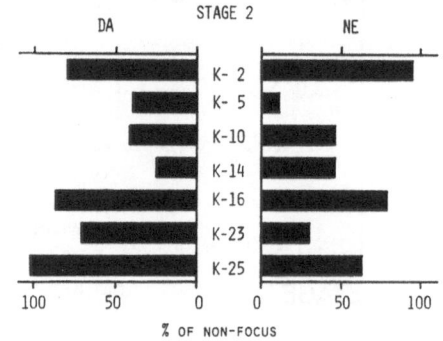

Fig. 4. Stage 2. See explanation in Fig. 3

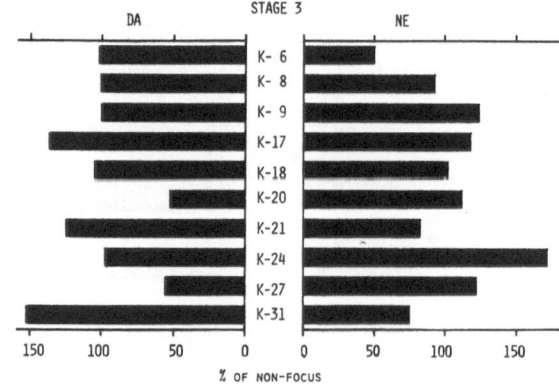

Fig. 5. Stage 3. See explanation in Fig. 3

mine and norepinephrine in the focus were significantly different from those of the non-focal cortex at the 5⁰/o level of probability.

In the second stage, norepinephrine also showed a significantly low level in the focal side at the 1⁰/o level of probability. But it was not for dopamine in statistical point of view. In the third stage, there were no differences of catecholamine levels in both cortices.

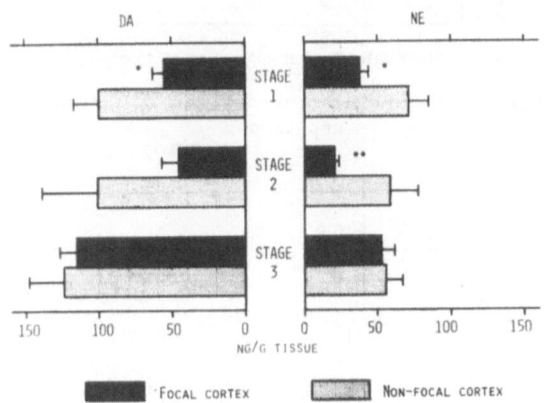

Fig. 6. Catecholamine levels (ng/g tissue) of the focal and non-focal cortex in the three stages. * p < 0.05, ** p < 0.01 (Mann-Whitney's U test)

2. Effect of Catecholamines and l-DOPA on Spike Activity

Bilateral rhythmic spike activity developed in constant frequency of 18–22 per minute at 20–25 minutes after the intracortical injection of penicillin. Spike activity was reduced by the topical application of dopamine in all epileptic animals. Fig. 7 shows an example of these cases. Inhibitory effect of dopamine was observed within 3 minutes after the application in all concentration of dopamine, and spikes disappeared at 3 minutes after 10^{-3} M dopamine. Just after washing out the brain surface by physiological saline, spike activity was recovered to control level within several minutes. On the other hand, no inhibitory effect was observed in the topical application of norepinephrine.

Spike activity was markedly reduced 15–20 minutes after the topical application of L-DOPA. The inhibitory effect of L-DOPA was also obtained even with the intravenous administration (Fig. 8). Spike counts were gradually reduced and its maximum effect was gained 13 minutes after the administration. And then spike counts gradually returned to the control frequency.

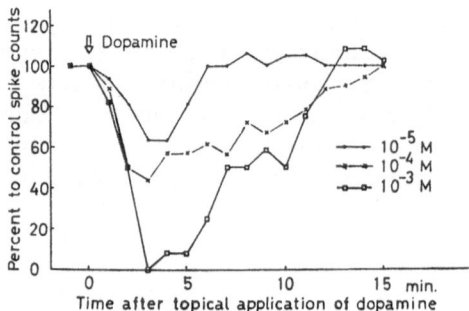

Fig. 7. An example of inhibitory effect of dopamine on penicillin spikes (topical application)

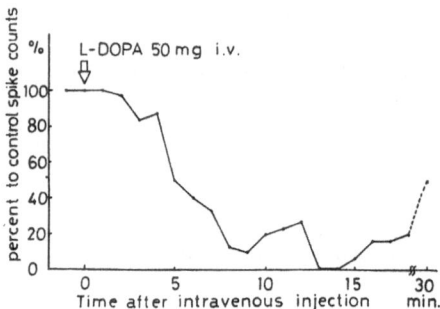

Fig. 8. An example of inhibitory effect of l-DOPA on penicillin spikes (intravenous injection)

Discussion

Billiet *et al.* (1970) studied the levels of caudate nucleus dopamine and whole brain norepinephrine and electroshock threshold in rabbits, and concluded that changes in the electroshock threshold were correlated not only with the caudate nucleus dopamine but also with the norepinephrine content in other areas of the brain. Laguzzi *et al.* (1970) related a reduction of the threshold for hippocampal seizure activity to diminished norepinephrine levels in hippocampus. However, in the majority of the reports concerning the relationship between catecholamine levels and epileptic seizures, the whole brain levels of catecholamine were measured in the experimentally induced epileptic process.

In the present study catecholamine levels of penicillin-induced epileptic focus were determined in the various stages of propagation. The levels of both dopamine and norepinephrine decreased in the

focus as compared with those of non-focus when spike activity localized in penicillin-treated cortex, but no differences existed in each
dopamine and norepinephrine levels between the focal and non-
focal cortex when spikes fully propagated to the non-focus. This
evidence suggests that catecholamine play an important role in the
development of seizure discharges. However, the information concerning which amine or amines may be most involved with the epileptic process can not be obtained.

On the other hand, dopamine, but not norepinephrine, showed
the inhibitory effect on penicillin-induced spike activity after the
topical application. l-DOPA also inhibited spike discharges after
the topical and intravenous application. This finding suggests that
l-DOPA was first metabolized to dopamine and then exhibited the
inhibitory effect on seizure activity. Latency of l-DOPA effect after
application could be the time for conversion of l-DOPA to dopamine.

Recently, some investigators (Thierry *et al.* 1973, Fuxe *et al.*
1974, Lindvall *et al.* 1974) reported the evidence for the existence
of dopaminergic neuron in the rat cerebral cortex. Therefore, it is
suggested that dopamine can play an important role in epileptic
process of penicillin focus, although further evidence is necessary
concerning the physiological function of dopamine in cerebral cortex.
De Schaepdryver *et al.* (1962), Goldberg and Salama (1970) and
Boggan and Seiden (1971) postulated an important role for dopamine
in the experimental seizures.

In conclusion, our data suggest that dopamine is directly involved
in regulating the development and the propagation of penicillin-
induced epileptic activity.

Summary

In 25 cats an unilateral epileptic focus was produced by intracortical injection of potassium benzyl penicillin and on the other
hemisphere, sham-operation was done by injection of the same
volume of saline solution without penicillin.

Catecholamine analysis was performed for each hemisphere separately.

In a second series of 15 cats, the effect of catecholamines and of
l-DOPA on penicillin-induced spike activity was examined.

In the first and second stage of propagation of penicillin-induced
spikes, dopamine and norepinephrine significantly decreased in the
focus. In the third stage no differences existed.

The penicillin-induced spike activity was reduced as well by the topical application of dopamine as of l-DOPA, whilst no inhibitory effect was observed in the topical application of norepinephrine.

Acknowledgement

We would like to thank Miss M. Hiramatsu and Miss Y. Shiraishi for their skilful technical assistance.

References

Azzaro, A. J., Wenger, G. R., Craig, C. R., Stitzel, R. E. (1972), Reserpine-induced alterations in brain amines and their relationship to changes in the incidence of minimal electroshock seizures in mice. J. Pharmacol. exp. Ther. *180*, 558—568.

Billiet, M., Bernard, P., Delaunois, A., De Schaepdryver, A. (1970), Induced changes in caudate nucleus dopamine and electroshock threshold. Arch. int. Pharmacodyn. *188*, 396—400.

Boggan, W. O., Seiden, L. S. (1971), Dopa reversal of reserpine enhancement of audiogenic seizures susceptibility in mice. Physiol. Behav. *6*, 215—217.

Chen, G., Ensor, C. R., Bohner, B. (1954), A facilitation action of reserpine on the central nervous system. Proc. Soc. exp. Biol. Med. *86*, 507—510.

De Schaepdryver, A. F., Piette, Y., Delaunois, A. L. (1962), Brain amines and electroshock threshold. Arch. int. Pharmacodyn. *140*, 358—368.

Fuxe, K., Hökfelt, T., Johansson, O., Jonsson, G., Lidbrink, P., Ljungdahl, Å. (1974), The origin of the dopamine nerve terminals in limbic and frontal cortex. Evidence for meso-cortico dopamine neurons. Brain Research *82*, 349—355.

Goldberg, M. E., Salama, A. I. (1970), Relationship of brain dopamine to stress-induced changes in seizure susceptibility. Eur. J. Pharmacol. *10*, 333—338.

Jobe, P. C., Picchioni, A. L., Chin, L. (1973), Role of brain norepinephrine in audiogenic seizure in the rat. J. Pharmacol. exp. Ther. *184*, 1—10.

Kilian, M., Frey, H.-H. (1973), Central monoamines and convulsive thresholds in mice and rats. Neuropharmacology. *12*, 681—692.

Kobinger, W. (1958), Beeinflussung der Cardiazolkrampfschwelle durch veränderten 5-Hydroxytryptamingehalt des Zentralnervensystems. Arch. exper. Path. u. Pharmakol. *233*, 559—566.

Laguzzi, R. F., Acevedo, C., Izquierdo, J. A. (1970), Seizure activity and hippocampal norepinephrine content. Arzneimittel-Forsch. 20, 1904—1905.

Lehmann, A. (1967), Audiogenic seizures data in mice supporting new theories of biogenic amines mechanisms in the central nervous system. Life Sci. *6*, 1423—1431.

Lessin, A. W., Parkes, M. W. (1959), The effects of reserpine and other agents upon leptazol convulsions in mice. Brit. J. Pharmacol. *14*, 108—111.

Lindvall, O., Björklund, A., Moore, R. Y., Stenevi, U. (1974), Mesencephalic dopamine neurons projecting to neocortex. Brain Research *81*, 325—331.

Thierry, A. M., Stinus, L., Blanc, G., Glowinski, J. (1973), Some evidence for the existence of dopaminergic neurons in the rat cortex. Brain Research *50*, 230—234.

Authors' address: Drs. K. Kobayashi, T. Shirakabe, H. Kishikawa, and A. Mori, Institute for Neurobiology, Okayama University Medical School, 2-5-1 Shikata-cho, Okayama, Japan.

Acta Neurochirurgica, Suppl. 23, 101—109 (1976)

Max-Planck-Institut für Hirnforschung, Neurobiologische Abteilung
(Direktor: Prof. Dr. R. Hassler), Frankfurt/Main, Federal Republic of Germany

Antivitamin B₆ Induced Ultrastructural Changes in the Hippocampus of the Convulsant Rabbit and Its Biochemical Correlates

C. Nitsch

With 3 Figures

Introduction

Although numerous attempts have been made to understand the mechanisms of epileptic seizure discharges (*e.g.* [7]), no satisfactory explanation is available concerning a causative factor resulting in the onset of generalized seizure [14]. One way of obtaining more information on this problem, is to study the supposed changes occurring just before the onset of the seizure, *i. e.* in the preictal period. For this purpose it is necessary to have a convulsant agent which acts with fairly constant time intervals, so that the moment at which the seizure starts can be predicted. This supposition is fulfilled by an antimetabolite of vitamin B_6, methoxypyridoxine (MP). By competitively displacing pyridoxalphosphate from its binding sites at the apoenzymes of decarboxylases and transaminases [15], MP imitates a strong vitamin B_6-deficiency, characterized by neuritis, ataxia, and spontaneous generalized convulsions [5]. One of the most susceptible B_6-enzymes is the glutamate decarboxylase [2], which controls the synthesis of the supposed inhibitory transmitter substance gamma-aminobutyric acid (GABA). Already preictally the enzyme activity is markedly reduced (Nitsch, in preparation), so that consumed GABA cannot be replenished. The regional change of the GABA-concentration after administration of convulsive agents has not yet been systematically studied in spite of the fact, that GABA-levels differ among brain regions [13]. Therefore the GABA-content was measured after MP time-dependently in 11 different brain structures.

In the first presentation on the convulsive properties of MP [16], it was demonstrated that the drug selectively induces degenerations of the pyramidal cells of the fields CA_3 and CA_4 of the hippocampus. Furthermore, we could demonstrate that after MP the seizure discharges start in the hippocampus, *i.e.* hippocampal discharges precede the cortical ones for about 10 seconds, suggesting a spreading of the hippocampal excitation to distant brain areas [6]. These facts and their possible correlation with the hippocampal sclerosis in the endblade gave the impulse for studying the early ultrastructural alterations occurring in this area after administration of MP.

Own Material

Methods

Rabbits of both sexes from a local strain, weighing between 2.5–3.5 kg, were used throughout the experiments. Invariably the rabbits were anaesthetized with ether during a tracheotomy for artificial respiration and during operation of the skull for the implantation of electrodes. After cutting ether anaesthesia, the animals were immobilized with gallamine triethiodide (Flaxedil®) under artifical respiration. When the cortical recordings indicated recovery from the effect of ether, 100 mg/kg MP was injected intravenously. Seizure discharges started 22 to 28 minutes after administration of MP.

The brain was removed from the skull before the injection of MP, and after 20 (preictally), 40, and 120 minutes. Regional areas were dissected out, weighed, and assayed for GABA-content [12].

For the ultrastructural investigations the rabbits were perfused with an aldehyde fixative according to the method of Sotelo and Palay [17]. Tissue blocks for thin sections were treated routinely. Freeze-fracture replicas were obtained by using the method of Moor and Mühlethaler [10].

Results

A. Regional Alterations of GABA-level after MP

In control animals the substantia nigra has the highest amount of GABA, followed by the hypothalamus, the superior colliculus, the thalamus, the caudate nucleus, and the putamen (Fig. 1 b). These six GABA-rich regions are collected in group A, because they show approximately similar patterns of GABA-decrease: in the first 20 minutes the GABA-content drops to about 69%, this is a decrease rate of 4.56 mM/kg/hr. The GABA-level further decreases to 61% after 40 minutes and reaches its lowest values after 120 minutes which range from 56% for putamen to 17% for substantia nigra. Thus, the ictal decrease rate is only 0.59 mM/kg/hr (Fig. 1 a).

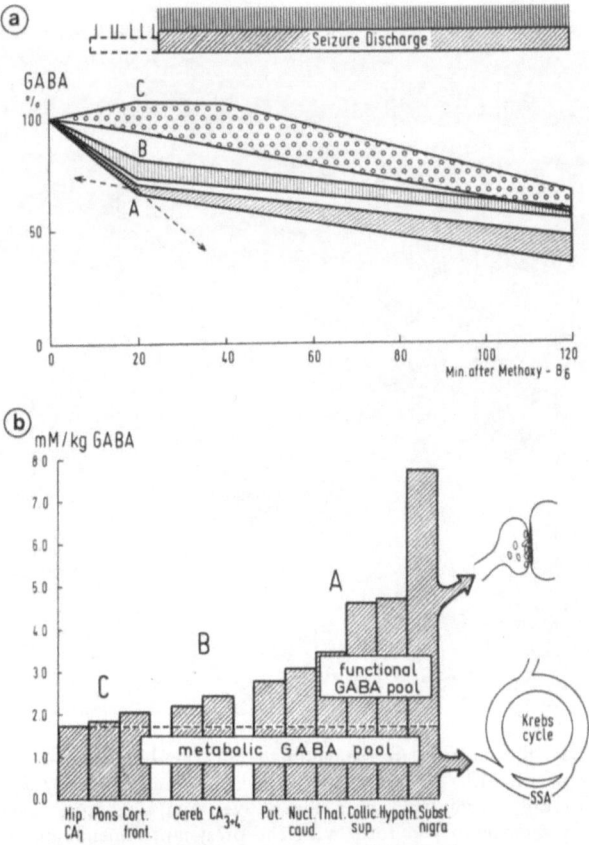

Fig. 1. a) Pattern of GABA decrease in the three groups of investigated brain structures. In GABA-rich regions (*A*) the preictal GABA decrease rate is high, in the GABA-poor regions (*C*) no decrease takes place during the first 40 minutes. The regions constituting group *B* lie between the two extremes. During the ictal period the decrease rate has slowed in group *A* and is now nearly identical in all brain regions. b) Schematic drawing of the regional distribution of GABA demonstrating that the metabolic pool is present in all brain structures. Metabolic GABA is consumed during the convulsions as a result of the high metabolic activity of the neurones. In the GABA-rich regions a functional pool is present in addition, which is used up already in the preictal period, thus giving rise to the seizure development (after Nitsch and Okada [12])

Group C consists of brain regions with low concentrations of GABA (gray matter of the frontal cortex, pontine reticular formation, regio superior of the hippocampus). In these GABA-poor regions practically no decrease can be found during the first 40 minutes. After 120 minutes an average decrease to 61% ist observed.

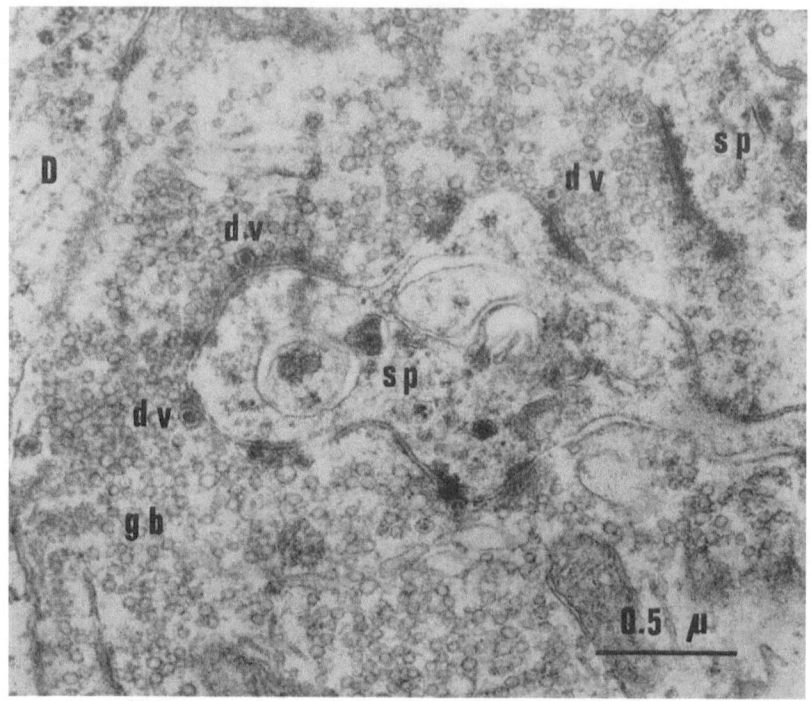

Fig. 2. Mossy fibre region in the endblade of the hippocampus 2 hours after administration of MP. A spine (*sp*) pierces a giant bouton (*gb*). Dense-core vesicles (*dv*) are accumulated near the active synaptic zones, several of them are fusing in a omegashaped form with the presynaptic membrane, ejecting their core into the synaptic cleft. *D* apical dendrite of a pyramidal cell

The mossy fibre region of the hippocampus and the cerebellar cortex, constituting group B, show a pattern of GABA-decrease which lies between the two extremes.

B. Ultrastructural Alterations in the Mossy Fibre System of the Hippocampus after MP

The axons of the granule cells of the dentate gyrus, the mossy fibres, expand to vast nerve terminals, the giant boutons, which make contact with spines of the apical dendrites of the pyramidal cells of the fields CA_3 and CA_4 [3]. In unanaesthetized animals it is possible to see sporadically omega-shaped fusions of dense-core vesicles with the presynaptic membrane of the active synaptic zones [11]. During MP-induced generalized convulsions the frequency of such fusions has increased considerably (Fig. 2). The whole synaptic zones

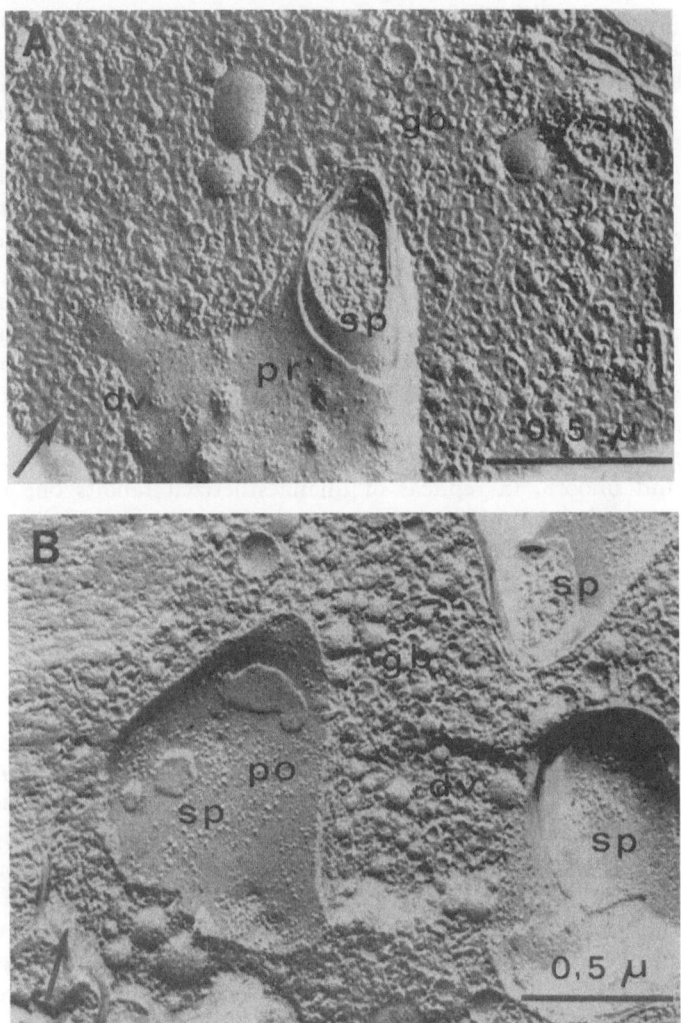

Fig. 3. Freeze-fractured replicas of the mossy fibre region of the hippocampus 45 minutes after administration of MP. The arrow indicates the direction of platinum shadowing. A) A spine (sp) lies inside a giant bouton (gb). The pre-synaptic membrane seen from the presynaptic side (pr) is filled of bumps, probably representing fusioned dense-core vesicles (dv). B) The postsynaptic side of a pre-synaptic membrane (po) is lying open. The reversals of the bumps are present, little holes or indentations. In addition the increased granulation is striking

are occupied by omega-shaped profiles, representing dense-core vesicles fusing with the presynaptic membrane. It looks as if the core of the dense-core vesicle is ejected into the synaptic cleft.

This finding led us to study more extensively the structure of the surface of the presynaptic membrane. For this purpose the freeze-etching method is very convenient, where one obtains platinum-carbon replicas of the broken surfaces of deep-frozen, aldehyde-fixed material. In convulsant rabbits active synaptic zones between the mossy fibre terminals and the spines of the apical dendrites of the pyramidal cells looked at from the presynaptic side are crowded with protuberances or bumps, about 1000 Å in diameter (Fig. 3 A). If one looks from the opposite side, from the postsynaptic side at the presynaptic membrane, the reversal of the bumps is present, i.e. small holes or indentations with a diameter between 800 and 1000 Å (Fig. 3 B). In freeze-fractured preparations of the anaesthetized animal the surface of the presynaptic membrane is even and smooth, in replicas of unanaesthetized rabbits one rarely observes single bumps [11].

Already after the first to the second generalized seizure discharge (40 minutes after administration of MP) the number of bumps, i.e. fusioned dense-core vesicles, increases tremendously.

Discussion

There is good evidence indicating that GABA is an inhibitory transmitter substance in the central nervous system [8]. The GABA-content of a brain region is probably a function of the number of GABA-containing boutons in the brain region, i.e. those brain regions with a high GABA-content possess more GABA-containing boutons per unit area than the GABA-poor regions. Since the inhibition of GABA-synthesis is approximately identical in all brain structures, the turn-over rate of GABA must be higher in the GABA-rich regions, or rather, there exist two GABA-pools in the same brain region which possess different turn-over rates. A high decrease-rate appears only in the GABA-rich regions, therefore it must be concluded that the pool with the high turn-over rate represents the functional GABA-pool with the GABA used for chemical transmission. As a result of the high turn-over rate in the functional pool it is rapidly exhausted, the balance between inhibition and excitation is shifted in favour of the excitation and, if a defined threshold is reached, uncontrolled discharges can take place.

In contrast to the functional pool, the size of the metabolic pool is nearly identical in all brain regions. GABA is an energy-donator through the GABA-shunt to the Krebs-cycle [9]. If, due to the decrease of the inhibitory transmitter, the generalized seizure discharges start, the energy-demand of the neurons is increased. As glucose and glycogen supply cannot cover all requirements, additional energy-sources are utilized as for example the GABA-shunt. This energy-demand which is identical for all regions causes the slow constant GABA-decrease during sustained epileptiform seizures.

In the hippocampus the functional GABA is localized in intrinsic neurons, in the basket cells, which contact the granule cells of the dentate gyrus as well as the pyramidal cells [1,18]. The preictal decrease of the hippocampal GABA results in a disinhibition of the granule cells, so that their nerve terminals, the giant boutons, can discharge unrestrained. As it is the case after long-lasting stimulation of the motor endplate where the number of vesicle in the bouton is decreased, and fusions of vesicles with the synaptic zone are observed [4], the same picture can also be elicited in giant boutons by epileptiform discharges.

This excessively increased excitatory input to the pyramidal cells which themselves no longer receive inhibitory input gives rise to the spreading of the hippocampal discharges to distant brain structures.

Summary

In rabbits epileptiform seizures were induced by systemic application of methoxypyridoxine, an antimetabolite of vitamin B$_6$. The regional distribution of GABA was measured in 11 brain structures, before the onset of the seizure and during the generalized convulsions. In brain regions with a high GABA level the GABA content drops already preictally, in contrast to the GABA-poor structures, where no preictal decrease takes place. From this it is concluded, that there exist two GABA pools, a functional one containing the GABA for chemical transmission, which is exhausted already preictally giving rise to the seizure discharges, and a metabolic one, which is utilized as an additional energy-source during the convulsions.

Due to the decrease of the hippocampal GABA, the endings of the dentate gyrus granule cells, the giant boutons contacting the apical dendrites of the pyramidal cells of CA$_3$ and CA$_4$, can discharge unrestrained. An ultrastructural correlate of the increased excitation is demonstrated. The dense-core vesicles of the giant boutons fuse in an omega-shaped form with the presynaptic membrane of the spines. This fusion-phenomenon is observed in ultrathin sections as well as in freeze-fractured replicas of this region.

References

1. Andersen, P., Eccles, J. C., Løyning, Y. (1964), Location of postsynaptic inhibitory synapses on hippocampal pyramids. J. Neurophysiol. 27, 592—607.
2. Bayoumi, R. A., Smith, W. R. D. (1973), Regional distribution of glutamic acid decarboxylase in the developing brain of the pyridoxine-deficient rat. J. Neurochem. 21, 603—613.
3. Blackstad, T. W., Kjaerheim, Å. (1961), Special axo-dendritic synapses in the hippocampal cortex. Electron and light microscopic studies on the layer of mossy fibres. J. Comp. Neurol. 117, 133—159.
4. Ceccarelli, B., Hurlbut, W. P., Mauro, A. (1972), Depletion of vesicles from frog neuromuscular junctions by prolonged tetanic stimulation. J. Cell Biol. 54, 30—38.
5. Coursin, D. B. (1960), Seizures in vitamin B_6 deficiency. In: Inhibition in the nervous system and GABA (Roberts, E., ed.), pp. 294—301. Pergamon Press.
6. Hassler, C., Hassler, R., Okada, Y., Bak, I. J. (1971), Pre-ictal and ictal changes of serotonin, GABA and glutamate contents in different regions of rabbit brain during methoxypyridoxine-induced seizures. Acta Neurol. Latinoam. 17, 595—611.
7. Jasper, H. H., Ward, A. A., Pope, A. (1969), Basic mechanisms of the epilepsies. Boston: Little, Brown and Co.
8. Kim, J. S., Bak, I. J., Hassler, R., Okada, Y., (1971), Role of γ-aminobutyric acid (GABA) in the extrapyramidal motor system. 2. Some evidence for the existence of a type of GABA-rich strio-nigral neurons. Exp. Brain Res. 14, 95—104.
9. McKhann, G. M., Albers, R. W., Sokoloff, L., Mickelsen, O., Tower, D. B. (1960), The quantitative significance of the γ-aminobutyric acid pathway in cerebral oxidative metabolism. In: Inhibition in the nervous system and GABA (Roberts, E., ed.), pp. 169—181. Pergamon Press.
10. Moor, H., Mühlethaler, K. (1963), Fine structure in frozen-etched yeast cells. J. Cell Biol. 17, 609—628.
11. Nitsch, C., Bak, I. J. (1974), Die Moosfaserendigungen des Ammonshorns, dargestellt in der Gefrierätztechnik. Verh. Anat. Ges. 68, 319—323.
12. Nitsch, C., Okada, Y. (1976), Differential decrease of GABA in the substantia nigra and other regions of the rabbit brain during methoxypyridoxine-induced convulsions. Brain Res. 105.
13. Okada, Y., Nitsch-Hassler, C., Kim, J. S., Bak, I. J., Hassler, R. (1971), Role of γ-aminobutyric acid (GABA) in the extrapyramidal motor system. 1. Regional distribution of GABA in rabbit, rat, guinea pig, and baboon CNS. Exp. Brain Res. 13, 514—518.
14. Prince, D. A. (1972), Topical convulsant drugs and metabolic antagonists. In: Experimental models of epilepsy (Purpura, D. P., Penry, J. K., Tower, D., Woodbury, D. M., Walter, R., eds.), pp. 51—83. New York: Raven Press.
15. Purpura, D. P., Berl, S., Gonzales-Monteagudo, O., Wyatt, A. (1960), Brain amino acid changes during methoxypyridoxine-induced seizure (cat). In: Inhibition in the nervous system and GABA (Roberts, E., ed.), pp. 331—335. Pergamon Press.
16. — Gonzales-Monteagudo, O. (1960), Acute effects of methoxypyridoxine on hippocampal endblade neurons: an experimental study of "special pathoclisis" in the cerebral cortex. J. Neuropath. exp. Neurol. 19, 421—432.

17. Sotelo, C., Palay, S. (1968), The fine structure of the lateral vestibular nucleus in the rat. I. Neurons and neuroglial cells. J. Cell Biol. *36*, 151—179.

18. Storm-Mathisen, J. (1972), Glutamate decarboxylase in the rat hippocampal region after lesions of the afferent fibre systems. Evidence that the enzyme is localized in intrinsic neurons. Brain Res. *40*, 215—235.

Author's address: Dr. med. Cordula Nitsch, Max-Planck-Institut für Hirnforschung, Neurobiologische Abteilung, D-6000 Frankfurt/Main, Federal Republic of Germany.

Acta Neurochirurgica, Suppl. 23, 111–118 (1976)
© by Springer-Verlag 1976

Department of Biochemistry and Neurosurgical Clinic, Medical Faculty and
Institute of Biochemistry, Comenius University, Bratislava, ČSSR

Formation of Glutamate and GABA
in Epileptogenic Tissue from Human Hippocampus
in Vitro

T. Turský, M. Laššánová, M. Šramka, and P. Nádvorník

With 4 Figures

Changes in the amino acid levels of epileptogenic foci of man were described by Van Gelder et al. (1972). Similar changes were found by Koyama (1972) during cobalt-induced epilepsy in rats. Changes of amino acid levels and of the activity of enzymes, involved in the brain amino metabolism, produced by convulsions were described by several investigators (Van Gelder 1974, Wiechert and Göllnitz 1970).

In tissues stereotactically removed from epileptogenic foci of the human hippocampus we tried to establish by experiments in vitro whether the amino acid metabolism was disturbed and where the eventual disturbance was localized. As controls we used nonepileptic tissues from human brains, mainly from the cortex, removed during neurosurgical operations.

The amino acid metabolism of brain has three characteristic features:

1. It is closely linked to the oxidation of compounds such as glucose or acetate, whereby carbon from the oxidatively degraded substrate is incorporated primarily into amino acids (Gaitonde et al. 1965).

2. In the course of these metabolic transformations the putative neurotransmitters stimulatory glutamate and inhibitory GABA are formed (Krnjević 1974).

3. Metabolic experiments demonstrate the compartmentation of amino acid metabolism in the brain. In 1961 Waelsch and coworkers (Berl et al. 1961) showed that at least two pools of glutamate exist in the brain. From the large glutamate pool GABA is formed, the

small one is the source of glutamine. Later on, Cremer (1964) showed that ^{14}C from glucose preferentially incorporates into the large glutamate pool. O'Neal and Koeppe (1966) found that the small glutamate pool incorporates the ^{14}C primarily from acetate.

Based on kinetic data many groups, including ours, have accepted the view, that the large glutamate pool is localized in neurons while the small glutamate pool is localized in glial cells (Balázs et al. 1973, Van den Berg 1973). In 1975 Minchin and Beart published the first direct experimental evidence supporting this view.

Materials and Methods

The localization of epileptogenic focus and its stereotactic removal was described by Nádvorník et al. (1975). Immediately after removal the tissue was rinsed in cold saline-glucose solution buffered to pH 7.4 with Tris buffer (Balázs et al. 1970). The tissue was cut in to 30–40 mg pieces and immersed into the same solution placed in Warburg vessels. In order to restore the normal metabolite levels the tissue was incubated at 37 °C in the atmosphere of pure oxygen for 30 minutes. Then 5 μCi of U-^{14}C-glucose or 1-^{14}C-acetate were added from the side arm of the Warburg vessel and the incubation was continued for exactly 10 minutes. The tissue was then filtered with suction on filter paper and homogenized in cold perchloric acid. From the sediment proteins and lipids were isolated and their radioactivity determined. The supernatant was neutralized with KOH and after removal of perchlorate the solution was poured through a column of Dowex 50 (H$^+$). The labelled glucose or acetate were washed out from the column by sufficient quantity of water. The amino acids bound to Dowex were liberated by diluted ammonia. The ammoniacal solution was evaporated and the amino acids were separated by paper electrophoresis. The radioactivity of amino acids was measured in a liquid scintillation spectrometer, their quantity was determined after ninhydrine reaction spectrophotometrically. The activity of glutamate decarboxylase was assayed by measuring the formation of $^{14}CO_2$ from 1-^{14}C glutamic acid according to Albers and Brady (1959). Pyridoxal kinase activity was measured by spectrofluorometric determination of formed pyridoxal phosphate according to Bonavita (1960).

Results and Discussion

No differences in oxygen consumption were found between the epileptogenic and control tissues. The same was true for the activities of glutamate decarboxylase, an enzyme catalysing the formation of GABA and for pyridoxal kinase catalysing the formation of pyridoxal phosphate.

The rate of incorporation of ^{14}C from glucose and acetate into proteins and lipids was equal from both substrates in each case, both in epileptogenic and normal tissue.

The levels of some individual amino acids in the examined tissues are given in Fig. 1. While the levels of glutamate and GABA did not change, the levels of glutamine in epileptogenic tissue decreased to approx. 80% and the levels of aspartic and neutral amino acids increased to 160 and 135% respectively. These differences could be caused by the fact that epileptogenic and control tissues were taken for experiments from different parts of the brain. Nevertheless, the unchanged levels of glutamate and GABA, but mainly the metabolic changes described below, suggest that the observed changes are most probably due to the pathogenic process.

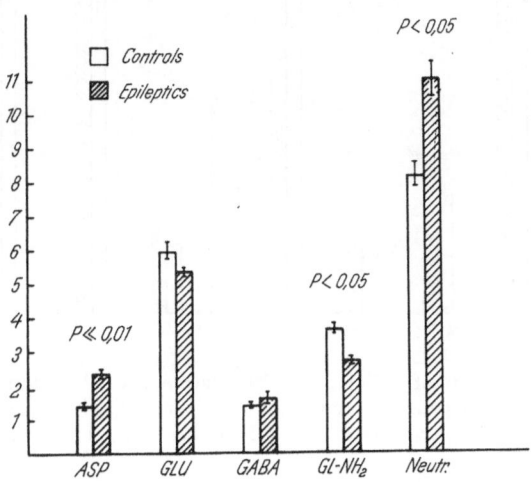

Fig. 1. The levels of amino acids (μmoles/g) in control (open bars) and epileptogenic tissue (hatched bars) after incubation. Mean values from 11–18 determinations ± S.E.M. *Asp* aspartic acid, *Glu* glutamic acid, *Gl-NH₂* glutamine, *GABA* gammaaminobutyric acid, *Neutr.* neutral amino acids (without glutamine and GABA)

Fig. 2 shows the incorporation of ^{14}C into amino acids as expressed in c.p.m. per gram of tissue. The epileptogenic tissue incorporated on the whole less activity than the controls. The incorporation from glucose was decreased to 80%, from acetate to 70%. The only difference in amino acid metabolism between the epileptogenic and control tissue was found in the incorporation of radioactivity into glutamine. In the case of glucose, which is a poor precursor of glutamine the decrease of incorporation was on the limit of statistical significance with $P = 0.05$ (evaluation by Student test). The incorporation into glutamine from acetate was markedly decreased in epileptogenic tissue. From the data shown in Fig. 2 the different fate of the ^{14}C atoms of the two used substrates can be clearly distinguished.

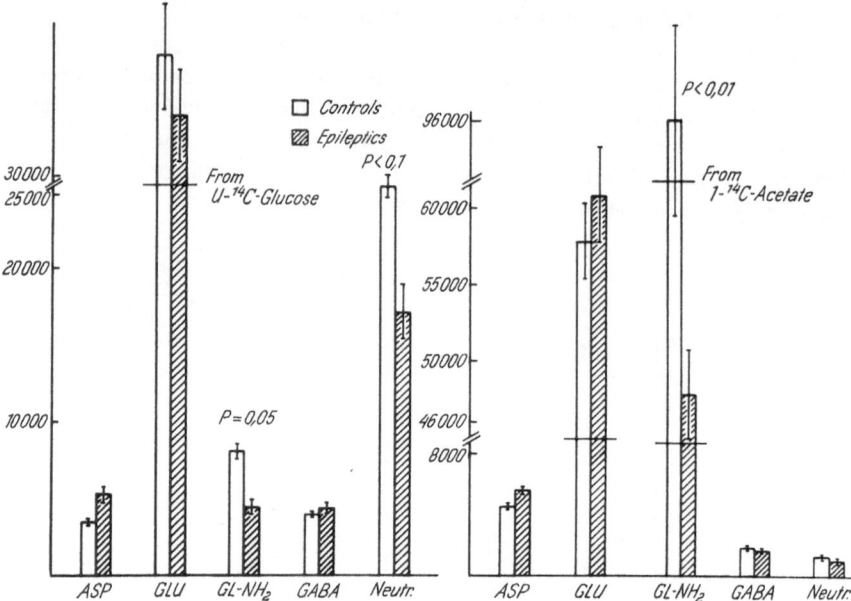

Fig. 2. Incorporation of ^{14}C from U-^{14}C-glucose and 1^{14}-C-acetate into amino acids expressed in c.p.m. per gram of control and/or epileptogenic tissue. Mean values from 3–9 determinations ± S.E.M. Other data are the same as in Fig. 1

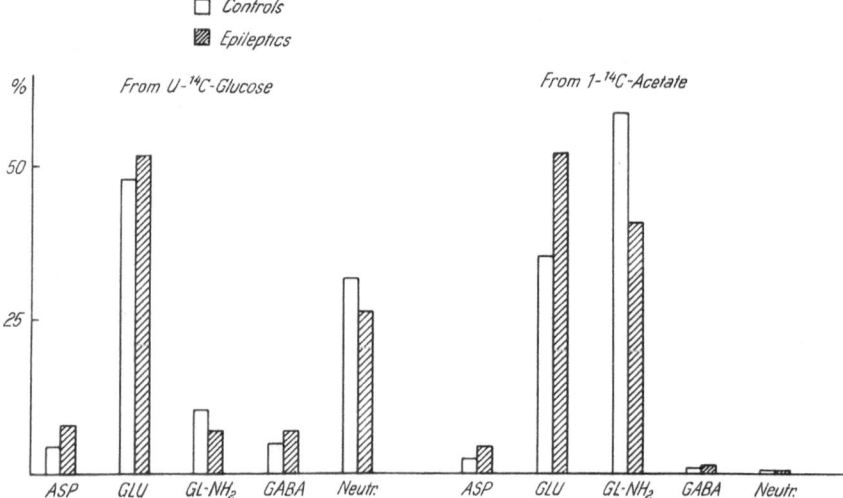

Fig. 3. Activities of amino acids after incorporation of ^{14}C from glucose and acetate expressed in %. Other data are the same as in Figs. 1 and 2

Assuming that the observed differences really reflect the properties of epileptogenic tissue we suppose that the key role at their origin is the decreased formation and lowered level of glutamine. The position of glutamine and GABA between two metabolic compartments was shown in the schemes of Van den Berg (1973) and Balázs et al. (1973). GABA passes from neurones to glia and glutamine is

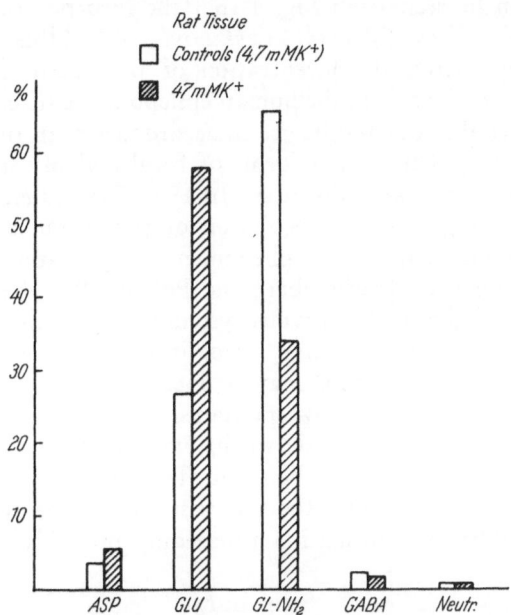

Fig. 4. Activities of amino acids in rat brain slices after incubation with 1-¹⁴C-acetate expressed in %. Open bars—normal medium, hatched bars—medium with increased concentration of potassium (47 mM)

transported from glia to neurones. Glutamine plays an important role in the metabolism of ammonia. At the site of its formation the ammonia is bound, at the site where glutamine is split the ammonia is released. The decreased formation of glutamine in glia could be associated with decreased decomposition of amino acids resulting in the increase of their concentrations.

The central position of metabolic transformations of glutamine in the observed changes in epileptogenic tissue is demonstrated in Fig. 3 where the radioactivity of the individual amino acids is expressed in %. In glial metabolism which preferentially utilizes acetate a marked difference in glutamic acid and glutamine was found. The

amounts of labelled glutamic acid formed from acetate in epileptogenic tissue was 20% higher when compared with controls, the level
of glutamine about 20% lower.

It is interesting to compare the effects observed in glial metabolism of epileptogenic tissue with the results obtained by following
the influence of increased concentration of potassium in the incubat-
ing medium on the metabolism of acetate in the cortex slices of rat
brain. It can be seen from Fig. 4 that the incorporation of acetate
in rat brain slices (Turský, Laššánová, unpublished results) is
influenced by increased concentration of potassium similar to the
incorporation of acetate in the human epileptogenic tissue.

We believe that our results are in accordance with the assumption
of Tower (1973) that certain forms of focal epilepsy may represent
glial rather than neuronal disorder. In 1966 Orkand et. al. described
participation of glia in the regulation of potassium levels in inter-
stitial spaces and named the phenomenon as "spatial buffering of
K+". The findings of Trachtenberg and Pollen (1970) have confirmed
this function of glia in the nervous system of mammals. They formed
the hypothesis that the reactive astroglia in the areas of gliosis in-
vesting epileptogenic neurons may be incapable of "spatially buffering" the potassium release by spontaneously firing neurons (Pollen
and Trachtenberg 1970). As shown in Fig. 3 and 4 our results could
support the hypothesis of Pollen and Trachtenberg. The increased
level of potassium in epileptogenic tissue could be related to the
decrease of glutamine formation proceeding probably in glial cells.

Summary

The levels of some amino acids and the incorporation rates of
^{14}C from glucose and acetate were estimated in control human brain
tissue and epileptogenic foci from human hippocampus incubated in
glucose-saline medium. In the epileptogenic tissue the level of glutamine and the incorporation of radioactivity from both substrates
into glutamine were lowered, mainly from acetate. These results
suggest damaged glial metabolism. The relative increase of glutamate and decrease of glutamate formation in epileptogenic tissue
were similar to the changes caused in rat brain slices by increased
concentration of potassium in the incubation medium.

References

1. Albers, R. W., Brady, R. O. (1959), The distribution of glutamic acid decarboxylase in the nervous system of the rhesus monkey. J. Biol. Chem. *234*, 926—928.

2. Balázs, R., Machiyama, Y., Hammond, B. J., Julian, T., Richter, D. (1970), The operation of the γ-aminobutyrate path of the tricarboxylic acid cycle in brain tissue in vitro. Biochem. J. *116*, 445—467.

3. — Patel, A. J., Richter, D. (1973), Metabolic compartments in the brain: Their properties and relation to morphological structures. In: Metabolic compartmentation in the brain (Balázs, R., and Cremer, J. E., eds.), pp. 167—184. London: Macmillan.

4. Berl, S., Lajtha, A., Waelsch, H. (1961), Amino acid and protein metabolism. VI. Cerebral compartments of glutamic acid metabolism. J. Neurochem. *7*, 186—197.

5. Bonavita, V. (1960), The reaction of pyridoxal-5-phosphate with cyanide and its analytical use. Arch. Biochem. Biophys. *88*, 366—372.

6. Cremer, J. E. (1964), Amino acid metabolism in rat brain studied with ^{14}C-labelled glucose. J. Neurochem. *11*, 165—185.

7. Gaitonde, M. K., Dahl, D. R., Elliott, K. A. C. (1965), Entry of glucose carbon into amino acids of rat brain and liver in vivo after injection of uniformly ^{14}C-labelled glucose. Biochem. J. *94*, 345—352.

8. Koyama, I. (1972), Amino acids in the cobalt induced epileptogenic and nonepileptogenic cat's cortex. Can. J. Physiol. Pharmacol. *50*, 740—752.

9. Krnjević, K. (1974), Chemical nature of synaptic transmission in vertebrates. Physiol. Rev. *54*, 418—540.

10. Minchin, M. C. W., Beart, P. M. (1975), Compartmentation of amino acid metabolism in the rat dorsal root ganglion: A metabolic and autoradiographic study. Brain Res. *83*, 437—449.

11. Nádvorník, P., Šramka, M., Fritz, G. (1975), Graphical representation of epileptic focus, Symposium on stereotactic treatment of epilepsy, Collection of Abstracts 15—16, Bratislava.

12. O'Neal, R. M., Koeppe, R. E. (1966), Precursors in vivo of glutamate, aspartate and their derivatives of rat brain. J. Neurochem. *13*, 803—810.

13. Orkand, R. K., Nicholls, J. G., and Kuffler, S. W. (1966), The effect of nerve impulses on the membrane potential of glial cells in the central nervous system of amphibia. J. Neurophysiol. *29*, 788—806.

14. Pollen, D. A., Trachtenberg, M. C. (1970), Neuroglia: gliosis and focal epilepsy. Science *167*, 1252—1253.

15. Tower, D. B. (1973), The role of astroglia as modulators of neuronal function in cerebral cortex: Comparative data and observations in vivo and in vitro on fluid, electrolyte and amino acid interrelationship. In: Problems of brain biochemistry, Vol. VIII (Bunjatian, H. Ch., ed.). Yerevan: Acad. Sci. Armenian SSR, pp. 269—288.

16. Trachtenberg, M. C., Pollen, D. A. (1970), Neuroglia: Biophysical properties and physiologic function. Science *167*, 1248—1252.

17. Van den Berg, C. J. (1973), A model of compartmentation in mouse brain based on glucose and acetate metabolism. In: Metabolic compartmentation in the brain (Balázs, and Cremer, J. E., eds.), pp. 137—166. London: Macmillan.

18. Van Gelder, N. M., Sherwin, A. L., Rasmussen, T. (1972), Amino acid content of epileptogenic human brain: focal versus surrounding regions. Brain Res. *40*, 385—393.
19. — (1974), Glutamate dehydrogenase, glutamic acid decarboxylase and GABA-amino transferase in epileptic mouse cortex. Can. J. Physiol. Pharmacol. *52*, 952—959.
20. Wiechert, P., Göllnitz, G. (1970), Stoffwechseluntersuchungen des cerebralen Anfallsgeschehens. J. Neurochem. *17*, 137—147.

Authors' address: Dr. T. Turský, Department of Biochemistry, Medical Faculty, Comenius University, Sasinkova 4, 80100 Bratislava, ČSSR.

Acta Neurochirurgica, Suppl. 23, 119—124 (1976)
© by Springer-Verlag 1976

Myerson Laboratory, Boston State Hospital, Boston, Mass., U.S.A.

Anatomical Rationale of Ablative Surgery for Temporal Lobe Seizures and Dyscontrol: Suggested Stereo-Chemode Chelate-Blockade Alternative

T. McLardy*

With 2 Figures

Summary

Anatomical data now strongly suggest that the common factor in curative ablative operations for the commonest (*i.e.* ammonshornsclerosis) form of temporal-lobe epilepsy is the cutting of the ipsilateral temporoammonic perforant path's "nozzle" where it leaves the entorhinal cortex to "spray" along the length of the ammonshorn. This substantially deafferences ipsilateral dentate granule-cells and hence the unsclerosed pyramidal neurons, notably in "resistant sector" CA2, which are probably the source of the seizures. Stereo-chemoding of long-lasting (experimentally tested) chelates along the zone of peculiarly zinc-rich synapses of the mossy fibre system should block the commissural as well as the ipsilateral inputs to these residual neurons, to give higher percentage cures, and could probably be performed bilaterally (where indicated, in adults) without endangering memory function.

Introduction

Good-to-excellent clinical results in 100% of those 17–20% of unilateral lobectomies for temporal-lobe epilepsy (TLE) where a hamartomatous lesion is found [1, 2] is readily understandable, since the primary pathological entity has been removed in the biopsy. Much less easily understandable is the attainment of good-to-excellent results in 68–75% of those 50–66% of cases where ammonshornsclerosis is found in the biopsy [1, 2], especially if, as seems neuropatho-

---

* Supported in part by Grant NS 09755-05 from the U.S.A. National Institute of Neurological Diseases and Stroke.

logically probable, the source of the seizures is centred within the residual island of CA 2 neurons. This CA 2 island,—so suggestively illustrative of Ward's pathogenic "aggregate of partially denervated neurons" [3], and possibly composed of slowly dying nerve cells [4],— almost always stretches throughout the axial extent of the ammons-horn ([5] and McLardy unpublished), yet classical lobectomy for TLE removes only its unco-proximost extremity, and the uncus itself contains no CA 2 elements [6]. This apparent paradox can now, I submit, be furnished a simple rationale in the light of new anato-mical data,—data which suggest possible non-ablative therapeutic alternatives.

(Ammonshorn is here defined as: hippocampus [CA] plus gyrus dentatus [GD].)

Data

Recent studies of the axonal connections of the entorhinal cor-tex in primates [7, 8] have re-emphasized the cytoarchitectonically established fact that this portion of the allocortex is restricted to a zone of parahippocampal gyrus adjacent to only the unco-ventral end of the ammonshorn. Neuroanatomical texts seldom make this clear, and the recent emphasis upon "lamellar" organization of much of the main axonal circuitry within the hippocampal formation perhaps tends to reinforce the misconception that the entorhinal cortex is coextensive with the ammonshorn.

Since the temporo-ammonic perforant path,—the heaviest main input from ipsilateral cortex to CA, via relay in the outer $2/3$ of GD's molecular layer,— originates only within entorhinal cortex [7, 9], it follows that this system of fibres must spray out from this portal almost axially up the subiculum (as illustrated in Fig. 1 a) if it is to reach mid and dorsal realms of GD—where electrophysiologists find evidence of its reaching (e.g. [11]). Van Hoesen and Pandya [8] have now shown by experimental neuroanatomical methods that this is indeed the case. Their focal entorhinal cortex lesions in macaques led to degeneration into the recognized termination zone of the per-forant temporo-ammonic path along the full axial length of GD. I have found that the "spray" can in fact be directly displayed in, especially parahorizontal, sections of normal brain. Fig. 1 b is such a section showing these axial elements coursing through the subiculum, (which IS coextensive with the ammonshorn). Horseradish-peroxi-dase studies in rats (McLardy, unpublished) furnish further anatomi-cal confirmation.

Classical temporal lobectomy for TLE [2], Crandall's modification

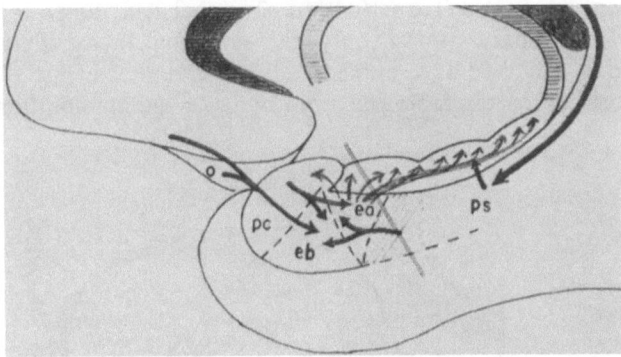

Fig. 1 a. Mesial view of inputs to, and some outputs from, entorhinal cortex (*ea* and *eb*) in primates. (Modified from Nauta [10] with permission of the author and the publishers)

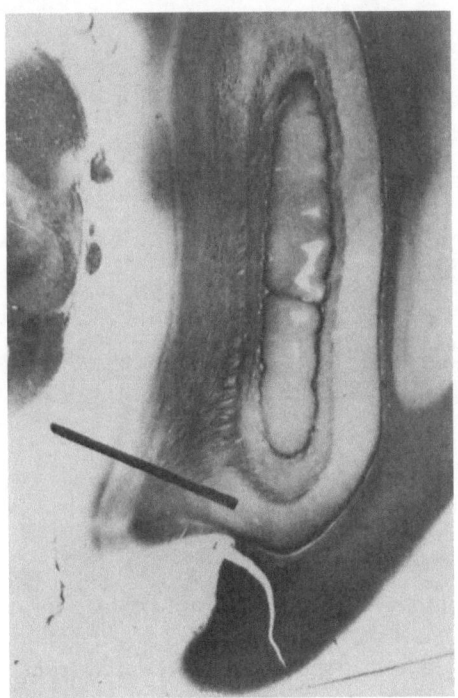

Fig. 1 b. Macaque; parahorizontal section along ammonshorn; Gros Bielschowski impregnation, ×7; ink-line through entorhino-subicular "nozzle" of temporo-ammonic perforant path

of it (^{1} p. 341), and Turner's "No. 2" focal leucotomy for TLE [12], anatomically share almost only the common factor that, besides transecting GD and CA immediately behind the uncus, they sever the entorhinal cortex from the main body of the ammonshorn. They

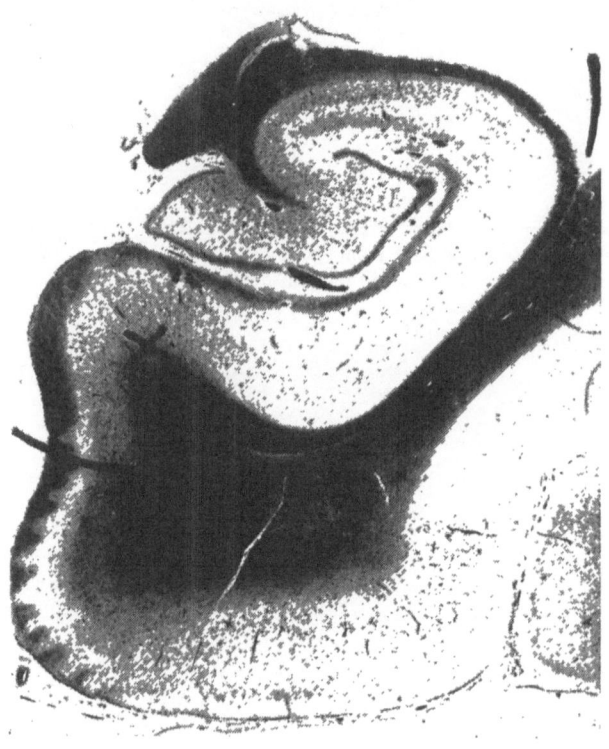

Fig. 2. Human; transverse section of hippocampal formation immediately posterior to uncus; Luxol stain, ×7; X in axial "spray" of perforant path through subiculum. Inked arc shows sweep of Turner's "No. 2" focal leucotomy [12]

cut across the "nozzle" of the perforant path's "spray" into the main body of the ammonshorn, as indicated by the oblique straight line in Fig. 1 a. No autopsy specimen is available from Turner's rotated 1 cm-blade leucotomy, but Fig. 2 shows a 1 cm-radius arc inscribed upon the area aimed at in his "No. 2" operation. All three operations therefore substantially de-afference the whole main body of GD, and hence its mossy-fibre-system's relay into the whole main body of CA.

Discussion

I submit that these ablative operations for TLE are therapeutically effective because they substantially de-afference the main body of GD/CA from entorhinal inputs. Potential positive-feedback "firing foci" within and among the residual unsclerosed neurons, especially CA 2, are thereby substantially de-activated, and seizures therefore abate. If this argument be valid, it should equally suffice to simply (stereotactically) ablate only the entorhinal "nozzle" zone.

Elsewhere, however, I [13] have propounded some probable advantages, over ablative surgery for TLE, of chelate-blockading the temporo-ammonic input to the CA 2 island further upstream, namely where the mossy-fibresystem relays onto the CA 2 pyramidals via peculiarly zinc-rich synapses. This would equally blockade also the commissural inputs from the contralateral temporal lobe (coming via relay in the innermost 1/3 of GD's molecular layer), thus even more thoroughly de-afferencing any ispilateral firing-focus within residual CA neurons. Such in-situ chemodic chelation should avoid the undesired side-effects (e.g. upon sperm and pancreatic islets) of systemically administered chelates. It should also permit bilateral treatment of bilateral firing-foci, in adolescents and adults, probably without endangering memory functions. This is because the permanently disabling effects of bilateral temporal lobectomy, due to loss of recent-experience recall, is almost certainly due to bilateral damage to entorhinal (and perhaps other parahippocampal) cortex, and not due to bilateral damage to GD and/or CA [14]. Such bilateral stereo-chelate-blockading should, of course, be tested first for efficacy and safety on the "baboon model" now becoming available [15]; and sophistication of chelates as to duration of blockade and apnoeic-anaesthetic factors in their penetration, should be determined through testings on in-vitro slices of hippocampal tissue [16]. The potential therapeutic efficacy of such chemode-chelating in TLE is not necessarily dependent upon the validity of my own emphasis upon CA 2. Unfortunately, there are no good observations of single cell activity from the region of CA 2 in human TLE brains (A. A. Ward, personal communication).

Elsewhere again, I [5] have posited that the rationale for good postoperative results in "dyscontrolled" behaviour in TLE patients lies in the fact that classical lobectomy, as well as Turner's "No. 1" focal leucotomy [12], cuts the only axonal and cellular connections between CA and the amygdala, namely 1. the myelinated fascicle between ventralmost alveus and posteriormost amygdala, and 2. the transition zone of neurons between uncal CA 3 and nucleus Asfcv of the amygdala [6]. Recent demonstration of concentrations of various heavy metals within normal amygdala [17] would suggest that stereo-chemoding of chelates directly into the amygdalae might also be a preferable alternative to ablative surgery for such TLE dys-control symptoms, as well as for other conditions featuring untoward aggressivity.

References

1. Brown, W. J. (1973), Structural substrates of seizure foci in the human temporal lobe. Epilepsy: its phenomena in man, pp. 339—374. London: Academic Press.
2. Falconer, M. A. (1970), Significance of surgery for temporal lobe epilepsy in childhood and adolescence. J. Neurosurg. 33, 233—252.
3. Ward, A. A. (1969), The epileptic neuron: chronic foci in animals and man. Basic mechanisms of the epilepsies, pp. 263—288. Boston: Little, Brown & Co.
4. Scheibel, M. E., Scheibel, A. B. (1973), The hippocampal pathology in temporal lobe epilepsy: a Golgi survey. Epilepsy: its phenomena in man, pp. 311—337. London: Academic Press.
5. McLardy, T. (1969), Ammonshorn pathology and epileptic dyscontrol. Nature 221, 877—878.
6. — (1963), Some cell and fibre peculiarities of uncal hippocampus. The rhinencephalon and related structures, pp. 71—88. Amsterdam: Elsevier.
7. Van Hoesen, G. W., Pandya, D. N., Butters, N. (1972), Cortical afferents to the entorhinal cortex of rhesus monkeys. Science 175, 1471—1473.
8. — — (1975), Some connections of the entorhinal and perirhinal cortex of the rhesus monkey. Brain Res., in press.
9. Hjorth-Simonsen, A. (1972), Projection of the lateral part of the entorhinal area to the hippocampus and fascia dentata. J. Comp. Neurol. 146, 219—231.
10. Nauta, W. J. H. (1973), Connections of the frontal lobes with the limbic system. Surgical approaches to psychiatry, pp. 303—314. Lancaster: Med. & Tech. Pub. Co. Ltd.
11. Lømo, T. (1971), Patterns of activation in a monosynaptic cortical pathway: the perforant path input to the dentate area of the hippocampal formation. Exper. Brain Res. 12, 18—45.
12. Turner, E. A. (1963), A new approach to unilateral and bilateral lobotomies for psychomotor epilepsy. J. Neurol. Neurosurg. Psychiat. 26, 285—299.
13. McLardy, T. (1974), Prolonged blockade by taurine of dentato-hippocampus synapses in rats. I.R.C.S. Med. Sci. 2, 1696.
14. — (1970), Memory function in hippocampal gyri but not in hippocampi. Internat. J. Neurosci. 1, 113—118.
15. Meldrum, B. S., Horton, R. W., Brierley, J. B. (1974), Epileptic brain damage in adolescent baboons following seizures induced by allylglycine. Brain 97, 407—418.
16. Skrede, K. Kr., Westgaard, R. H. (1971), The transverse hippocampal slice: a well-defined cortical structure maintained in-vitro. Brain Res. 36, 589—593.
17. Danscher, G. (1975), Personal Communication, Brain Res., in press.

Author's address: T. McLardy, M.D., F.R.C. Path., F.R.C. Psych., Myerson Research Laboratory, Boston State Hospital, Boston, MA 02124, U.S.A.

Acta Neurochirurgica, Suppl. 23, 125—128 (1976)
© by Springer-Verlag 1976

2nd Department of Neuropsychiatry,
Semmelweis Medical School, Budapest, Hungary

Carotis Hexobarbital Test; a Method for Investigation of Interhemispherical Synchrony in Generalized Spike-Wave Mechanisms

P. Halász, A. Balogh, and P. Rajna

With 2 Figures

We have observed a strong activating effect of Hexobarbital on the clinical and EEG symptoms of petit mal (PM) epilepsy and recently we have modified the intracarotid Amytal and Metrazol tests elaborated by the Montreal school, by administering intracarotidly Hexobartital.

The patients examined went through detailed electroclinical investigations including PEG, CAG, serial EEG-s while awake and during induced and night sleep. The intracarotid Hexobarbital administration was performed through a catheter introduced percutaneously into the internal carotid artery up to the first cervical vertebra under radiological control. The effect on the contralateral hemisphere via communicating arteries was disclosed by angiography. The contrast material was given in the same quantity and at the same rate as Hexobartital.

Ten of the patients were characterized by 3 c/s spike-wave (s-w) mechanism and petit mal-grand mal epilepsy while four showed the symptoms of epileptic encephalopathy with slow s-w mechanism.

Intracarotid administration of small doses of Hexabarbital had a strong activating effect on the s-w mechanism. The activating effect of unilateral injection was either bilateral or only homolateral. At the same time as the EEG activation a clinical seizure or absence can be also present. The hemispherical threshold of the bilateral trigger effect was found to be between 5–20 mg., most frequently 10–15 mg. A hemispherical latency in the development of the bilateral reaction could be established below 1.5 seconds and frequently even below 0.5 sec. The latency of the whole reaction was between 1–2 seconds (Fig. 1).

Larger doses 100–200 mg while inducing temporary hemispherical functional disturbances (paresis and aphasia) inhibited the s-w seizures activated by the small doses.

Considering the elicitability of bilateral responses, the hemispherical latency, the required doses, the presence or absence of a clinical

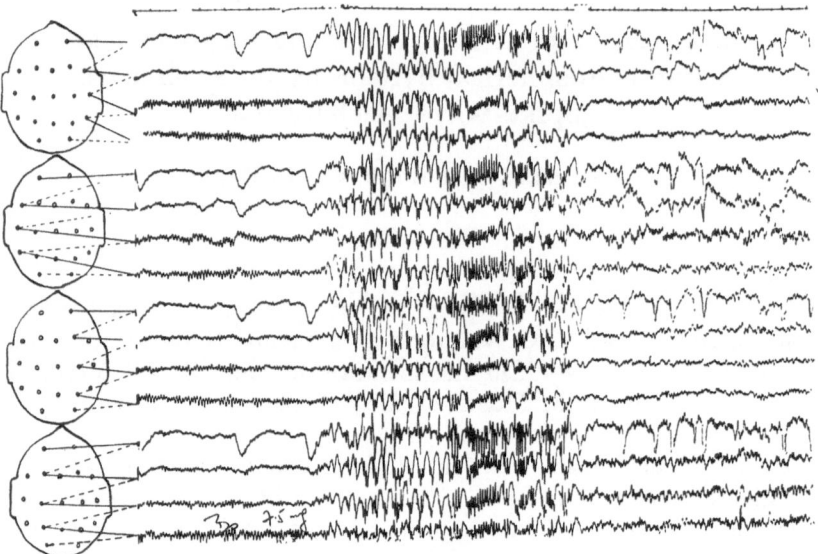

Fig. 1. Activating effect of 7.5 mg. Hexobarbital given into the left internal carotid artery. The latency of the homolateral effect is 1.5 seconds while of the contralateral 2.5 seconds. Hemisperial latency of the right side 1.0 seconds. Time of injection marked on the time signal

seizure, the possibilities of inhibition fine differences could be detected between the two hemispheres. With this method the participation of each hemisphere in the mechanism could be studied and it enabled us to specify the trigger hemisphere and the degree of interhemispherical synchrony.

The effect of unilateral injections can be divided into 10 groups (Fig. 2) producing a continuum the two end points of which are the ideal bilateral synchronisation on the one hand, and the only unilaterally reproducible s-w mechanism on the other hand. From our 14 patients the intracarotid injections elicited s-w paroxysms from either side in 9 cases. Bilateral paroxysms were elicited only from one side in 5 cases. With one exception absences were also elicited from either side in all of 3 c/s s-w mechanism cases, while in the slow s-w cases seizure was elicited only from one side or neither. The hemispherical differences suggested by the previously known electroclinical data and by the test, pointed to the same hemisphere as to trigger side in 8 cases. In 3 patients the test gave some hint to a trigger side although previous data did not indicate it.

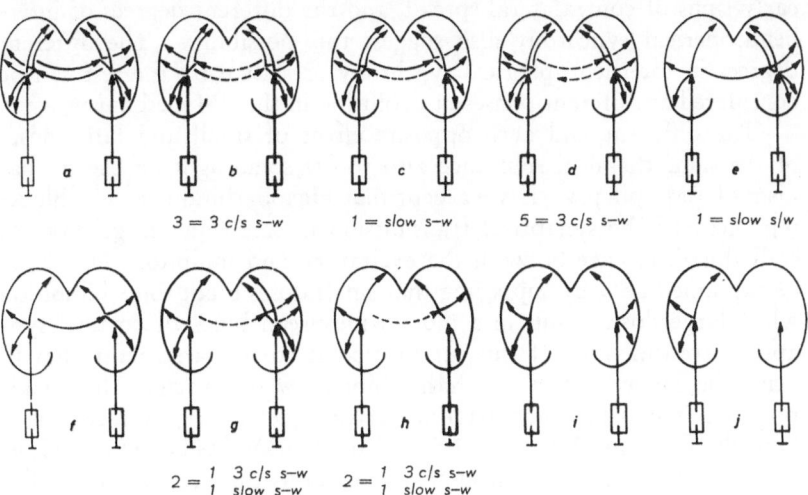

Fig. 2. Interhemisperial synchronization in spike-wave mechanism revealed by the activating effect of intracarotid Hexobarbital.

a Ideal interhemisperial synchrony: bilateral effect from either side injection without latency (unbroken arrow). (Has not been observed in our material.) *b* High degree of interhemisperial synchrony: bilateral effect from either side injection with similar latency (broken arrow). *c* Hemisperial difference in the elicitability of bilateral effect evoked without latency from one side while with latency from the other. *d* Hemispherial difference in the elicitability of bilateral effect evoked with different latency (represented by the different length of the broken arrows). *e* and *g* Bilateral effect is evoked only from one side injection, with or without latency. The contralateral injection results in uni(homo)lateral effect. *f* Perfect synchrony from one side injection while without even homo(uni)-lateral effect from the other side. (Has not been observed in our material.) *h* Same as in *g* but without homolateral activation. *i* and *j* Without any sign of inter-hemisperial synchrony. From either side (*i*) or only from one side (*j*) uni(homo)-lateral effect. (Only theoretical possibilities without real manifestation)

In two cases the test did not show any hemispherical differences in spite of EEG evidence of so-called focal signs.

Beyond the practical value of establishing the trigger hemisphere the effect of intracarotid Hexobarbital gave further insight into the mechanism of petit mal epilepsies.

Intracarotid Hexobarbital can evoke a bilateral s-w paroxysm without reaching the contralateral hemisphere through the vascular bed. Since the internal carotid artery does not supply the midline projection systems the bilateral effect can be explained only by trans-hemispherical neural spread or transneural induction. The phenomena of hemispherical latency, the dose dependency of this latency, the early signs of contralateral spread, and the different degrees of inter-hemispherical synchrony also suggest this possibility. The different degrees in interhemispherical synchrony as shown by the test can be considered as different phases of evolution in the PM mechanism.

The different and even opposite effect of small and large doses of the same chemical substance also throw some light on the mecha-nism of PM epilepsy. If we accept that Hexobarbital acts as a block-ing agent of the synaptical transmission in small and large doses as well this difference between the excitatory and inhibitory effect can be explained only by supposing that small doses block some inhibition while large doses result in a more widespread block of cortical syn-aptical transmission. If this supposition is correct a structure has to exist, the cortical effect of which inhibits s-w paroxysms. The inhibi-tion of this structure must have an activating effect on s-w mechanism. Our observations (Halász 1972) and the work of Gloor *et al.* (1974) suggest that the reticular arousal system fulfils these requirements. The great barbiturate sensitivity of the reticulo-cortical transmission further supports the possibility that small doses are effective before wide-spread cortical synaptical effects develop. In summary the aforesaid phenomena of intracarotid Hexobarbital effect emphasize two impor-tant features of the s-w mechanism; namely the different degree of interhemispherical synchronization and the role of functional depres-sion of the reticular activating system in the occurrence of an actual seizure.

References

Gloor, P., Testa, G. (1974), Electroenceph. clin. Neurophysiol. *36*, 499—515.
Halász, P. (1972), Acta Physiol. Acad. Sci. Hung. *42*, 293—314.

Authors' address: Dr. P. Halász, Dr. A. Balogh, and Dr. P. Rajna, 2nd De-partment of Neuropsychiatry, Semmelweis Medical School, Budapest, Hungary.

Acta Neurochirurgica, Suppl. 23, 129—133 (1976)
© by Springer-Verlag 1976

A. L. Polenov Neurosurgical Institute, Leningrad, USSR

Anatomo-Physiological Variability of Deep Brain Structures and Stereo-Neurosurgery of Epilepsy

K. V. Grachev, T. S. Stepanova, S. L. Jatsuk, and **V. A. Rogulov**

With 2 Figures

One of the basic problems of clinical stereotaxis and, particularly, of the stereoneurosurgery of epilepsy is the individual variability of deep brain structures in man. Brain atlases available demonstrate limited anatomical material which does not enable us to make adequate statistical conclusions; the use of contrast x-ray graphical methods may, in our opinion, bring about only a partial solution. The indetermination of brain structures localization cannot be overcome by the most perfect stereotactic devices nor by using electronic computer for calculation purposes. This situation may well be helped by a new approach to a stereotactic atlas elaboration.

Anatomo-topometrical investigation of 200 human brain preparations (K. V. Grachev, T. S. Stepanova, S. L. Jatsuk, 1973; K. V. Grachev, T. S. Stepanova, V. A. Rogulov, 1976) showed that the frequency-distributions of brain structure coordinates of basic importance in the stereotactic treatment of epilepsy are the bell-like form similar in indexes of asymmetry, excess and significant levels to the normal form. The evaluation of variation series according to Pearson criterion confirms this. In all cases, the value χ^2 did not reach the level corresponding to 95% probability difference of both the obtained and theoretical Gauss distribution. Assuming the forms normal, each group of topometrical parameters was fully characterized by two values, viz. arithmetic mean ($\bar{x}$) and standard deviation (σ). Calculations showed the statistical errors of mean ($\overline{xm}$) to be small and within the range of practical calculation performed on brain sections. The error values are relatively larger in choosing ventricle brain structures for intracerebral registration points because of their considerable variability.

The classification of the initial material according to the cephalic

index, hemisphere side and sex made it possible to investigate the
importance of these characteristics for stereotactic calculations. Significance of distribution differences of each of the parameters for
subgroups have been analysed using t-criterion of Student. The calculations made did not show any marked differences whatsoever of the
topography of brain structures studied nor any laws of the distribution of such differences for brachy-, meso- and dolychocephals,
right and left-hand hemisphere, males or females; in some of the
structures (such as n. caudatus) they have not been mentioned in
neither subgroup. The identical character of the conclusions we obtained in two separate samples made it possible to us to assume the
difference as practically negligible. Further mathematical evaluations
showed that the unified frequency-distributions of the stereotactic
coordinates are also close to normal ones and may well be characterized by simple statistics: $\bar{x}$ and σ resp. The general characteristics
of the material reduces considerably the number of investigations
which appears to be necessary for obtaining statistically significant
results. In agreement with our data (K. V. Grachev and T. S. Stepanova, 1969), 95% significance may well be obtained at an average
presence of 40 identical brain sections.

The statistical characteristics obtained in this way are quite exact,
but because of a complex and intricate metric work, they are only
found for a few of the most characteristic points of each structure (marginal points of the border, centre and the like, Fig. 1)
that is why they have only been used in orientating calculations.
Exact evaluations of intracerebral position of the stereotactic instrument depends on the knowledge of full continuous brain structure
outlines. To obtain them we used the analogue method of coherent
signal accumulation enabling us to determine the middle brain outline
("useful signal") on the background of individual variability of its
position ("noise"). The suggested method of graphical statistical treatment of anatomo-topographical brain data (K. V. Grachev and T. S.
Stepanova, 1969) enabled us to obtain practically without any calculations, the average position of continuous brain structures as well as
significant borders of its variations or meaning of the average square
deviation in any outline point whatsoever (Fig. 1). This method
appears to be quite a simple one; the period needed for obtaining a
full outline of the structure is much less than that needed for
measurement of variables and calculation of the statistical parameters
of just one of its points.

The statistical analysis performed showed that in several structures the variability proves to be so high that it is impossible to
obtain on some sections all three outlines (except the outher border).

This refers, particularly, to n. lentiformis, some nuclei of thalamus and n. caudatus. In these cases, outlines of larger nuclei including the given structures had to be determined. This kind of factors showes the necessity of strict consideration of statistical significance of topometrical parameters used in stereotactic calculations. At the same time, they point to the importance of auxiliarly investi-

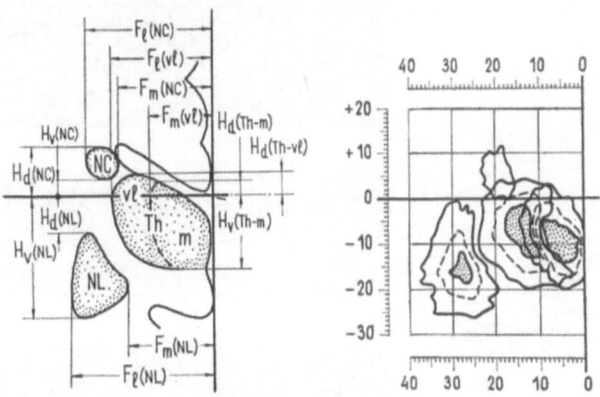

Fig. 1. Fragment of frontal brain section of man on 14 mm behind foramen Monroe. Ortogonal coordinates system: medially sagittal line and the one passing along the inferior medial part of corpus callosum

Left-hand figure: Scheme of main topographical parameters of n. ventrolateralis (*vl*), and medialis (*m*) thalami (*Th*), n. caudatus (*N.C.*), n. lentiformis (*N.L.*), determined by direct statistical calculations

Right-hand figure: Statistically significant (P 0.95) brain section in the same system of coordinates: dotted lines—central outline of structures, full lines—significant borders

gation of deep brain structures identification. Not to describe in the present paper the particular appearance of intracerebral epileptic foci and the character of their correlations, we would wish to refer to the basic possibilities of neurophysiological localization of some of the brain structures.

Our experience with the registration of the summarized electro-subcorticogram (ESCG) in 400 patients suffering from epilepsy and hyperkineses in the course of one-stage stereotaxis and the using multicontact implanted electrodes indicates the absence of specific spontaneous activity in deep brain structures as well as the complexity of their reliable identification as to character of the background biopotentials (T. S. Stepanova and K. V. Grachev, 1972). At the same time, reaction changes of ESCG and EEG may reliably be referred to appropriate brain structures. Thus, both the theta-rhythm of hyppocampus and the low-modulated fast amygdala activity, known from the experiment, arise in these structures as the reaction to the sensory stimulation which rapidly fades. In the course of one-stage operations, such phenomena could be observed in mechanical irritation of these structures immediatly after electrode

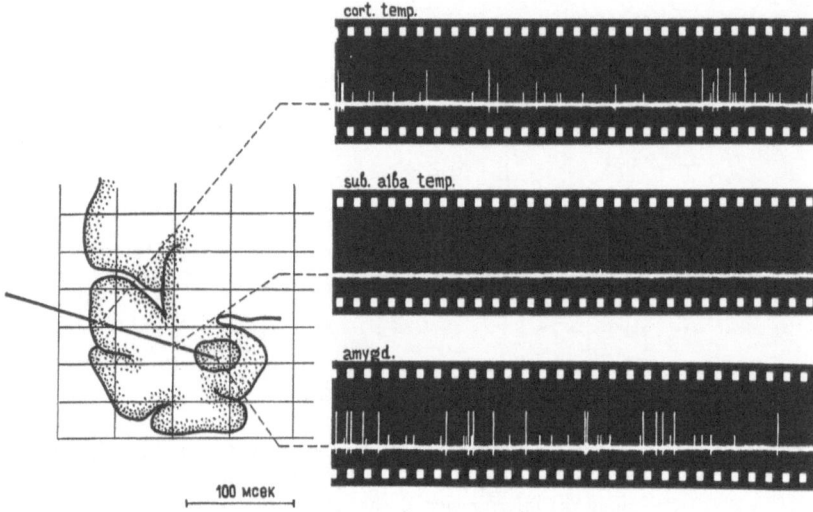

Fig. 2. Dynamics of impulse activity of neuron charge along the line cortex—white matter in using temporal approach. Extracellular outlet

insertion. The recording of evoked potentials on light, tactile irritators and electrostimulation may be useful in thalamus investigation. In the process, there is the characteristic phase inversion of the secondary response along the thalamus-cortex line, multimodal impulsation convergency in medial nuclei (CM), somatotopical correspondence of primary responses in relay nuclei (VL). Among the effects of electrical stimulation of brain structures for differentiation of specific and non-specific thalamic nuclei, generalized cortical (EEG) recruiting reactions, augmenting response or desynchronizations depending on the structure stimulated and the stimulation parameters are of greatest importance. The recording of impulse activity (extracellular) during stereotactic operations facilitates differentiation of the white and grey brain matter (Fig. 2), and often, more exact differentiation. So, according to our data (T. S. Stepanova and K. V. Grachev, 1971), in both frontal thalamus and the hippocampus of man slow frequency fluctuations with minute periodicity ("seesaw activity") may be observed as well as the evoked activity of phase character in response to light flashes and acoustic clicks in non-specific thalamus and hippocampus.

The use of statistically significant map-sections and special neurophysiological approaches makes it possible to overcome, to a large extent, the difficulties connected with the individual variability of the human brain which appear to be one of the factors causing poor results in stereotactic surgery. Additional failure in the stereoneurosurgery of epilepsy may arise due to the seeming incomparability of the diagnostic observations in the same patients. This is associated with functional instability of homologous brain points manifesting itself in frequency and variability of electrosubcortical stimulation effects and their thresholds. In this situation, the use of multicontact implanted intracerebral electrodes enables simultaneous physiological control of a large volume of brain and may prove very useful in a variety of functional conditions for obtaining statistically significant diagnostic data.

References

1. Grachev, K. V., Stepanova, T. S. (1969), Metod statističeskoj obrabotki dannych metričeskich issledovanij individualnoj variabil'nosti topografii golovnogo mozga. Arch. anat. 56, 6, 72—76.
2. — — Jacuk, S. L. (1973), Statističeskije dannyje o topografii blednogo šara čeloveka primenitel'no k stereotaksisu. Arch. anat. 64, 3, 33—40.
3. — — Rogulov, V. A. (1976), Topografija zritel'nogo bugra, chvostatogo i čečeviceobraznogo jader mozga čeloveka na frontal'nom sreze. Arch. anat. 70, 2, 81—87.
4. Stepanova, T. S., Gračev, K. V. (1971), Impul'snaja aktivnost' perednego talamusa u čeloveka. V sb.: Fiziologija i patofiziologija limbikoretikul'arnogo kompleksa. Izd. "Nauka", Moskva, 71—74.
5. — — (1972), Novye dannye o funkcional'nom nejrofiziologičeskom kontrole v processe stereotaksičeskich operacij po povodu epilepsii. V sb.: 3-ja konferencija nejrochirurgov Pribaltijskich respublik. Riga, 192—195.

Authors' address: K. V. Grachev, Ph.D., T. S. Stepanova, M.D., S. L. Jatsuk, M.D., V. A. Rogulov, M.D., A. L. Polenov Neurosurgical Institute, Leningrad, USSR.

Acta Neurochirurgica, Suppl. 23, 135—140 (1976)

Laboratory of Neurophysiology, Nencki Institute, Warsaw,
Department of Neurosurgery, Polish Academy of Sciences, Warsaw, Poland

Some Electrophysiological Characteristics of the Spontaneous Activity of the Amygdala and Effect of Hypothalamic Stimulation on the Amygdalar Units Responses

R. Tarnecki, E. Mempel, E. Fonberg, and J. Łagowska

With 2 Figures

Introduction

Several interesting papers have recently appeared concerning the amygdalo-hypothalamic interrelations in the control of various behavioural, electrophysiological and neurochemical reactions. From the morphological point of view the amygdala is divided into several nuclei, whose different functional roles are not yet fully elucidated. For many years the amygdaloid complex was treated as an entity and given a general modulatory role upon the other structures of the limbic circuit. During the last decade however several authors have differentiated the functions of particular nuclei.

The morphological differentiation into the baso-lateral and dorsomedial parts was made on the basis of ontogenetic and phylogenetic studies (Crosby and Humprey 1941).

Physiological experiments confirm this differentation. According to Fonberg (1974) the dorsomedial part plays an excitatory and the basolateral an inhibitory role both in defensive and alimentary functions. Recently the results of electrophysiological experiments showed similar dichotomy (Murphy 1972, Dreifuss 1972). Other authors point out further subdivisions according to the characteristics of the electrophysiological responses (Egger 1972). The aim of the present paper was to find the difference between the patterns of spontaneous firing of neurons located in various parts of the amygdaloid complex, as well as their responses to the stimulation of different hypothalamic regions. Our experiments were designed to demonstrate the characteristics of spontaneous activity of the amygdala neurons in both parts of amygdala (basolateral and dorsomedial), and their responses to stimulation of the anterior and posterior hypothalamus.

Material and Method

The experiments were performed on 10 cats lightly anaesthetized with nembutal or chloralose. The animals were paralysed with gallamine triethiodide (flaxedil) and passively artificially respired. The preparation was fixed in a stereotaxic apparatus; the stimulating concentric electrodes were inserted stereotaxically to the anterior and posterior hypothalamus. The electrodes were 2 mm apart from one another in the sagittal plane. Single rectangular pulses or trains of 3–5 pulses (50–500 µA duration 100 msec) were used for stimulation. Unitary activity from the amygdala complex was recorded by glass micropipette inserted stereotaxically. Action potentials were recorded photographically. Interval histograms of spontaneous activity and poststimulus histograms were constructed using "ANOPS"-digital computer. The location of the electrodes was subsequently confirmed histologically.

Results

The electrical activity of 69 amygdala neurons was analyzed. Analysis included: a) Frequency of spontaneous firing, b) Pattern of firing in response to hypothalamic stimulation.

In dorsomedial amygdala in most cases neurones fired irregularly out 10–20 spikes/sec (Fig. 1 A). 17 Spikes were investigated during hypothalamic stimulation.

Anterior hypothalamus stimulation changed the rate of firing of 12 neurons. Four types of responses to stimulation of anterior hypothalamus were observed.

a) Obvious increase of firing frequency in two neurones (from average 30/sec to 60/sec in one case, from 30–178/sec in another one). The latency of these responses was less than 12 msec and duration 12 msec and 80 msec respectively (Fig. 1 B).

b) Initial increase of rate firing followed by decrease (3 neurones). Latencies of the excitatory response were also short—less then 12 msec, and its duration 40–60 msec, with firing rate 80–120 spikes/sec. The following inhibitory period lasted 40–50 msec, the decrease of firing was close to zero (Fig. 1 C).

c) Initial decrease of firing followed by increase (two cells). Latency of the inhibitory response was less than 12/sec, and the duration 120 msec. Further excitation period appeared after about 110–100 msec with duration 30–100 msec (Fig. 1 D).

d) Decrease of firing (5 neurons). Latency of inhibition was shorter than 12 msec, its duration 100 msec or more. The inhibition of firing was almost complete (Fig. 1 E).

e) No effect (2 neurones).

Stimulation of posterior hypothalamus changed the activity of 14 cells in dorsomedial amygdala. Three of them reacted by excitation, one after the short latency less than 12 msec and two after the latency about 30 msec. The duration of these reactions was about 50 msec and preferred activity was 80–130 spikes/sec. In all three cases after the first excitation took place the next similar reaction

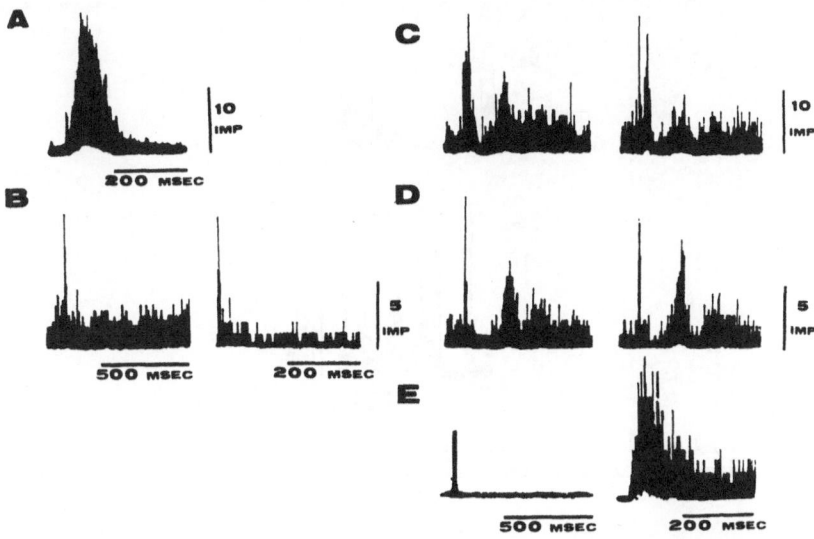

Fig. 1. The pattern of responses recorded of amygdala neurons. A) Interval-histogram (spontaneous activity). B) PSH—short latency, short duration response. C) Short latency excitation followed by decrease of firing rate. D) Decrease of firing rate followed by a long latency excitation. E) Left-site: complete inhibition of spontaneous firing; right-site: interval histogram responding distribution of spontaneous firing (E represent the same unit)

had latency 150 : 250 msec. Three cells reacted by excitation-inhibition. The latency of the excitation was short and its duration was not longer than 12 msec, with preferred activity 40–90/sec. The inhibition had latency 30–55 msec, duration 40–100 msec and the preferred activity 0–5 spikes/sec. One cell reacted by inhibition-excitation, when the latency of the inhibition was about 50 msec, its duration about 12 msec the excitation took place with latency about 100 msec, lasting 60 msec. Seven cells reacted with a very short latency inhibition, lasting 80–400 msec. Two cells were not influenced by stimulation of posterior hypothalamus. It seems that any kind of responses took place with the cells with spontaneous activity more than 15 spikes/sec.

In the lateral amygdala there were generally two kinds of cells: regularly firing cells with a low rate of spontaneous activity (less than 10/sec) and rather small cells, with fast spontaneous activity very difficult to analyze because they deteriorated very easily. Therefore almost all analyses were made on the basis of the first group of neurones. Some of those neurons reacted to sensory stimulation

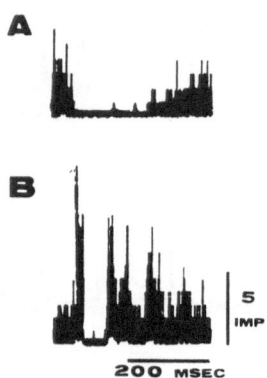

Fig. 2. A) Example of inhibition execreted by electrical stimulation of posterior hypothalamus. B) Another cell with short inhibition followed by long-lasting excitation

viz light, sound, touching of vibrisa and mouth. 31 cells were analyzed from this part of amygdala, 15 were not influenced by stimulation of either parts of the hypothalamus. 12 cells responded to stimulation of the anterior hypothalamus. Only one, with spontaneous activity—about 8 spikes/sec reacted by excitation, lasted about 20 msec. Two cells responded by excitation followed by inhibition. In both cases latency was short—less than 12, duration 15 and 60 msec. Inhibition lasted 40 and 70 msec and was not complete. Nine cells responded with short latency, long lasting—inhibition.

After stimulation of the posterior hypothalamus 9 cells from the lateral amygdala were completely inhibited for a period of 30–100 msec (Fig. 2 A). In one case the inhibition was short and was followed by longlasting excitation (Fig. 2 B).

Generally cells from the dorso-medial amygdala responded to stimulation of the hypothalamus by inhibition or were not influenced by stimulation. We conclude, that in the dorsomendial amygdala rather irregularly firing neurones exist with spontaneous activity 10–30 spikes/sec, responding to stimulation of hypothalamus by excitation, inhibition or both.

In the lateral amygdala units with regular slow spontaneous activity were analyzed which reacted by inhibition to stimulation of the hypothalamus or were not influenced by such stimulation.

Discussion

The results of the experiments showed that the spontaneous activity of the amygdala neurons as well as their responses to hypothalamic stimulation reveal different features. The observed evoked responses were excitatory, inhibitory and combined (although the neurones with various characteristics are intermixed in different amygdala nuclei most of the very active neurones with high frequency were located in the medial part of amygdala and most of the slow "unreactive" to hypothalamic stimulation neurons were located in the lateral amygdaloid nucleus).

The convergency of different modalities is in accordance with the experiments of Sawa and Delgado (1963).

Our results of the effect of hypothalamic stimulation on the amygdala neurones showed that besides the efferent connections of amygdala to hypothalamus by stria and WEF, there also exist afferent connections from hypothalamus to amygdala. This is in agreement with experiments on cats by Happel and Bach (1969). These authors showed that the pattern of evoked responses depends upon whether they are recorded in cortico-medial or baso-lateral part of amygdala. Moreover, these responses have a different pattern depending on whether stimulation concerned the lateral or ventromedial hypothalamus. According to Happel and Bach these afferent influences are, similar to efferent ones conducted by stria terminalis and ventral diffuse system. The results of our experiments on cats in general are in accordance with the results of other authors.

Our data indicate that the population of units located in the medial part of amygdala have a rich spontaneous activity and are more sensitive to hypothalamic stimulation than units located in the lateral part of amygdala. These results indicate that the medial part of amygdala could play an important role in epileptic processes.

References

Crosby, E. C., Humpray, T. (1941), Studies on the vertebrate telencephalon. J. Comp. Neurol. 74, 309—352.

Dreiefuss, J. J. (1972), Effect of electrical stimulation of the amygdaloid complex on the ventro-medial hypothalamus. In: The neurobiology of amygdala, p. 295—317. New York: Plenum Press.

Egger, M. D. (1972), Amygdaloid-hypothalamic neurophysiological interrelation-
    ships, The neurobiology of amygdala (E. Eleftherioun, ed.), p. 319—342. New
    York: Plenum Press.
Fonberg, E. (1969), Effects of small dorsomedial amygdala lesions on food intake
    and acquisition of instrumental alimentary reactions in dogs. Physiol. and
    Behav. *4*, 739—743.
— (1974), Amygdala functions within the alimentary system. Acta Neurobiol.
    Exp. *34*, 435—466.
Happel, L. T., Bach, L. M. N. (1969), Amygdalopedal fiber influences upon
    excitability of amygdaloid nuclei. Fed. Proc. *29*, 392 (No. 829), Abstract.
Murphy, J. T. (1972), The role of the amygdala in controlling hypothalamic out-
    put. In: The neurobiology of amygdala, p. 371—395. New York: Plenum
    Press.
Sawa, M. J. M., Delgado, J. (1963), Amygdala unitary activity in the unrestrained
    cat. EEG Clin. Neurophysiol. *15*, 637—650.

Authors' addresses: R. Tarnecki, M.D., E. Fonberg, M.D., and J. Łagowska,
M.D., Laboratory of Neurophysiology, Nencki Institute, 3 Pasteur str., Warsaw,
and E. Mempel, M.D., Department of Neurosurgery, Polish Academy of Sciences,
16 Barska str., Warsaw, Poland.

Acta Neurochirurgica, Suppl. 23, 141—144 (1976)

Medical Post-Graduate Institute, Neurosurgical Department, Leningrad, USSR,
Research Laboratory of Clinical Stereotaxy at Neurosurgical Department,
Comenius University, Bratislava, ČSSR

Contribution to Surgical Terminology in Epilepsy

A. G. Zemskaja, P. Nádvorník, and M. Šramka

Introduction

Though denoted by the common term „epilepsy", various forms of epileptic attacks in both the organic and functional brain damages show various clinical manifestations. In spite of the uniform diagnostic designation, we can meet with epilepsy in different pathologico-anatomical brain changes, as well as with various changes of bio-electrical brain activity. It stands to reason that even in repeated electro-encephalographic examinations, therapy and prognosis of epileptical disease are not identical. It is, therefore, not quite easy to unify all aspects asserting themselves useful in epilepsy. The efforts to integrate the different aspects of epilepsy lead to various suggestions of classification schemes, the best known nomenclatures being those of the World Health Organization, Gastaut [1], Symonds [5] and Saradshishwili [4]. This classification refers to five fundamental aspects of epilepsy as disease, clinical picture, anatomical and EEG changes predetermining both the therapy and prognosis.

According to these classifications, epilepsy may basically be divided into two big categories, namely those of generalized and partial epilepsies. In the classifications, however, the neurological view is preferred to the surgical with the main attention being focused particularly on medical treatment and not on the possibility of surgery. The first attempt to develop a surgical classification of epilepsy was made by Penfield. He divided epilepsy into central and focal and pointed out that temporal epilepsy responded well to surgery in contrast to central epilepsy where classical surgery was generally ineffective.

The development of stereotactic techniques offered new possibilities for the electro-physiological study of epilepsy, so that together with the radical treatment of epilepsy, the surgical epilepsy nomenclature comes again into the foreground. At present, some new terms of classification, such as multifocal epilepsy, modified epilepsy, and iatrogenic epilepsy appear. The individual terms are motivated in different ways.

Multifocal epilepsy belongs, as a rule, to the category of generalized epilepsies. The original electro-encephalographic view is enriched by those obtained from the stereoelectroencephalographic records of deep brain structures. Since epileptic activity was found to show a larger amount of both cortical and subcortical formations, the term „multifocal epilepsy" is justified and necessary. With the stereotactic treatment of epilepsy carried out in our laboratories, deep brain structures are examined invariably along with scalp records or immediately in the course of electro-corticography from the brain surface. Some of the surgical procedures are combined and made by means of both the stereotactic and classical techniques or during a single operation when simultaneous superficial and depth electro-corticography is being carried out. Thus the designation "multifocal epilepsy" is solved by means of several EEG data in multi-lesion surgery (Tab. 1).

Modified epilepsy appears to be another term justified by the results and sequence of surgical performances. The original clinical picture of epilepsy may change owing to damage of brain structures which may result in the disappearance of adversions or removal of only the partial form of the attack. The generalized form may, however, persist, or, conversely, only the aura remain, after which no more attacks occur or, the structure of the epileptic attack changes after surgery in individual patients. In our laboratories modified forms of epilepsy were observed in 23%, representing the intermediate results of successive epilepsy treatment. The clinical picture remains within the classification schemes of epilepsy, but post operative conditions changed. Following individual surgery, the epileptic manifestations may vanish, reappearing, after a period of time, in a modified form. Even in simular cases, we may consider a modified form of epilepsy which we encounter several times, in our own material.

Iatrogenic epilepsy may be the result of surgery carried out on indication other than for epilepsy, for instance removal of cerebral tumour, or following surgery carried out close to hippocampus, after tentorial herniation, various injuries and in topectomies in psychosurgery. A new, so far clinically quite unknown cause of iatrogenic epilepsy may be the production of epilepsy after brain stimulation of the kindling type [2].

It is to be expected that, in connection with the wide use of the

Table 1

Patient	SEEG Exploration	I. Surgery	II. Surgery	III. Surgery
A. J. f. 41 yrs.		6. 4. 1971 A–G. hp bilat.	3. 11. 1971 Resection of G. hp dx	
Č. L. f. 17 yrs.	5. 9. 1969 A–G. hp dx Cng dx	17. 10. 1969 Resection of Cng dx	14. 4. 1969 H_2 dx P dx A dx	20. 4. 1972 Dm. h dx
H. š. m. 49 yrs.	23. 6. 1969 A–G. hp bilat.	12. 11. 1969 A bilat.	6. 7. 1972 A–G. hp dx	
H. V. m. 31 yrs.	24. 6. 1969 A–G. hp bilat.	13. 2. 1969 A–G. hp sin	6. 5. 1970 A–G. hp bilat.	
J. M. f. 20 yrs.		24. 2. 1972 A–G. hp bilat.	10. 3. 1972 Scaritication of N. Vagi. bilat.	
M. J. m. 20 yrs.		13. 1. 1972 A sin Cm. a sin		
M. M. f. 17 yrs.		16. 2. 1972 Dt bilat.	25. 6. 1972 Ru sin	
M. J. m. 22 yrs.		12. 2. 1972 H_2 sin Rt sin	7. 2. 1971 A dx P dx	
O. J. m. 13 yrs.		10. 2. 1971 P dx Fx dx	11. 5. 1971 A sin	
R. J. m. 13 yrs.		4. 6. 1970 H_2 dx Rt dx A dx	21. 4. 1971 A sin	
S. M. m. 19 yrs.	3. 3. 1971 A bilat.	11. 11. 1971 Cm. a bilat.		
S. E. f. 15 yrs.		9. 3. 1971 Rt sin H_2 sin	5. 1. 1971 Ce sin La. m sin	
S. I. m. 23 yrs.		2. 3. 1972 A–G. hp sin	6. 10. 1972 Resection of G. hp sin	
V. M. f. 18 yrs.		27. 1. 1971 A sin Lpo dx, Voa dx	23. 3. 1972 Cd sin	

surgical treatment of epilepsy, another aspect will arise affecting classification of epilepsy. Thus, with the simultaneous introduction of examination of biopsied individual brain structures enabling biochemical, histological, histochemical and ultramicroscopical investigations, the present epilepsy classification will possibly have to be completed or changed to determine different forms of epilepsy.

Summary

The classifications of the World Health Organization used in epileptology do not contain any aspects of surgical treatment. The introduction of stereotactic techniques make it necessary to include in the classification such terms as multifocal epilepsy, modified epilepsy and iatrogenic epilepsy.

Epilepsy classification will most likely be affected also by the neuro-histological changes found from epileptogenic zones with biochemical analysis of brain structures as well as from the zone of epileptic focus.

References

1. Gastaut, H. (1954), The epilepsies. Electro-clinical correlations. Springfield, Ill.: Ch.C Thomas.
2. Goddard, V. G. (1967), Development of epileptic seizures through brain stimulation at low intensity. Nature *214*, 1020—1021.
3. Penfield, W., Erickson, T. (1941), Epilepsy and cerebral localization. Springfield, Ill.: Ch.C Thomas.
4. Saradshishwili, P. M. (1972), Klasifikacia epileptičeskich pripadkov. Tbilisi: Mecniereba.
5. Symonds, Ch. (1955), Classification of the epilepsies. Brit. med. J. 21, 1038.
6. Zemskaja, A. G. (1972), Focal epilepsy (uni and multifocal) in children and some aspects of its surgical treatment in Kunc, Fusek Present limits of neurosurgery, p. 409—410. Prague: Avicenum.

Authors' addresses: Dr. A. G. Zemskaja, Medical Post-Graduate Institute, Neurosurgical Department, Leningrad, USSR, Prof. Dr. P. Nádvorník and Dr. M. Šramka, Research Laboratory of Clinical Stereotaxy at Neurosurgical Department, Comenius University, Bratislava, ČSSR.

Acta Neurochirurgica, Suppl. 23, 145—146 (1976)

Neurochirurgische Klinik der Karl-Marx-Universität
(Direktor: Prof. Dr. Niebeling), Leipzig, German Democratic Republic

Conventional Surgery in Epilepsy

W.-E. Goldhahn

The following report summarises the results of 75 patients with sufficient data for analysis suffering from epilepsy, operated on from 1951 to 1971. The report is intended to answer the question, which method of conventional surgical approaches can be performed with any chance of success, and what kind of surgery must be improved.

The following methods are used in our institution:

Scar excision	Cortical lysis
Undercutting	Topectomy
Ventricle aperture	Excision of temporal lobe
Dural plastic	Hemispherectomy.

In some approaches different methods were combined. In the tables a numeral arrangement of the main procedure is given.

Excision of brain-dural scar was done after positive electocorticography. The pia was not touched, if possible. Excision areas are always greater in the frontal and temporal region than in the central region or in the speech area respectively and in other functionally important areas.

In 28.6 percent we achieved complete loss of seizures, and in 42.9 percent the frequency of seizures was reduced. Excisions in the temporal area were more successful than in the frontal area.

Corticolysis was the main approach in 15 cases, often combined by dural plastic. We preferred to use the patient's own fascia. In a few cases lyophilized cadaver dura was used. Results: 33.3 percent seizurefree, 26.7 percent seizure-reduction, 40.0 percent no improvement.

Undercutting is possible after exact corticographical localization of the affected area. So that no scars are visible on the surface. In 25 percent we achieved a complete disappearance of seizures and in 25 percent the frequency of seizures was remarkably reduced.

Puncture of the lateral ventricle was done in the opinion that a posttraumatic enlargement of ventricles causes disorders in cerebrospinal fluid flow and, therefore, that an artifical pathway between the internal and external cerebrospinal fluid space could result in an improvement. In most cases this method was combined with excision of brain-dural scar. Puncture alone was done in the frontal area. Nevertheless, in 56.2 percent a positive result was achieved (18.7% seizure free, 37.5% seizure reduction).

Excision of temporal lobe or pole was necessary in 14 cases, limited in the dominant hemisphere by the great vein of Labbé: *i.e.*, the middle of the second temporal gyrus. Releated structures of the uncus were also excised. 28.6 percent of our patients were rendered seizurefree, in 35.7 percent the frequency and severity of seizures was improved.

In three cases treated by *hemispherectomy*, one died postoperatively, one was free from symptoms, and the last was improved.

Topectomy never resulted in any disappearance of seizure although the frequency of discharges was reduced.

The following observations can now be made:

1. Scars between brain and dura with foreign bodies (particular gun shots wounds with indriven bone fragments) are excised, followed by autologous plastic repair with patient's own fascia. In shallow scars a cortical lysis is satisfactory but the decision must depend on corticography.

2. Undercutting is useful in cases of limited corticographical foci.

3. The main indication for resection of temporal lobe and related uncus areas are in cases of heavy psychomotor discharges.

4. Hemispherectomies are useful in cases of accompanying epileptic seizures.

5. Because of the rate of posttraumatic epilepsy after open brain lesions conventional approaches are less frequently performed.

6. From this reason we even hesitate to introduce in our clinic stereotactic operations against epilepsy.

Author's address: Dr. sc. med. W.-E. Goldhahn, Neurochirurgische Klinik der Karl-Marx-Universität Leipzig, DDR-701 Leipzig, German Democratic Republic.

Acta Neurochirurgica, Suppl. 23, 147—151 (1976)
© by Springer-Verlag 1976

Medical Post-Graduate Institute, Neurosurgical Department, Leningrad, USSR

Application with Classic Craniotomy in the Treatment of Focal Epilepsy

A. G. Zemskaja, Ju. A. Garmashov, and N. P. Ryabukha

With 1 Figure

Introduction

Both the search for new methods of surgical treatment of epilepsy and improvement of the contemporary ones depends on attempts to improve the results of surgical treatment itself. The introduction of stereotactic methods into the surgical practice of epilepsy treatment in the early fifties was stimulated by the experimental works of Jasper et al.[2], Kopeloff et al.[4] who demonstrated the possibility of obtaining experimental epilepsy from a focus in the brain situated in deep brain structures. In the following years, epilepsy investigation by means of chronic electrodes in man demonstrated the possibility of introducing epileptogenic charge in subcortical structures with the secondary appearance of epileptogenic discharges in different zones of the cortex. In this respect, particular interest was focused on the paper by Pagni[5] concerned with stereo-encephalographical observation in psychomotor temporal attacks, where the epileptogenic focus was shown to occur in mediobasal structures of temporal lobe following which the secondary invasion of new cortex is followed by clinical manifestation of epileptic attack.

Own Material and Discussion

Our wide experience with open surgical performances made for focal epilepsy shows that repeated epileptic attacks, as a result of such procedures arise most frequently in patients lacking any visible morphological cortical changes. There is justification for the presumption that in some of these patients, the epileptic cortical focus was not the primary but the secondary one depending on cortex activation as a reaction to a strong impulsed proceeding along spe-

10*

cific trajectories from subcortical structures. The removal of such a secondary cortical epileptogenic focus does not therefore lead to the desired therapeutic result. One of the first ways of overcoming these objections was the division of the surgery into two stages, open operation on the cortical focus and stereotactic destruction of the subcortical nucleus associated by trajectories with the pathway of the cortical epileptogenic focus.

The sequence of both the stereotactic and open stages is determined individually. In temporal epilepsy, the stereotactic stage is performed first as a rule.

The following difficulties have been met. It is well known that both the localization and the dimensions of the epileptic focus found on scalp EEG and in the course of electro-corticography, differ from each other. The final solution of cortical epileptogenic epilepsy localization may be brought about on the basis of electrocorticographical data. The data of EEG represent the preliminary topical diagnosis. However it is not always justified to destroy this or of other subcortical structure on the basis of EEG. This circumstance offers two solutions, the former being the open surgical performance which should invariably precede the stereotactic one. The cortical focus is detected accurately in the first stage which then determines the subcortical target for stereotactic destruction. The latter consists in performing, in one stage, both the open and stereotactic performances. The technical possibilities of such an approach were presented in 1973 by Riechert [6] at the International meeting of neurosurgeons in Japan for removing foreign bodies lying in brain depths, and approaching other deep lesion of vascular tumours. We have suggested the same approach for multifocal epilepsy treatment.

The open craniotomy is preceded by pneumo-encephalography with the working wheel of the stereotactic apparatus placed on the head of the patient, and two calculation photographs in side and direct projections. After that, the apparatus with the wheel firmly fixed on the patient's head, is moved to the operation room, where intubation and anaesthesia are carried out. This is followed by the second stage consisting of open craniotomy and electrocorticography to precisely localize the epileptogenic focus. In the course of open craniotomy, stereotactic calculations on a few subcortical structures are made according to clinical data and preoperational EEG examination. If the position of the focus on superficial EEG coincides accurately with that on the electroencephalogram, the electrode is introduced via open brain section into the chosen subcortical structure. If a new focus appears on the electroencephalogram, it is necessary to carry out fresh calculations according to the new data. This is followed by electrosubcorticographical stages and stimulation of subcortical structures, in the course of which the functional conjunction between the chosen target and the cortical epileptic focus is established. The degree to which these cortical and subcortical procedures are determined depends on the data obtained. The presence of epileptogenic activity on electro-corticogram and its absence on electrosubcorticogram determine the need of surgical performance on the cortical epileptical focus only. When quite a clear association is found between the pathological activity of brain cortex and the subcortical structure the subcortical nucleus is destroyed and then preserving the epileptic activity in the cortical area, subpial resection in the region of the epileptic focus is made. Isolated destruction of subcortical nucleus is carried out only, if the cortical epileptic focus occurs in functionally important cortical area after whose removal major neurological anomalies may be expected.

Theoretical grounds for the choice of subcortical targets in cortical foci in various areas of brain cortex are based on the data obtained by Hassler [1] that major specific thalamic neurons show synaptical associations with numerous cortical regions of 3 and 4 cortex layers. From deeper cortical layers, activity is carried away back into the appropriate thalamic nuclei. With respect to the diagram showing thalamo-cortical projections of Walker [8], Jakovlev [2], and Sarkisov [7], it may be seen that the nuclei of the thalamus show projection bonds with certain cortex areas. The appropriate localization of the cortical epileptic focus serves as a means for the choice of the particular subcortical target. In localizing the epileptic focus in the range of temporal lobe structures, the temporal and more frequently amygdalae nucleus or hippocampus gyrus are chosen as subcortical targets.

We are aware of the simplified and conditional nature of such a choice of subcortical targets for the purpose of investigation. Firstly, the topographical correlation of the nuclei of thalamus with cortex areas as show by the aforementioned authors is carefully studied, some divergencies of projection topography might be detected. Secondly, the pathway of the projection zone in oral dorsal direction from sufficiently wide cortex areas is very long. Thus, for instance, cortex zones 8, 9, 10, 11 and 12 of Brodman's fields project into the medial group of nuclei along almost the whole of the oral-caudal length of the thalamus [8]. This circumstance had previously been determined and the results obtained in the course of 6 surgical procedures combined in our patients. In two of the patients only we detected during operation electrophysiological correlations between the chosen subcortical structure and cortical epileptogenic focus. In these cases, operation was carried out both in the cortical focus and in the subcortical structure. In all of the remaining cases, the operation was carried out on the cortical epileptogenic focus with no destruction whatsoever of the subcortical structures.

· Case Report

We now present a few clinical observations, where we determined during the operation an association between cortical epileptogenic focus and subcortical structures.

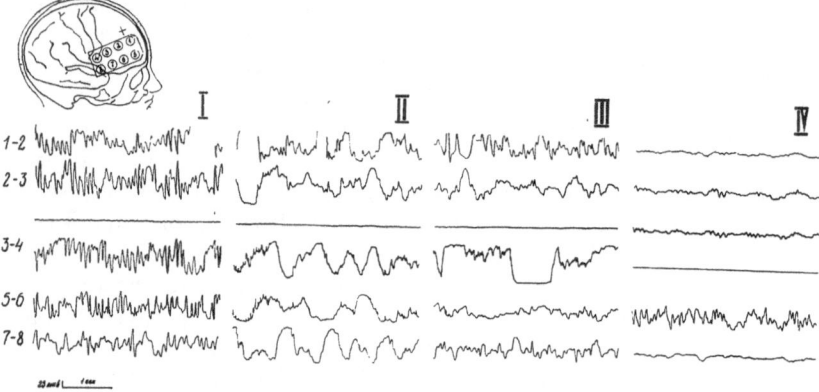

Fig. 1. Stages of ECoG in patient K. during combined operation. Explanations given in the text

The patient K., 12 years old, received a head injury from a blunt projectile entering the right-hand hemisphere. The patient had a well developed epileptic status which was controlled with difficulty by medication. After one month the epileptic status reappeared. No focal neurological symptoms were found but marked behavioural changes, such as hyperactivity, argumentiveness, and aggressiveness. X-rays showed many bone fragments in the region of the entrance wound. Preoperative EEG detected general changes of biological activity, indication of both the dysfunction of middle structures and the presence of epileptogenic focus in the frontal skull area. On November 23, 1973, a combined operation was carried out namely osteo-plastic trepanation of the right-hand cranio-temporal region and stereotactic destruction of frontal sections of the right medial dorsal nucleus of optical thalamus. In the course of electrocorticographic examination a focus of epileptogenic activity was found at the circumference of a brain scar in the region of right convexity. Stereotactic introduction of an electrode into the frontal sections of medial dorsal nucleus of right thalamus was performed. In the electrostimulation of this nucleus quite a marked increase of high-voltage slow activation in the focus (Fig. 1) was observed. Following nuclear destruction, there were amplitude decreases and slowing of rhythms of bioelectrical activity in the cortical focus. After resection of cortical epileptogenic focus, the epileptic phenomena disappeared from the electrocorticogram. Over the following 17 months, there were no further attacks observed, and there was a marked improvement in the patient's verbal responses.

The present paper is aimed at submitting the first experience made with a new approach to the surgery of multifocal epilepsy. Just like any other new approach, its results have to be carefully checked. Its prospects, however, seem good for the most serious category of patients, in whom multifocal epilepsy so frequently results in serious disability.

Summary

A new method of surgical treatment in dealing with severe forms of multifocal epilepsy—stereotactic intervention on subcortical structures during open craniotomy—is proposed. The method allows stereoelectrographic examinations to be performed during open operative interventions, helps discover subcortical epileptogenic foci, establish functional interrelationship of the chosen subcortical structure and the cortical epileptogenic focus and to undertake a differentiated intervention on the cortical, subcortical and both these foci at the same time.

References

1. Hassler, R. (1959), Anatomy of the thalamus. In: Introduction to stereotaxis with an atlas of the human brain, Vol. 1, p. 234 (Schaltenbrand, G., Bailey, P., eds.). Stuttgart: Thieme.
2. Jakovlev, P. (1959), In: Walker, A. E., Introduction to stereotaxis with an atlas of the human brain, Vol. 1, p. 306 (Schaltenbrand, G., Bailey, P., eds.). Stuttgart: Thieme.
3. Jasper, H., Droogleever-Fortuyn, J. (1946), Experimental studies on the functional anatomy of petit mal epilepsy. Ass. Res. Nerv. Ment. Dis. Proc. 26, 272—298.
4. Kopeloff, N., Whittier, J. R., Pacella, B. L., Kopeloff, L. (1950), The epileptogenic effect of subcortical alumina cream in the rhesus monkey. Electroencephalog. Clin. Neurophysiol. 2, 163—168.
5. Pagni, C. A. (1966), Stereo-electroencephalographic observations in the psychomotor seizure. Confin. Neurol. 27, 1—3, 137—143.
6. Riechert, T. (1973), The stereotactic method combined with classical craniotomy—a new operative procedure. 5th International Congress of Neurological Surgery. Amsterdam, 1973, p. 27.
7. Sarkisov, S. A. (1964), Očerki po strukture i funkcii mozga. Moskva: Medicina.
8. Walker, A. E. (1959), In: Introduction to stereotaxis with an atlas of the human brain, Vol. 1, p. 306 (Schaltenbrand, G., Bailey, P., eds.). Stuttgart: Thieme.

Authors' address: Dr. A. G. Zemskaja, Dr. Ju. A. Garmashov, Dr. N. P. Ryabukha, Medical Post-Graduate Institute, Neurosurgical Department, Leningrad, USSR.

Acta Neurochirurgica, Suppl. 23, 153—158 (1976)

A. L. Polenov Neurosurgical Institute, Leningrad, USSR

Stereotactic Treatment of Epilepsy in the Light of Pathophysiological Disease Concept

V. M. Ugriumov, T. S. Stepanova, K. V. Grachev, V. A. Shustin, S. L. Jatsuk, V. A. Rogulov, and G. A. Dolgopolova

With 2 Figures

The prospects of further development of stereotactic neuro-surgery, as well as the increase of its efficiency are determined not only by the technical improvement of the method but, particularly, by the best possible use of the data presented by contemporaneous neurophysiology and by the continuous accumulation of new information on functional anatomy and physiology of human brain achieved for the purpose.

We carried out 109 stereotactic procedures in patients suffering from focal (temporal) and generalized (grand mal, petit mal) epilepsies. Patients were selected for stereotactic treatment after unsuccessful drug therapy with appropriate clinico-electrophysiological phenomena. The issue of the terms of conservative therapy has lately been revised and shortened up to 1–1.5 years, since the efficiency of stereotactic surgery does depend on the development stage of the pathological process. The target was individual in all cases and was chosen on the basis of a clinico-electrophysiological and otho-neurophysiological data, which considering cerebral anatomo-functional correlations encouraged a concept on the leading pathological links. Together with the systemity of epileptic brain disease (T. S. Stepanova, K. V. Grachev, 1968, 1971; V. M. Ugriumov, T. S. Stepanova, K. V. Grachev, 1969), in the presence of complex inter-focal relations on a cortico-subcortico-stem level, the local destructions may be aimed at both the elimination of the epileptic focus (foci) and the interruption of the pathological impulsation chain. The concept of balanced correlations of both epileptogenic and antiepileptogenic systems in the brain, which we are now developing, justifies the use of therapeutic electro-subcortical stimula-

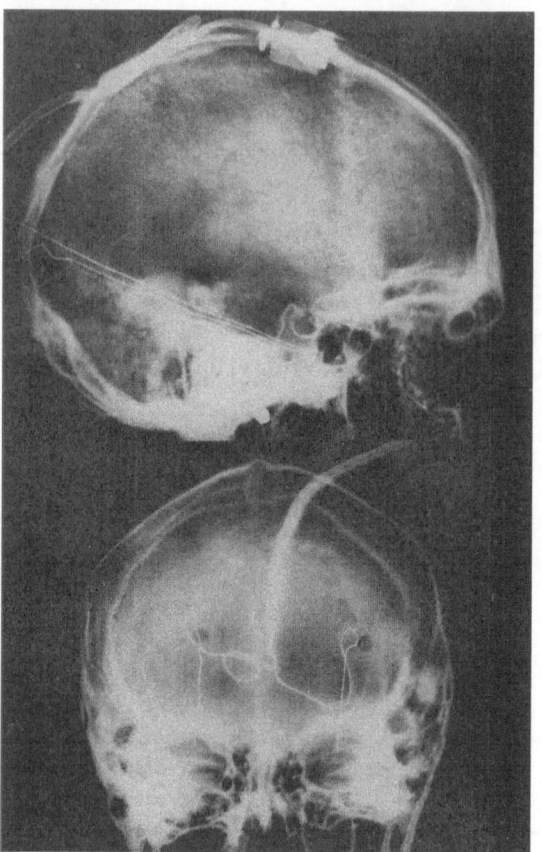

Fig. 1. Implanted multicontact electrodes introduced via occipital longitudinal approach into hippocampal structures bilaterally. Top: lateral roentgenogram, bottom: anterior-posterior roentgenogram

tions (TES) aimed at the restoration of intracentral relations by means of competing inhibitory system activation. Therefore, the number of structures subjected to stereotactic surgery included, in the forms of epilepsy investigated, the thalamus, zona incerta, campus Forelii, globus pallidus, hippocampus, corpus amygdaloideum, gyrus cinguli, nucleus caudatus and the like. In several cases, destruction of several structures or destruction of some of them and TES of the others proved to be effective. Depending on the localization of stereotactic targets the operations were carried out using temporal, parietal or occipital approaches (Fig. 1, 2). It should be noted that the latter is particularly adequate if manipulations on hippocampal structures are necessary.

We carried out two types of stereotactic operations: one-stage procedures and chronic procedures with implanted intracerebral electrodes. Experience showed that implantation of multicontact electrodes is justified in the case of complex, wide spread and bilateral brain damages. One-stage operation imply less flexible neurosurgical tactics,

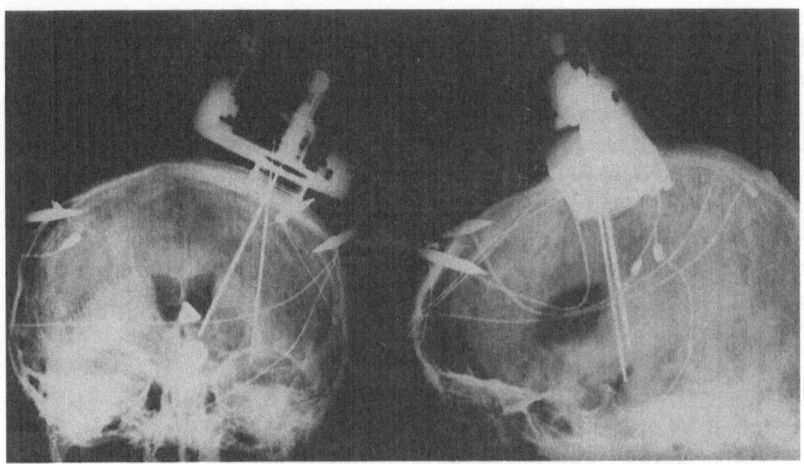

Fig. 2. Variant of one-stage stereotactic top approach surgery on structures not lying on a single trajectory. Left: anterior-posterior pneumoencephalogramme, right: lateral pneumoencephalogramme

i.e. destruction of the prechosen target. However, our variant of one-stage stereotactic surgery using electrodes with flexible sliding polyethylene insulation makes it possible to manipulate, in the course of a single performance, on structures which do not lie on a single trajectory (Fig. 2).

Long-term experience based on the study of diencephalic and limbic brain structures in man made it possible to elaborate a system of neurophysiological control (T. S. Stepanova and K. V. Grachev, 1972), which being compared with the data of stereotactic atlases as well as with special statistically significant topographo-anatomical section cards of brain permitted in individual approaches. The method of the layer-by-layer registration of bioelectrical parameters under the conditions of direct electrode-brain contact made it possible to obtain "the section" of both the grey and white brain substance around the target. The simultaneous electrosubcorticogram (ESCG), registration of nuclear population activity, steady potential level, convexity EEG and vegetative parameters (ECG, pneumogram, psychogalvanic reflex) and application of electrostimulation enabled an exact localization of the electrode with respect to brain formations. This enabled us to determine the space distribution and the extent of the epileptic zone, to obtain the maximum of information on structural functional relations in deep brain structures.

By means of neurophysiological investigations, the participation of basal ganglia and diencephalic structures (T. S. Stepanova and K. V. Grachev, 1972) in attack paroxysms was established and thus the basis formed for combined operation *i.e.* amygdalopallidotomy and amygdalothalamotomy. In the generalized forms of epilepsy, thalamotomy proved to be effective; in some patients, subthalamic structures participated in the pathological process. In both the temporal and the generalized epilepsies, it proved necessary to investigate, simultaneously, both the diencephalic and the mediobasal temporal and frontal structures. This was achieved by means of multicontact chronical electrodes or using a modification of onestage procedure on the structures not lying on a single trajectory.

Our data showed that the epileptic foci might occur in intricate hierarchical relations to each other, changing in various stages of disease development. The possible existence of the correlations of the type domination-subordination, sometimes transient and instable, determined the importance detection of leading foci, since the sequence of stereotactic effects on the links of epileptic system proved important. In this respect, important diagnostic data may be obtained in subsequent applications of electrical polarization of brain tissue in "working" points and evaluation of its electrophysiological and clinical effects.

Depending on the morphological and functional characteristics of the targets and their involvement in the pathological process, the method of getting sufficient destruction appears to be different. Local electrolysis through very thin implanted electrodes (60–100 μ) may be important in operations on highly differentiated formations with clear somato-topical representation and definite limited epileptogenic foci, *i.e.* on diencephalic structures. Minimum destructions are also justified to prevent undesirable clinical phenomena, for example Klüver-Bucy syndrome in bilateral stereotactic operations for bitemporal epilepsy. In one-stage procedures or through manipulation on relatively monomorphous structures, particularly on mediobasal temporal formations, such "point like" destructions do not always give the expected effect. Increase of destruction volume is obtained by means of highfrequency coagulation via large-diameter electrode; according to the indications several subsequent destructions are possible. The polarization test produces structural damages of nuclear units close to the electrode (V. P. Kurkovski and K. V. Grachev, 1967) and may only be used directly before therapeutical destructions; its application prior to TES might irreversibly change both the physiological and biophysical parameters of the electrode-contacted brain tissue and considerably decrease or eliminate the benefits of this procedure.

The facts obtained in the course of these investigations underline the necessity of an individual approach in the stereotactic treatment of patients suffering from epilepsy in all of its stages: determination of indications and conditions of operation, choice of targets as well as of type of stereotactic surgery, volume of destruction or therapeutic electrostimulations and the like.

Stereotactic surgery implies the practical realization of the principle of sparing brain performances; the local stimulations for the purpose of inhibitory (antiepileptogenic) systems activation should be considered a serious aspect of nearly atraumatic functional neurosurgery. On the basis of neurophysiological methods application, stereotaxis establishes conditions for further and more detailed detection of intimate mechanisms of patho-physiological reactions in epilepsy.

References

1. Kurkovski, V. P., Gračev, K. V. (1967), Nekotoryje nabljudenija nad morfologičeskimi izmenenijami golovnogo mozga krolikov pri dejstvii slabych postojannych tokov čerez glubinnyje elektrody. V. Sb.: Nejrochirurgija 2, Leningrad, 31—40.

2. Stepanova, T. S., Gračev, K. V. (1968), Nekotoryje osobennosti električeskoj aktivnosti glubokich struktur mozga pri epilepsii. Z. nevropatol., psichiatr. 68, 2, 1593—1599.

3. — — (1971), Elektrofiziologičeskije ocenki epileptogennych očagov v kortikal'-nych i subkortikal'nych strukturach pri chirurgičeskom lečenii bol'nych epilepsiej. V sb.: Chirurgičeskoje lečenije epilepsii. Trudy 1 Vsesojuzn. sjezda nejrochirurgov 3. Moskva, 138—141.

4. Stepanova, T. S., Gračev, K. V. (1972), Novyje dannyje o funkcional'nom nejrofiziologičeskom kontrole v processe stereotaksičeskich operacij po povodu epilepsii. V sb.: Trudy 3 konferencii nejrochirurgov Pribaltijskich respublik. Riga, 192—195.

5. Stepanova, T. S., Gračev, K. V. (1972), Elektrofiziologičeskije charakteristiki nekotorych podkorkovych struktur golovnogo mozga čeloveka v uslovijach prjamych intracerebral'nych otvedenij. Tezisy simpoziuma "Bazal'-nye ganglii i povedenie". Leningrad, 63—64.

6. Ugrjumov, V. M., Stepanova, T. S., Gračev, K. V. (1969), Funkcional'naja organizacija podkorkovych struktur golovnogo mozga čeloveka i nejrochirurgičeskaja klinika. V sb.: Glubinnyje struktury mozga (anatomija, fiziologija, patologija), I, Moskva, 128—144.

Authors' address: Prof. V. M. Ugriumov, T. S. Stepanova, M.D., K. V. Grachev, Ph.D., Prof. V. A. Shustin, S. L. Jatsuk, M.D., V. A. Rogulov, M.D., G. A. Dolgopolova, M.D., A. L. Polenov Neurosurgical Institute, Leningrad, USSR.

Acta Neurochirurgica, Suppl. 23, 159—165 (1976)

Department of Surgery, Kinki University, Osaka,
Department of Neurosurgery, Osaka University, Osaka,
and Institute for Neurobiology, Okayama University, Okayama, Japan

Forel-H-Tomy for the Treatment of Intractable Epilepsy

D. Jinnai, J. Mukawa, and K. Kobayashi

Introduction

The latest clinical results of Forel-H-tomy [1—3, 5, 6] for the treatment of epilepsy are summarized in this report.

Cases and Method

Sixty four patients with intractable epilepsy composed of 13 idiopathic and 51 symptomatic, were treated by Forel-H-tomy. There were 38 male and 26 female patients aged 2–33 years at the time of operation. The follow-up period was 1–12 years.

Bilateral operations was initially performed with an interval of 0–2 weeks, but, in recent years, the interval has routinely been over 6 months which seems to be long enough to evaluate the postoperative course of the first operation. The target point is located 2 mm posterior to the midpoint of the AC-PC line, 4 mm ventral to the line and 4.5 to 5 mm lateral to the 3rd ventricle wall. The criteria of clinical evaluation and location of lesion are the same as already reported [3]. Two cryogenic lesions were made at the beginning and, later, with radiofrequency electrocoagulation method.

Clinical Results

1. Clinical Seizures:

As summarized in Table 1, strategically placed lesions produced better results both in the idiopathic and symptomatic groups. If the lesion missed the target point, the effectiveness was decreased. It is to be noted that some of the cases of unilateral surgery have remained under observation awaiting surgery on the opposite side, especially in the symptomatic group, for example in cases with the Lennox syndrome.

Table 1. *Clinical Evaluation of Forel-H-Tomy Correlating with the Completeness of Forel's H Lesion*
Effect on clinical seizures
(idiopathic epilepsy)

	Lesions	Excellent	Good	Poor or no effect
Bilateral surgery (7)	Bilaterally well placed	3	1	
	Others		2	1
Unilateral surgergy (6)	Complete	2	1	1
	Poorly placed or out of target		1	1

(symptomatic epilepsy)

	Lesions	Excellent	Good	Poor or no effect
Bilateral surgery (20)	Bilaterally well placed	2	5	4
	Others	1	2	6
Unilateral surgery (31)	Complete	13	3	11
	Poorly placed or out of target			4

Others mean well-placed on one side but poorly placed on the other, poorly placed on both sides or out of the H field altogether.

Table 2. *Effect on Clinical Seizure Types*
(11 symptomatic cases with bilaterally well placed lesions)

Generalized convulsion	Abolished	6
	Diminished	1
Focal convulsion	Abolished	2
	Diminished	2
Lennox syndrome	Abolished	2
	Diminished	2
Reflex epilepsy	Abolished	1
Psychomotor	Unchanged	3
Total		19

2. Seizure Types:

In 4 idiopathic cases with well-placed bilateral lesions, grand mal seizures were abolished in 2 and diminished in 1 case, and myoclonic seizures were abolished in 1 and diminished in 2 cases.

In 11 symptomatic cases with well-placed bilateral lesions, generalized, hemi- and focal convulsions, Lennox syndrome and reflex epilepsy were controlled, but not psychomotor seizures (Table 2).

Table 3. *Effect on Clinical Seizure Types*
(28 symptomatic cases with unilaterally well placed lesion)

Generalized convulsion	Abolished	14
	Diminished	3
Hemiconvulsion	Abolished	2
	Diminished	1
Focal convulsion	Abolished	10
	Diminished	2
Akinetic	Diminished	2
Psychomotor	Unchanged	6
Lennox syndrome	Abolished	1
	Diminished	1
	Unchanged	5
Petit mal	Diminished	1
Total		48

In 28 symptomatic cases with well-placed unilateral lesions (Table 3), generalized, hemi- and focal convulsions were controlled. Psychomotor seizures were not controlled. The Lennox syndrome was slightly controlled by a unilateral lesion. One case of status petit mal which was operated unilaterally had an excellent result, but the seizures although controllable, recurred 1 year later but without status epilepticus for 4 years.

3. Electroencephalographic Changes:

As reported in a previous paper[6], an increase of background activity and improvement of abnormal discharges were found after Forel-H-tomy, although there was no direct correlation with the clinical course. There was no evidence to indicate epileptogenicity produced by the lesion of Forel's H field.

4. Other Symptoms:

Unstable behaviour, especially aggression were markedly improved in 3 cases. Motivation was improved in 4 cases of Lennox syndrome together with seizure improvement. Cerebellar signs were completely abolished in one patient which enabled him to stand and walk without disturbances of balance after operation. Stridor, one of the most uncontrollable symptoms often causings respiratory infection in severely debilitated children was cleared up in 2 cases of postmeningitic epilepsy.

Table 4. *Social Evaluation*
(Over 3 years after surgery)

Bilateral operation with well placed lesions (8 cases)	
Improved (5)	Reschooling (1)
(2 without anticonvulsants)	Employment (1)
	Housekeeping (1)
	CP-Rehabilitation (2)
Unchanged (1)	Hospitalization (1)
	Myoclonus Ep.
Dead (2)	Myoclonus Ep. (1)
	(1 year after surgery)
	Heart Failure (1)
	(6 years after surgery)
Unilateral operation with well-placed lesion (13 cases)	
Improved (13)	Reschooling (3)
(2 without anticonvulsants)	Reemployment (8)
	Housekeeping (1)
	CP-Rehabilitation (1)

Table 5. *Side-Effects* (3 cases)

Motor disturbance (2) Akinetic type		
K. Ch.	(13 years, male)	CP and Idiocy
N. M.	(11 years, male)	CP and Idiocy
Disturbance of speech and swallowing (2)		
N. M.	(11 years, male)	CP and Idiocy
K. K.	(18 years, female)	Myoclonic Ep.

5. Social Evaluation:

Social evaluation was carried out in cases with well-placed lesions over 3 years after operation (Tab. 4). Except for one case which was unchanged and 2 deaths, 18 out of 21, composed of 5 bilateral and 13 unilateral operations, were obviously improved from the social standpoint. Four of them have remained well without the necessity of anticonvulsant medication.

6. Side-Effects:

Side-effects were observed in 3 cases (Tab. 5). An akinetic type of motor disturbance and disturbances of speech and swallowing were found in 2 cases. These 3 cases were operated by bilateral Forel-H-tomy. Psychometric tests revealed no intellectual deficit following operation. The deficits appear, therefore, to be due to extrapyramidal lesions.

Discussion

Forel-H-tomy was originally designed to interrupt the pathway of epileptic discharge at the level of Forel's H field between the lenticular nucleus and substantia nigra as summarized in the previous paper [4]. However, the control of seizures was found to be due not only to interrupting the descending convulsive impulses but also by elevating seizure threshold, possibly by interrupting the corticosubcortical reverberating circuit [5].

Clinically, this is explained by the improvement of electroencephalographic abnormalities, especially of seizures discharges [6]. As mentioned above, the improvement of "Other symptoms" such as aggression and motivation was found after operation irrespective of drug dosage. Stridor was also cleared up by the operation. These behavioural and respiratory abnormalities are often found in severe epileptic patients, and the improvements coincide with clinical course of the seizures.

There have been many reports describing psychoneurological abnormalities in epilepsy, but correlation is difficult from the clinical point of view, as to whether these abnormalities are primary or secondary to the seizures. It is reasonable to postulate, from our surgical experiences, that some of them are directly associated with seizures and some with clinically latent seizure episodes, and the improvement in these psychoneurological abnormalities immediately following operation indicates the improvement of epileptic disturbance of the nervous system.

The problem is how to determine the stereotaxic coordinates in epileptic patients. As summarized in Tab. 6, most of our cases have dilatation of the lateral and third ventricles. Normal range of VC-index (less than 0.25) is found only in 12 out of 50 cases (minimum 0.22). The same number of cases have definite dilatation (over 0.3 based on Evans criteria: maximum 0.57). On the other hand, normal range of the width of the third ventricle (less than 5 mm) is found only in 4 cases (minimum 4 mm) out of 50 cases based on Taveras criteria. Marked dilatation (over 10 mm) is found in 11 cases (maximum 17 mm). The lateral distance between the target point and the

Table 6. *Ventricular Dilatation*
(50 cases)

1) Lateral Ventricle

VC-Index (0.22~0.57)
0.2~   12 cases
0.25~   26 cases
0.3~   12 cases

Index/Side	LT (0.16~0.61)	RT (0.20~0.63)
0.15~	2 cases	0 cases
0.2~	18 cases	25 cases
0.25~	18 cases	17 cases
0.3~	12 cases	8 cases

2) IIIrd Ventricle (4~17mm)

2.5 mm~   4 cases
5   mm~   24 cases
7.5 mm~   11 cases
10   mm~   8 cases
12.5 mm~   3 cases

lateral ventricle wall is, therefore so, usually set 4.5–5 mm in adult so as not to involve the hypothalamus and internal capsule. It is to be noted that there is no direct correlation between the surgical effect and ventricular dilatation, and also ventricular dilatation is not a contraindication to surgery.

Side-effects were found in 3 cases of bilateral surgery, although there were no discouraging complications in unilateral surgery. The symptoms were akinetic motor disturbance and disturbances of speech and swallowing. As previously mentioned, the evidence of no post-operative intellectual deficit shows that these disturbances are due to extrapyramidal lesions. Two of them were cases of cerebral palsy with idiocy, whose preoperative motor deficit including speech and swallowing difficulty might aggravate the disturbances after surgery.

With regard to age distribution, 25 cases were 2–10 years of age at the time of operation. Intractable childhood epilepsy mostly demonstrate the so-called Lennox syndrome, that is childhood epileptic encephalopathy with diffuse slow spike and wave (Gastaut *et al.* 1966). Eleven such patients were operated by Forel-H-tomy. Excellent results were obtained in 2 out of 4 bilateral operations and 1 out of 7 unilateral operations. These data encourage us to carry out this type of stereotaxic surgery before epileptic brain damage and personality changes have been so widely and uncontrollably built up in these children.

Conclusions

Sixty four cases of intractable epilepsy were operated on by Forel-H-tomy and analyzed from the clinical point of view.

1. Lesions should be made at the target point accurately, 2 mm posterior to the midpoint of the AC-PC line, 4 mm ventral to the line and 4.5–5 mm lateral to the 3 rd ventricle wall.

2. Forel-H-tomy resulted not only in seizure control, but also in improvement of electroencephalographic abnormality and associated psychoneurological abnormalities.

3. Side-effects are found in 3 cases of bilateral surgery: akinetic motor disorder and disturbances of speech and swallowing, which are due to extrapyramidal lesions.

4. When surgery is indicated, it is considered essential to carry out stereotaxic surgery before epileptic brain damage and personality changes have become irreversible.

References

1. Jinnai, D., Nishimoto, A. (1966), Stereotaxic destruction of Forel-H for the treatment of epilepsy. Neurochirurgia 6, 164—175.
2. Jinnai, D. (1966), Clinical results and the significance of Forel-H-tomy in the treatment of epilepsy. Conf. neurol. 27, 129—136.
3. Jinnai, D., Mukawa, J. (1970), Forel-H-tomy for the treatment of epilepsy. Conf. neurol. 32, 307—315.
4. Mukawa, J., Jinnai, D. (1971), The propagation of focal cortical epilepsies and its modes. Acta Neurol. Latinoamer. 17, 613—643.
5. Jinnai, D., Mukawa, J. (1973), Surgery for Epilepsy. In Krayenbühl, Maspes and Sweet: Progress in Neurological Surgery, Vol. 5, p. 222—296. S. Karger.
6. Mukawa, J., Kimura, T., Nagao, I., Kobayashi, K., Iwata, Y., Koshino, K., Ikeda, T., Kamikawa, K., Mogami, H., Jinnai, D. (1975), Forel-H-tomy for the treatment of intractable epilepsy. Special reference to postoperative electroencephalographic changes. Conf. neurol. 37, 302—307.

Authors' addresses: D. Jinnai, M.D., Professor and Director, Department of Surgery, Kinki University Hospital, Sayama-cho, Minami-Kawachi-gun, Osaka, J. Mukawa, M.D., Department of Neurosurgery, Osaka University, Osaka, and K. Kobayashi, M.D., Institute for Neurobiology, Okayama University, Okayama, Japan.

Acta Neurochirurgica, Suppl. 23, 167—175 (1976)

Departamento de Neurocirugia, Hospital Clinico Universitario, Valencia, Spain

Stereotactic Fornicotomy in Temporal Epilepsy: Indications and Long-Term Results

J. L. Barcia-Salorio and J. Broseta

With 3 Figures

The purpose of stereotactic fornicotomy was, initially, to isolate the temporal lobe with the aim of avoiding the spread of the epileptic focus. In previous papers [6, 8, 9] and in our own experience it has been observed that in those patients whose main problems were epileptic seizures the results were rather incomplete and eight years ago, Barcia-Salorio [2] developed the theory that fornicotomy should be used primarily in those patients with sporadic seizures in which the main clinical problem was behavioural disturbance. Since then most of our patients have been of this pattern, of usually in children, the so-called infantile epileptic psychoses (Annell [1] and Barcia [2]).

Clinical Material and Methods

1. Clinical Material

There were 42 patients, 30 male and 12 female, with ages ranging from 3.9 to 57 years, 52% of whom were children.

The commonest findings were: the clinical features of epilepsy in 73% with severe behavioural disturbance and the EEG record of a temporal lobe epileptic focus.

The aetiology was asphyxia at birth (11 cases), head injury (6 cases), infections (2 cases), expandings intracranial lesion (2 cases) and idiopathic (21 cases).

All the patients had grand mal epileptic fits, occasionally alternating with other types of seizure (absences, equivalents, etc.). The attacks usually occurred daily, showing a tendency to increase in frequency. Lumbar air encephalography revealed focal atrophy in 3 patients. The EEG always demonstrated a temporal lobe focus with unilateral spike complexes. In some instances we could not find the temporal lobe focus by conventional electroencephalography, and it was necessary to implant deep electrodes for localization. There were no significant differences in the frequency of the involved hemisphere.

A rich variety of pathological behavioural manifestations appeared in 31 patients. We have selected the fourteen most representative symptoms, according to its frequency. These were nocturnal fear, heteroaggression, autoaggression, escapism, somniloquy, psychomotor anxiety, insomnia, anorexia, extravagant behaviour, affective lability, pathological masturbation, enuresis, fits of temper and thefts. The I.Q. (Wechsler's scale) was studied in these patients and we found that 82% of them were below normal, with some cases of mental deterioration and well defined oligophrenia.

2. Indications for Operation

We have observed that the our best results with fornicotomy have been achieved in patients who have the following characteristics, they are young, frequently children, their EEG has an unilateral temporal lobe focus, the behavioural disturbances are severe but the other epileptic manifestations are well controlled by drug treatment (Landolt's phenomenon of reciprocal induction), the I.Q. is within normal limits and finally, psychiatric treatment failed to improve their condition.

In our view these conditions fits into the so called infantile epileptic psychoses [4], of which we have 20 patients in our records. This group is clearly separate from the others which we have called encephalopathy with epilepsy and pure epilepsy without behavioural disturbances.

According to Barcia [3] these three groups can be differentiated by the frequency of each symptom as well as by their I.Q. and bioelectrical alterations. In this way by giving to each symptom its statistical value or weighting by means of Bayes' Law, we can determine which patient will be improved by fornicotomy.

3. Surgical Technique

The target is placed on the bend of the fornix upon the anterior comissure, attempting to make a lesion in both structures.

We use the Barcia's stereoencephalotome, mod. IV, with pneumotomoencephalography (Fig. 1). The target is localized by means of a computerized programme based upon the conformal transformation. Once the coordinates have been placed on the frame, the elec-

trode is introduced under TV control. It is a monopolar electrode of
1 mm diameter with a thermocouple inside. The lesion is made by
radiofrequency at 75 degress C, producing a lesion of 5 mm diameter.

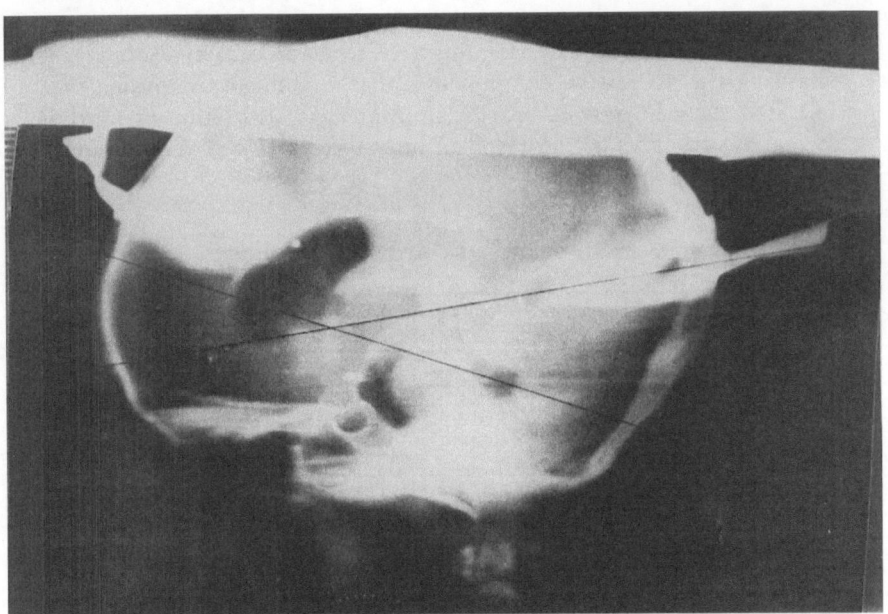

Fig. 1. Barcia's stereoencephalotome, mod. IV. Pneumotomoencephalography.
Method of calculation of the target, trough the numbered scales

Results

The follow-up period varied between 6 months and 13 years, with
an average of 8.6 years.

In 43% the epileptic symptomatology disappeared, although the
majority still require antiepileptic drug therapy. In the rest of the
patients fits persist with a frequency and intensity similar to the
preoperative ones. We have had no morbidity or mortality from the
operative procedure. The fornicotomy has always been homolateral.
In three patients with poor results, there was an associated contralateral amygdalectomy [7], and in one case homolateral temporal
lobectomy.

The EEG is not modified immediately although it is possible to
see in some instances that the focus does not spread as it did before

the operation (Fig. 2). In about two months, in those patients who return to normal [12], the record becomes desynchronized until the focus disappears, coinciding with the improvement of convulsive attacks. In the rest of the patients dysrhythmia persists or new foci appear on the contralateral side, or even at other sites.

Behavioural disturbances improve in 58% and usually immediately after the operation and much earlier than the bioelectrical changes. Tab. 1 shows the rate of improvement for each symptom, emphasising the aggressive component and the ambient adaption. The I.Q. is slightly improved, bearing in mind that alleviation of psychological disturbances would result in improved attention and co-operation.

In order to evaluate the results, we used the following criteria:

Rank	Evaluation	Definition
4	Excellent	Disappearance of behavioural and neurological symptomatology. Satisfactory familial, social and school adaptation. Normal EEG. No drugs needed.
3	Good	Clinical picture similar to 4, but the patient needs drug therapy. EEG without focal localization but persistence of paroxysmal activity.
2	Mild	Persistance of either neurological or behavioural disturbances. Drug treatment needed. Abnormal social adaptation. EEG as in 3.
1	Poor	Behavioural and neurological symptomatology without improvement on the preoperative state. EEG with focal activity.
0	Deterioration	Increase of the preoperative symptomatology.

According to these criteria we have had the following results in 42 patients: Excellent 6, Good 7, Mild 20, Poor 8, and Deterioration 1. However as has been emphasised in the surgical indications, we feel that the group with infantile epileptic psychosis constitutes the main indication for fornicotomy. We have 20 patients with this clinical entity and in Tab. 2 in shown the difference between preoperative and postoperative symptomatology. Thus reviewing only the infantile epileptic psychosic group, the results are: Excellent 5, Good 6, Mild 6, Poor 3, and Deterioration 0. In this way it is evident that there are significant differences in the results obtained in the infantile epileptic psychosic group and in the rest of the series, which confirms our preoperative indications.

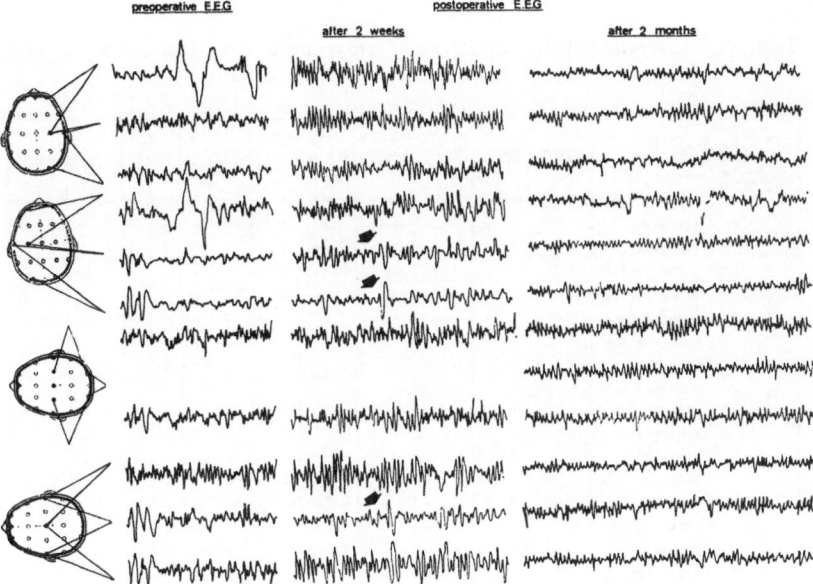

Fig. 2. Preoperative EEG showing a temporal lobe focus. EEG, two weeks after fornicotomy, shows the focus yet, but there is not generalization. EEG, two months after fornicotomy, shows bioelectric hypoactivity but within the normal limits

Table 1. *Frequency of Improvement of Behavioral Disturbances Improvement of the Psychic Symptomatology* (in 31 cases)

Symptoms	Frequency	Improvement
Nocturnal fear	3 cases (9.6%)	3 cases (100 %)
Heteroaggression	27 cases (87.0%)	23 cases (85.1%)
Autoaggression	11 cases (35.4%)	9 cases (81.8%)
Escapes	12 cases (38.7%)	8 cases (66.6%)
Somniloquy	3 cases (9.6%)	3 cases (100 %)
Psychomotor anxiety	31 cases (100 %)	20 cases (64.5%)
Insomnia	6 cases (19.2%)	2 cases (33.3%)
Anorexia	3 cases (9.6%)	3 cases (100 %)
Extravagant behavior	26 cases (83.8%)	19 cases (73.0%)
Affective lability	16 cases (51.6%)	10 cases (62.5%)
Masturbation	7 cases (25.5%)	3 cases (42.8%)
Eneuresis	3 cases (9.6%)	2 cases (66.6%)
Fits of temper	31 cases (100 %)	21 cases (67.7%)
Thefts	6 cases (19.2%)	3 cases (50.0%)

Table 2. *Preoperative (White Lines) and Postoperative (Grey Lines) Symptomatology in the Infantile Epileptic Psychosis*

Cases 1–10 (each case: left = preoperative, right = postoperative)

CASES	1.a.l.r		2.a.c.o		3.a.c.l		4.e.m.b		5.a.a.b		6.a.a.a		7.a.a.p		8.f.a.c		9.a.r.g		10.e.s.p	
AGE/SEX	3.9/m		9.11/f		6/m		14/m		14.10/m		7.11/f		9.11/f		11.10/m		13.11/m		10.7/m	
NEUROL.S epileptic fit	+	−	+	+	+	−	+	−	+	−	+	−	+	+	+	+	+	−	+	+
type	g.m	−	g.m	g.m	g.m	−	g.m	−	g.m	−	g.m	−	g.m	g.m	g.m	p.m	g.m	−	g.m	g.m
frequency	d	−	d	d	d	−	d	−	d	−	d	−	d	d	d	d	d	−	d	d
tendency	↑	−	↑	↑	↑	−	↑	−	↑	−	↑	−	↑	↑	↑	↑	↑	−	↑	↑
ELECTROENCEPHALOGRAM	t.f	n	t.f	i.r	t.f	i.r	s.d	n	t.f	i.r	t.f	n	t.f	i.r	t.f	t.f	t.f	i.r	t.f	i.r
PSYCHIC.S nocturnal fear	+	−	−	−	−	−	−	−	+	−	+	−	−	−	−	−	−	−	+	+
heteroagression	+	−	−	−	+	−	+	−	+	−	+	+	+	−	+	+	+	−	+	+
autoagression	+	−	−	−	+	−	−	−	+	−	+	−	+	+	+	−	+	−	−	−
escapes	+	−	−	−	+	−	−	−	+	−	+	−	+	+	+	−	+	−	+	+
somniloquy	+	−	−	−	−	−	−	−	−	−	−	−	−	−	+	−	−	−	−	−
psychomotor a.	+	−	+	−	+	−	+	−	+	+	+	−	+	+	+	+	+	−	+	+
insomnia	+	−	−	−	−	−	−	−	+	−	−	−	+	+	−	−	−	−	+	+
anorexia	+	−	+	−	−	−	−	−	+	−	−	−	−	−	−	−	−	−	−	−
extrav. behavior	+	−	−	−	+	−	−	−	+	−	+	−	+	+	+	−	−	−	+	+
affec. lability	+	−	↑	−	+	−	−	−	+	−	−	−	+	+	+	−	−	−	−	−
masturbation	−	−	−	−	−	−	−	−	+	+	−	−	+	+	+	−	−	−	+	+
eneuresis	+	−	−	−	−	−	−	−	+	−	−	−	−	−	+	−	−	−	−	−
fits temper	+	−	+	−	+	−	+	−	+	+	+	−	+	+	+	−	+	−	+	+
thefts	−	−	−	−	+	−	−	−	−	−	+	−	+	+	−	−	−	−	−	−

Cases 11–20 (each case: left = preoperative, right = postoperative)

CASES	11.j.t.r		12.a.v.l		13.i.b.s		14.p.p.r		15.r.s.e		16.m.b.p		17.r.c.r		18.m.g.g		19.h.g.s		20.j.p.s	
AGE/SEX	13/m		11/m		12.2/m		15/m		14.1/f		8.3/m		8/f		12.6/f		29/m		15.9/m	
NEUROL.S epileptic fit	+	+	+	−	+	−	+	−	+	+	+	−	+	−	+	−	+	−	+	−
type	g.m	g.m	g.m	−	g.m	−	g.m	−	g.m	g.m	g.m	−	g.m	−	g.m	−	g.m	−	g.m	−
frequency	d	w	d	−	d	−	d	−	d	d	d	d	d	−	d	−	d	−	d	−
tendency	↑	↑	↑	−	↑	−	↑	−	↑	↑	↑	↑	↑	−	↑	−	↑	−	↑	−
ELECTROENCEPHALOGRAM	t.f	i.r	t.f	i.r	t.f	s.d	t.f	i.r	t.f	i.r	t.f	n	t.f	i.r	t.f	n	t.f	n	t.f	n
PSYCHIC.S nocturnal fear	−	−	−	−	−	−	−	−	−	−	−	−	−	−	−	−	−	−	−	−
heteroagression	+	−	+	−	+	−	+	−	+	−	+	−	−	−	+	−	−	−	+	−
autoagression	−	−	−	−	−	−	−	−	−	−	−	−	+	+	−	−	−	−	−	−
escapes	−	−	+	+	−	−	+	−	−	−	−	−	−	−	−	−	+	−	−	−
somniloquy	−	−	−	−	−	−	−	−	+	−	−	−	−	−	−	−	−	−	−	−
psychomotor.a	+	−	+	−	+	+	+	−	+	−	+	+	+	−	+	−	+	−	+	−
insomnia	−	−	−	−	−	−	+	−	+	−	−	−	−	−	−	−	−	−	−	−
anorexia	−	−	−	−	−	−	−	−	−	−	−	−	−	−	−	−	−	−	−	−
extrav. behavior	+	−	+	−	+	−	+	−	+	−	+	+	−	−	+	−	+	−	−	−
affec. lability	−	−	−	−	+	−	+	−	+	+	−	−	−	−	+	−	−	−	−	−
masturbation	−	−	+	−	+	−	−	−	−	−	−	−	−	−	−	−	−	−	−	−
eneuresis	−	−	−	−	−	−	−	−	−	−	−	−	−	−	−	−	−	−	−	−
fits temper	+	−	+	−	+	−	+	+	+	+	+	+	−	−	+	−	+	−	+	−
thefts	−	−	−	−	−	−	+	+	−	−	−	−	−	−	−	−	−	−	+	−

Abbreviations: *g.m.* grand male, *p.m.* petit male, *d* daily, *w* weekly, *t.f.* temporal lobe focus, *i.r.* irritative record, *s.d.* subcortical dysfunction, *n* normal.

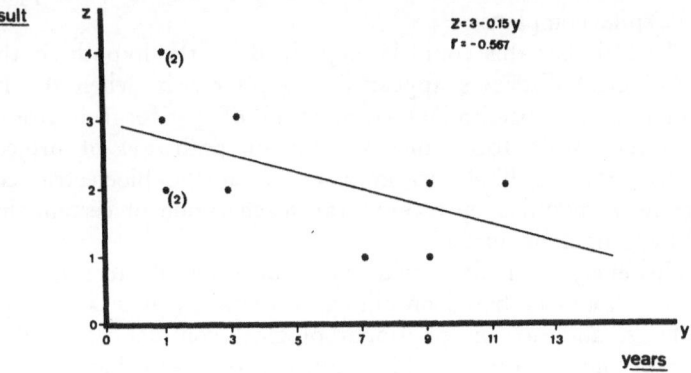

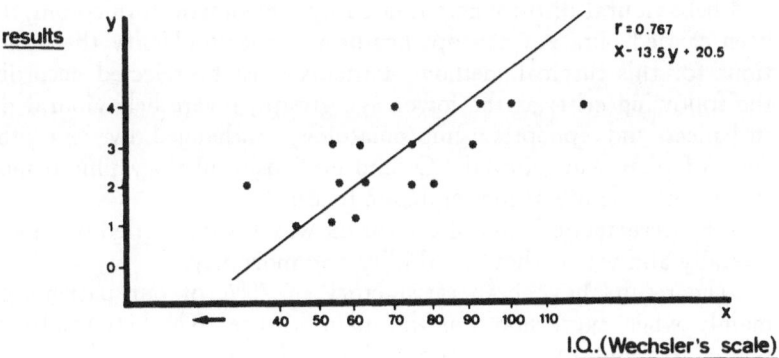

Fig. 3. a) Relation between duration of clinical history and results. b) Relation between I.Q. and results

Discussion

Studying the postoperative evolution we can define two stages. At first, immediately following the operation, behaviour begins to improve, although the EEG remains unchanged or perhaps shows a precise focal localization.

Then, about two months after the operation seizures decrease in frequency and the EEG shows desynchronization and dissappearance of the spike complexes.

We feel that this could be explained by the hypothesis that the psychological disorders appear in the intercrisis, when the EEG is normal, due to subliminal stimulation of perifocal neurons from which the fornix forms one of its main pathways of projection [5]. Finally, fits are likely to improve when the bioelectric cerebral response is modified by transneural degeneration of certain thalamic and hypothalamic nuclei [6].

However, we believe that the indications of stereotactic fornicotomy should be based on clinical criteria, as in infantile epileptic psychosis, and not on physiopathological considerations which are not well known. Even in this group it is observed that improvement is more evident when the period between the onset of symptoms and the operation is short and when the I.Q. is high (Fig. 3).

Summary

An analysis of the long-term results of 42 patients with epilepsy and behavioural disturbances treated by stereotactic fornicotomy has been carried out. An attempt has been made to classify the indications for this surgical method. Patients must be selected according the following criteria: the lower age groups, severe behavioural disturbances and epileptic symptomatology unchanged by any other form of treatment, normal I.Q. and electroencephalographic demonstration of a temporal lobe epileptic focus.

The stereotactic lesion of the fornix was always carried out homolaterally and was without morbidity and mortality.

The results have been satisfactory in 70% of our patients but mainly when aggression was the main feature. The best results are related to a high I.Q. and a short clinical history.

References

1. Annell, A. L. (1963), The prognosis of psychotic syndromes in children. Acta psychol. scand. 39, 2.
2. Barcia-Salorio, J. L., Barcia, D. (1967), Indicaciones psicoquirúrgicas de la fornicotomia estereotáxica. Rev. Esp. Oto-Neuro-Oftal. 26, 51—57.

3. Barcia, D., *et al.* (1971), Problemas psiquiátricos y sociales de la epilepsia infantil. Ponencia al II Congreso de Neuropsiquiatria Infantil, Madrid.
4. Broseta, J., Barcia-Salorio, J. L., Barbera, J. (1972), Resultados a largo plazo de 33 casos de fornicotomia. Rev. Esp. Oto-Neuro-Oftal. *30*, 31—37.
5. Gastaut, H. (1958), A propos des symptoms cliniques rencontrés chez les epileptiques psychomoteurs dans l'intervalle de leurs crises. In: Bases physiologiques et aspects cliniques de l'epilepsie. Paris: Masson et Cie.
6. Hassler, R., Riechert T. (1957), Über einen Fall von doppelseitiger Fornicotomie bei sogenannter temporaler Epilepsie. Acta Neurochir. *5*, 330—340.
7. Narabayashi, H. (1966), Long-term results of stereotactic amygdalectomy for behavioral disorders. Confin. Neurol. *27*, 121—123.
8. Umbach, W. (1957), Versuche zur Epilepsiebehandlung durch gezielte Tiefenausschaltungen. Acta Neurochir. *5*, 341—349.
9. Umbach, W. (1966), Long-term results of fornicotomy for temporal epilepsy. Confin. Neurol. *27*, 121—123.
10. Umbach, W. (1972), Follow-up study on stereotactically treated patients with abnormal behavior. In: Psychosurgery. Springfield, Ill.: Ch.C Thomas.

Authors' address: Dr. J. L. Barcia-Salorio and J. Broseta, Departamento de Neurocirugia, Hospital Clinico Universitario, Valencia, Spain.

Acta Neurochirurgica, Suppl. 23, 177—182 (1976)
© by Springer-Verlag 1976

Department of Stereotactics and Neuronuclear Medicine
(Medical Director: Prof. Dr. F. Mundinger)
Departmental Group: Neurochirurgische Universitätsklinik, Freiburg im Breisgau,
Federal Republic of Germany

Late Results of Stereotactic Surgery
of Epilepsy Predominantly Temporal Lobe Type*

F. Mundinger, P. Becker, E. Groebner, and G. Bachschmid

With 4 Figures

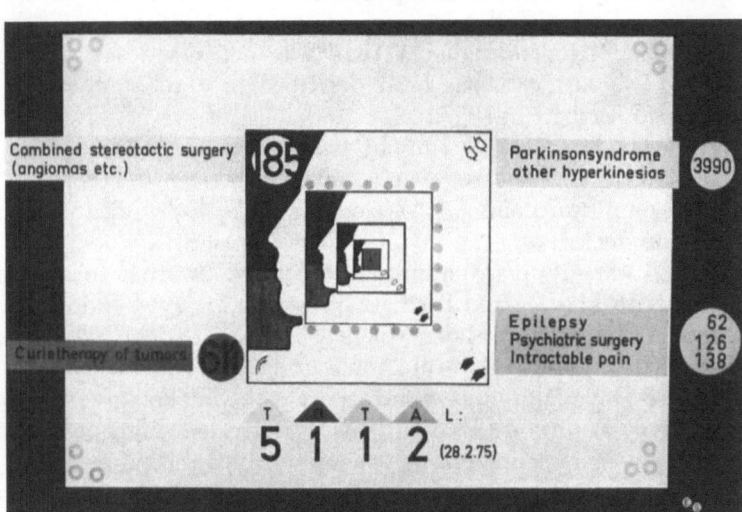

Fig. 1

On January 21, 1951 the Freiburg group (Hassler, Mundinger, Riechert) performed the first stereotactic operation for epilepsy [1, 4, 7]. The case in question was a centrencephalic epilepsy. During the following years we performed 62 further interventions from a total of 5,120 stereotactic operations primarily in treating temporal lobe epilepsy while maintaining strict control of indications (Fig. 1).

* With support of the Special Research Division—Brain Research and Physiology of the Senses (SFB 70 E₂) of the Deutsche Forschungsgemeinschaft (Bad Godesberg).

We shall report here the long-term evaluation of up to 24 years for 33 operated cases. Mean post-operative observation time amounted to 5.83 ± 2.25 years. Apart from 4 cases of centrencephalic epilepsy we were able to evaluate pre- and post-operatively using the EEG of 24 cases of temporal lobe epilepsy, 9 of which had one dominant focus and 15 bilateral seizure foci. Problems in obtaining records prevented complete follow up of all 33 cases.

The majority of the patients suffered psychomotor seizures and petit mal as well as generalised attacks. In all cases drug therapy failed: for some, at the outset, for others after long-term treatment.

8 patients showed epileptic personality changes ranging from slight to severe, 24% showed serious behavioural disturbances.

5 of the 33 patients observed post-operatively have succumbed: 2 died from unknown causes; 2 under circumstances having nothing to do with the operation; 1 female patient died 7 days after the operation following serious vegetative crises caused by a diencephalic oligodendroglioma that was not diagnosed until the autopsy. This last case has been described in a separate paper by Hassler and Riechert in 1957.

The coagulated target sites of the lesions are shown in Fig. 2. In the majority of the cases we performed either a fornicotomy or an anterior commissurotomy [2, 3, 5]—alone or combined with a unilateral amygdalotomy [5, 6].

One of our group (Mundinger) performed the first fornicotomy together with Hassler and Riechert on March 23, 1954 following the suggestion of Jung and Maier-Mikeleit [2, 3, 5]. 6 patients were reoperated: 3 with a bilateral fornicotomy and commissurotomy, 1 using a bilateral amygdalotomy—which moreover, did not give rise to a Klüver-Bucy syndrome. Two patients were treated subsequently with a temporal lobe resection one of whom improved thereafter.

There were relatively few complications: one case each of transient paresis of the oculomotor nerve, facial nerve and arm paresis. Two of the three patients mentioned who underwent bilateral fornicotomies and commissurotomies experienced a temporary condition of confusion with short-period memory and confabulation as noted in cases of Korsakow's syndrome.

We have divided the evaluation time of up to 24 years into 3 periods: the first encompassing the first three months following the operation, the second the first 2 years and the third exceeding the two-year limit. We have in fact ascertained that a meaningful evaluation of the operational effect should not be expected before the end of the first year. In many cases there is indeed an improvement during the first three months but this is followed by a regression in

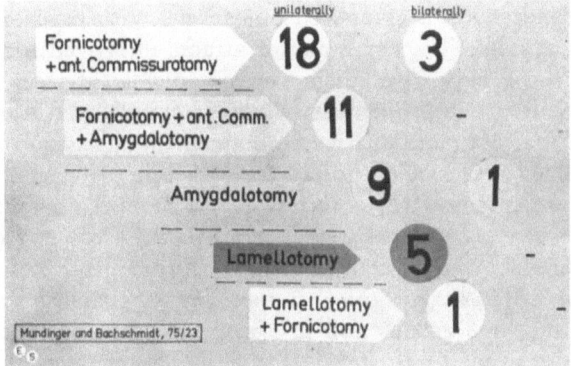

Fig. 2. Coagulated structures of 33 cases of epilepsy (1951—1954)

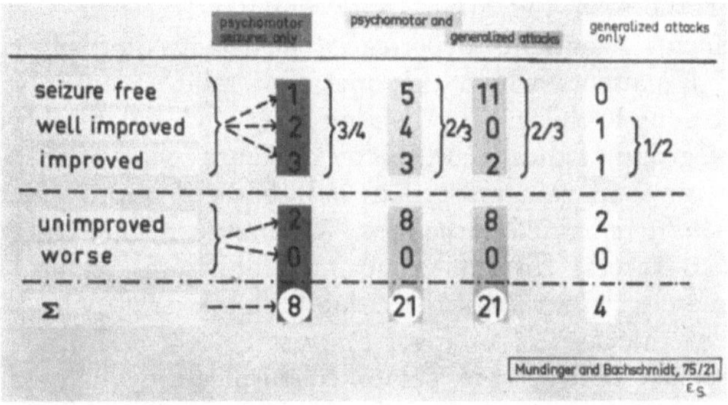

	psychomotor seizures only	psychomotor and generalized attacks		generalized attacks only	
seizure free	1 } 3/4	5 }	11 } 2/3	0	
well improved	2	4 } 2/3	0	1	} 1/2
improved	3	3	2	1	
unimproved	2	8	8	2	
worse	0	0	0	0	
Σ	8	21	21	4	

Fig. 3. Results of long-term follow up ($\bar{x}$ = 5.83 ± 4.1 years) of 33 stereotactically operated cases of temporal lobe epilepsy predominantly

the next months. After a year the operational effect has been stabilised and can thus serve as a basis for evaluation.

The long-term evaluation of clinical improvement classified according to the type of seizure reveals that 3/4 of the patients in the first group with psychomotor fits alone improved; 1/8 of them were fully free of fits, 1/4 showed a significant reduction in the frequency of their seizures, and 1/3 showed some improvement. There was no instance of a worsening of the patient's condition, i.e. of an increase in intensity or frequency of the fits or a change in the type of fit (Fig. 3).

12*

The second group is composed of patients with psychomotor and generalised attacks. The psychomotor attacks improved for $2/3$ of the patients in this group; $1/4$ of them were completely fit-free, $1/5$ showed good, $1/7$ moderate improvement, while $2/5$ experienced no change in their condition. Better results were obtained for this group as regards ·the generalized attacks: $2/3$ showed long-term improvement and half of these were entirely free of attacks. $1/10$ showed no improvement and for $2/5$ no effect was registered. Half of the 4 cases of centrence-phalic seizures showed good or moderate improvement.

We find it worthy to note that there was no case of a regression in any of the three groups and in a sense this can be regarded as a positive result as well. However, all of the patients continue to need anticonvulsive therapy. For 62% the EEG improved. Based on the results relating to the EEG focus we derived the following:

The EEG reports were evaluated pre- and post-operatively for 24 patients.

$7/9$ of those in the group with unilateral seizure foci showed improvement. 2 patients experienced no change in their condition. 4 of the 6 patients whom the operation relieved entirely of their seizures belong to this group; the remaining 2 had bilateral foci.

In the group of those with bilateral seizure foci 8 of the 15 operated cases, or somewhat more than half, showed improvement, while the other half remained unchanged. We may conclude from this that operational success for the group with unilateral seizure foci was approximately twice that of the group with bilateral foci.

In 9 of the cases of bilateral seizure foci we performed a forni-cotomy or, respectively, a combined fornico-amygdalotomy. This operation brought improvement for $2/3$ (6 patients), while $1/3$ (3 patients) were left unimproved.

In 6 cases of bilateral seizure foci we carried out only an amyg-dalotomy or thalamotomy. This led to an improvement for $1/3$ of the patients (2) while $2/3$ (4 patients) showed no improvement.

In summary therefore, the EEG-tracings demonstrated that:

in 15 cases there was an improvement of the post-operative EEG ($2/3$),

in 7 cases EEG findings remained constant (ca. $3/7$),

in 2 cases there was a worsening (ca. $1/6$).

We could not discover any correlation between the clinical improvement and an improvement in EEG findings.

Results depend on target structure and type of attack (Fig. 4). In this connection, of course, the individuality of each case and the relatively small number of cases produce considerable difficulties in evaluation. For the centrencephalic attacks we consistently performed a thalamic coagulation which brought for a quarter of the patients a uniform improvement of the generalized and petit mal attacks, while in a further quarter of the cases the generalized attacks improved considerably.

Fornicotomy, usually performed in combination with the anterior commissurotomy, brought about an improvement in $^3/_4$ of the cases; combined with the amygdalatomy in $^7/_{10}$; and following the amygdalatomy performed alone in $^2/_3$. Our collection of cases shows the

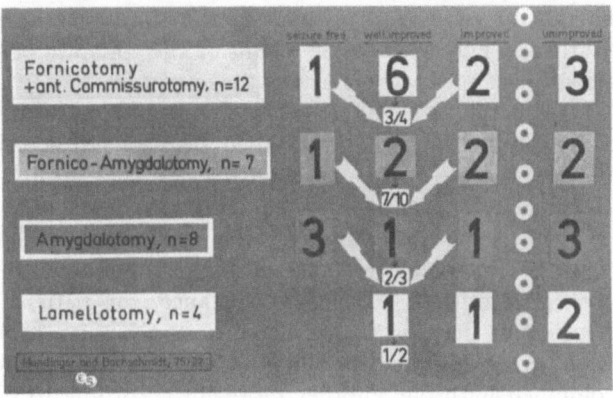

Fig. 4. Long-term results ($\bar{x} = 5.83 \pm 4.1$ years) of 33 cases of temporal lobe epilepsy predominantly depending on coagulated structures

following trend as regards the influence of operation on the type of attack:

The combination of fornicotomy and anterior commissurotomy produces the best results for both types of attacks — the generalized more frequently than the psychomotor attacks. Psychomotor attacks alone are influenced more effectively using the amygdalotomy or the combination amygdalotomy-fornicotomy than with just the fornicotomy. However, the fornicotomy should always be included as a supplementary coagulation when there is also a seizure focus of the contralateral temporal lobe.

As concerns the personality and behavioural changes, we have noted improvements such as loss of depression or ill humour, reduction of irritability and aggressivity, and a more extraverted attitude—in one case voracity disappeared.

The 8 patients who showed slight epileptic personality changes were not fundamentally influenced by the operation; one patient only felt psychologically freer; in another case family difficulties and alcoholism led to a deterioration of both his socio-professional situation and the state of his fits. One patient was pensioned at 29 years of age despite good improvement of his attacks.

3 of the 8 patients in the group with serious personality changes showed a progression of their psychic disturbances and worsening of their socio-professional situation. One of them had to be placed in a mental hospital 15 years after the operation due to his very aggressive behaviour and progressively paranoid development. Another patient was interned in mental hospitals from time to time.

For the most part professional and social rehabilitation does not depend on the improvement attained in the status of the patient's attacks. Rather, it is related to the extent of the epileptic personality and behavioural changes present before the operation.

The 6 patients who showed no noticeable psychological disturbances preoperatively could all continue their professional activities following the operation — or as the case may be successfully finished their professional training — independently of the status of their attacks. However, we must not overlook the fact that, due to the high level of social security in the Federal Republic of Germany with many opportunities for public assistance, the patient is freed of any necessity to develop initiative and responsibility for himself.

Hence we may say that stereotactic amygdalotomy and fornicotomy combined with one another represent according to our experiences of up to 24 years an effective instrument for treating both generalized epileptic attacks and psychomotor attacks as well.

References

1. Birg, W., Mundinger, F. (1973), Computer calculations of target parameters for a stereotactic apparatus. Acta Neurochir. (Wien) 29, 123—129.
2. Hassler, R., Riechert, T. (1957), Über einen Fall von doppelseitiger Fornicotomie bei sogenannter temporaler Epilepsie. Acta Neurochir. (Wien) 5, 330—340.
3. Hassler, R., Riechert, T. (1957), Beitrag zur Behandlung der temporalen Epilepsie durch gezielte Fornicotomie. Zbl. ges. Neurol. 140, 10.
4. Hoefer, Th., Mundinger, F. Birg, W., Reinke, M., Computer calculation in localizing subcortical targets in native X-rays for stereotactic surgery. 6th Symposium of the International Society for Research in Stereoencephalotomy, Tokyo, 12.—13. 10. 1973.
5. Mundinger, F. (1975), Stereotaktische Operationen am Gehirn. Stuttgart: Hippokrates.
6. Narabayashi, H. (1963), Stereotactic amygdalotomy for behavior disorders. Arch. neurol. 9, 1—16.
7. Riechert, T., Mundinger, F. (1956), Beschreibung und Anwendung eines Zielgerätes für stereotaktische Hirnoperationen (II. Modell). Acta Neurochir. (Wien) 3, 308—333.

Authors' address: Prof. Dr. F. Mundinger, Dr. P. Becker, Dr. E. Groebner and Dr. G. Bachschmid, Neurochirurgische Universitätsklinik, Hugstetter Straße 55, D-7800 Freiburg im Breisgau, Federal Republic of Germany.

Acta Neurochirurgica, Suppl. 23, 183—191 (1976)
© by Springer-Verlag 1976

Department of Neurological Surgery, University of Zürich, Switzerland

Stereo-Electroencephalographic Exploration and Epilepsia Partialis Continua

J. Siegfried and C. Bernoulli

With 5 Figures

Epilepsia partialis continua of Koževnikov is rare in children and in their extensive study in the literature, Löhler and Peters [6] mention that children less than 10 years represent less than 10% of the 162 cases reported. In 1972 we had the opportunity to collect 2 infantile cases of true epilepsia partialis continua and in 1974 1 case of focal sensorimotor epilepsia with up to 200 fits a day. In these 3 cases, after eliminating neuroradiologically a space occupying lesion, we decided to explore stereo-electroencephalographically the suspected cerebral structures and we will report here the findings and the results of surgery.

Cases Report

Case 1 (Sc. Br.): This 5 years old girl had her first generalized attack without loss of consciousness when she was 4½ years. One month later she developed focal motor fits on the left side and 2 months later started the epilepsia partialis continua on the left foot and during the night Jacksonian fits on the left leg. On neurological examination, a discrete left hemiparesis, more pronounced in the leg, was found. On EEG, a large epileptogenic area was constantly recorded from the right postcentral region. The neuroradiological examination showed no unusual findings and all the usual drugs were given without success. Five months after the onset of the epilepsia partialis continua, stereotactic neuroradiological exploration was done and 4 days later, 4 electrodes with multiple contacts were implanted under general anaesthesia from the precentral to the postcentral region. During the 4½ hours exploration, besides the jerks, 22 fits were recorded. The main epileptogenic activity was demarcated on the medial precentral and postcentral regions. At operation, a very limited excision of this focus was performed, but the fits persisted after surgery. Reoperation was necessary and more extensive medial cortectomy was done (Fig. 1). During the 3 years follow-up period, with the patient still under antiepileptic drugs, no epileptic fits were observed and the EEG now shows no more spike activity, but pronounced rhythmic discharges. The postoperative hemiparesis which was more marked in the left leg improved slowly. The child leads a physically normal life, but is mentally retarded. The histological examination of the excised cortex showed marked gliosis.

Case 2 (Ma. An.): This 3½ years old girl had a family history of epilepsy. At the age of 3, she had gastro-enteritis and soon after during the febrile period she had facial jerks on the right side. A few hours later a generalized tonic-clonic fit occurred followed by an other one limited to the right side. A right-sided hemiconvulsion with hemiparesis developed rapidly. The convulsions were not controlled with medications, the facial jerks persisted and 2 months later there

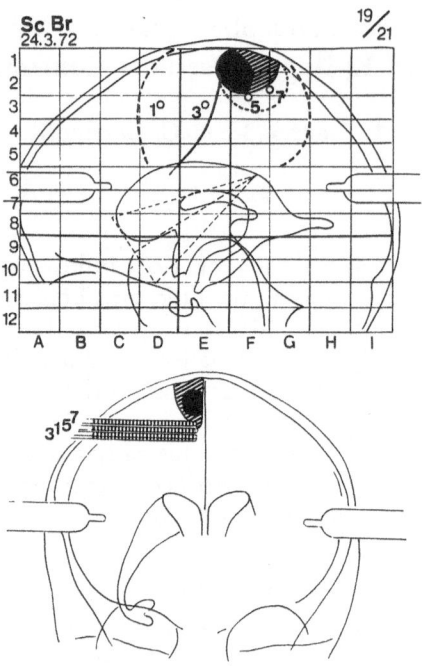

Fig. 1. Case 1 (Sc. Br.). Placement of depth electrodes and sketch of medial cortectomy made in two stages. The black area corresponds to the marked gliosis which was already seen macroscopically

were episodes of absences. After about 3 months, jerks and Jacksonian fits, marked on the right leg and slight on the right arm, were again noted to occur constantly. The hemiparesis increased. On EEG the main focus was seen in the left central region. The neuroradiological examination was normal. Five months after the beginning of the disease, we performed the stereo-electroencephalographic examination with 4 depth electrodes and, besides the jerks, 33 fits were recorded (Figs. 2 and 3). The focus could be demarcated in the medial part of the precentral and postcentral regions. Due to the general anaesthesia, verification of the somatotopy was not possible. At operation, a large portion of medial cortex was resected. The epilepsia partialis continua disappeared and in the 2 year follow-up period, facial jerks reappeared occasionally, but are now under control with medication. Absences still persist, but occur rarely. The hemiparesis of the right foot has improved but the neglect of the right arm is unchanged. Histologically, inflammatory signs were described in the specimen of the excised cortex.

Case 3 (Va. La.): This 8 year old girl suffered from borderline epilepsia partialis continua, but due to the similarity of location of the primary focus, can be presented here. When she was 8 months old, she had Sabin-vaccination. On the following day paresis of the left arm was observed but disappeared

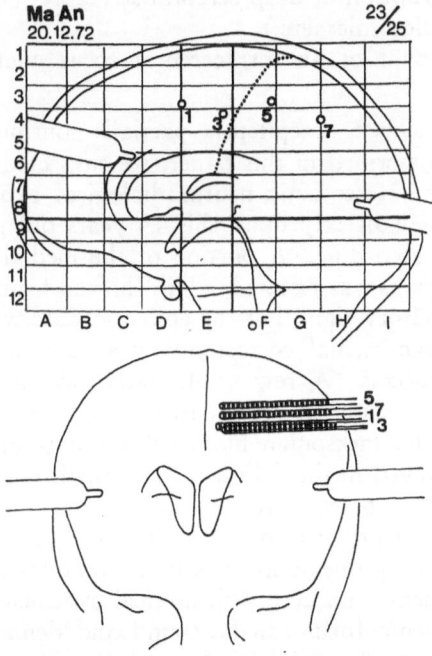

Fig. 2. Case 2 (Ma. An.). Placement of depth electrodes. Electrode *1* LSMA to LA 6 lat, Electrode *3* LA 4/6 med to LA 4 lat, Electrode *5* LA 4 med to LA 1–3 lat, Electrode *7* LA 1–3 med to LA 5–7 lat

within 24 hours. The first seizure started at the age of 6 and daily complex sensorimotor fits up to 200, developing to a focal epileptic status, were observed since then, despite many antiepileptic drugs. The girl developed a slight hemiparesis on the right side. EEG showed a large epileptogenic area of the left central and parietal region. The neuroradiological examination was normal. First exploration with 6 electrodes was unsuccessful, because, due to the general anaesthesia, no fits could be obtained during the many hours of recording. Therefore, we repeated the exploration 6 weeks later with the patient awake and this time several spontaneous and induced seizures were recorded (Fig. 5). A main focus on the medial part of the precentral and postcentral region was demarcated. This focus was excised surgically (Fig. 4). No more fits were seen postoperatively and the hemiparesis improved rapidly. One year later, the condition of the girl was very good and EEG was normal. The histological examination of the removed cortex showed no remarkable abnormality.

Discussion

The conservative treatment of epilepsia partialis continua is very disappointing. Three surgical approaches can be proposed:

1. The removal of a space occupying lesion (tumor, abscess, intracerebral haematoma, etc.).

2. The interruption of deep cerebral structures (stereotactic thalamotomies, capsulotomies, etc.).

3. The removal of an intracerebral focus confirmed by depth recording.

In 1970 in a case of epilepsia partialis continua similar to the first two cases described in this paper, we suspected a space occupying lesion at the stereotactic neuroradiological exploration. Therefore, we operated directly upon this 14 years old girl without preliminary depth recording. A portion of the medial prerolandic and postrolandic regions was resected, which showed histologically marked chronic inflammatory signs, but the epileptic state was not improved. A more extensive medial cortectomy was performed, also without postoperative success. A few weeks later, we decided to make a stereotactic coagulation of the ventrolateral part of the thalamus. The jerks and the Jacksonian fits disappeared completely, but EEG examination showed in the follow-up an impairment of the epileptic activity. Since then, we are of the opinion that a preliminary exploration with depth electrodes is indispensable.

If a space occupying lesion has been eliminated and if the conservative treatment is unsuccessful, surgical treatment is most effective if the epileptogenic focus can be found and demarcated preoperatively. The stereo-electroencephalographic exploration is the only useful method to obtain safely enough information on the location of the focus in order to propose the therapeutical surgical approach.

The first stereo-electroencephalographic exploration of cases of epilepsia partialis continua seems to have been made by Bancaud et al.[2]. In 1970, these authors[1] report 6 well documented cases, out of which 4 were operated on and an anatomo-pathological study was made in 2 cases. Only 2 children belong to this category: one 7 years old girl with anatomo-pathological evidence of an inflamma-

---

Fig. 3. Case 2 (Ma. An.). Jacksonian fit starting soon after having stoped the fluothane-narcosis. The jerks of the right foot ceases before the Jacksonian fit. The first 16 channels correspond to the depth electrodes in accordance with Fig. 2. Channels 17 to 28 record surface EEG. The last 4 channels correspond to EMG of the right m. deltoid, of the right thigh and the right foot (flexor and extensor)

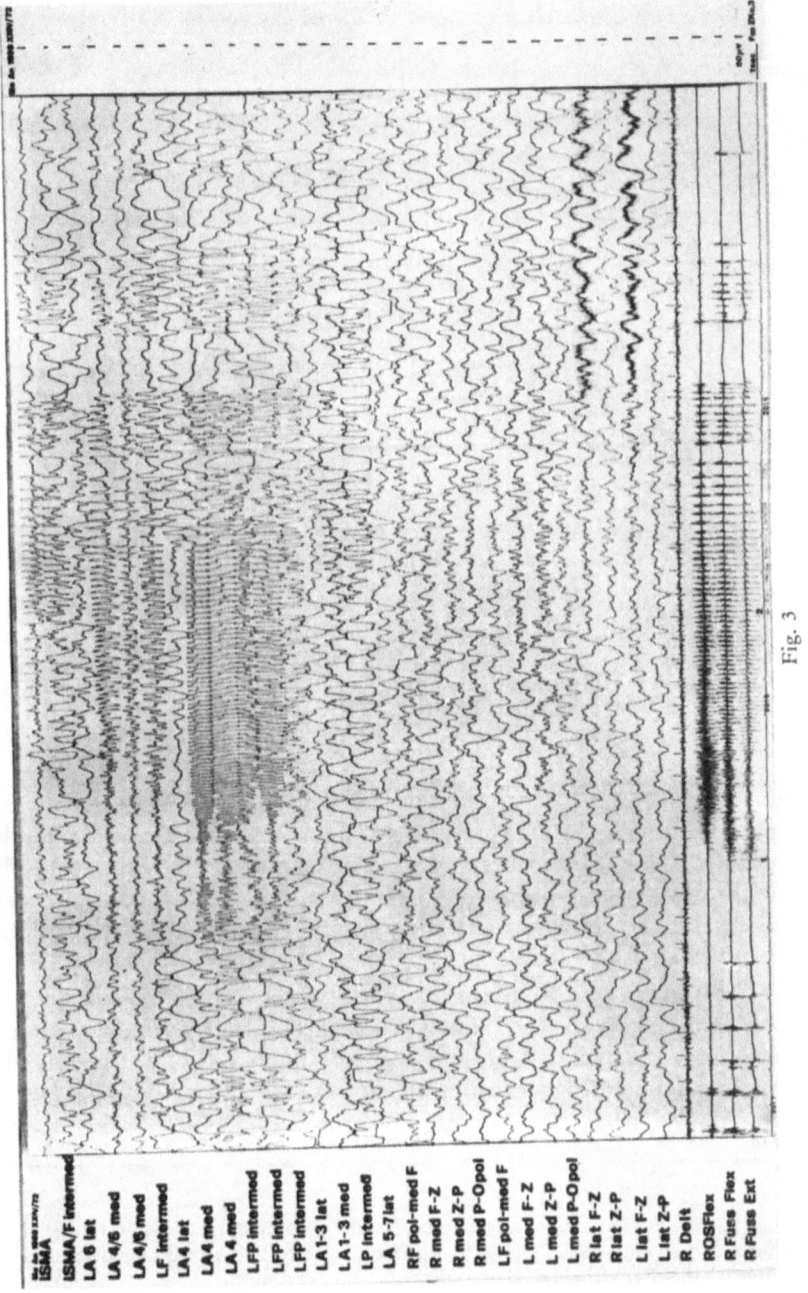

Fig. 3

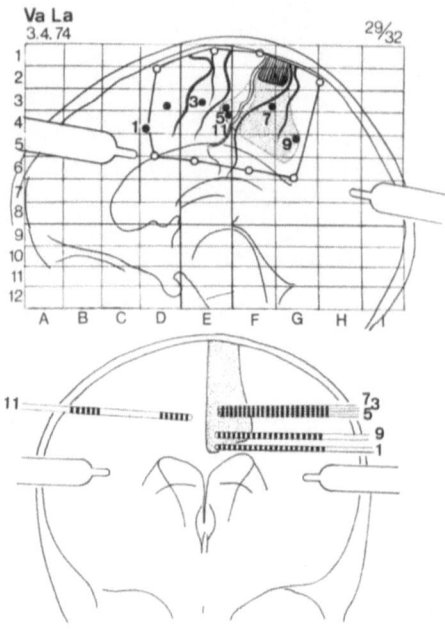

Fig. 4. Case 3 (Va. La.). Placement of depth electrodes. Electrode *1* LSMA ant to LF 2, Electrode *3* LSMA post to LA 4 lat, Electrode *5* LA 4 med to LA 1–3 lat, Electrode *7* L Praecuneus ant to L lob par sup, Electrode *9* L Praecuneus post to L lob par inf, Electrode *11* RA 4 med to RA 1–3 lat

tory origin and a 10 year old boy. In their clinical and electrophysiological study [1], the authors did not mention the therapeutic results of their stereo-electroencephalographic explorations and the results of the cases operated on. Later on, Talairach and Bancaud [7] reported 12 cases of epilepsia partialis continua operated on after exploration with depth electrodes but no details were given.

Therefore, our 3 infant patients, who were stereo-electroencephalographically explored and subsequently, after having demarcated a focus, were operated on and cured or improved, are probably the first cases described in detail in the literature.

Fig. 5. Case 3 (Va. La.). Sensorimotor seizure with complexe bilateral semeiology during hyperventilation. The ictal discharge starts in LA A med and L Praecuneus ant. In the EEG change in activity, but no ictal discharge is recorded. Same parameters as in Fig. 3

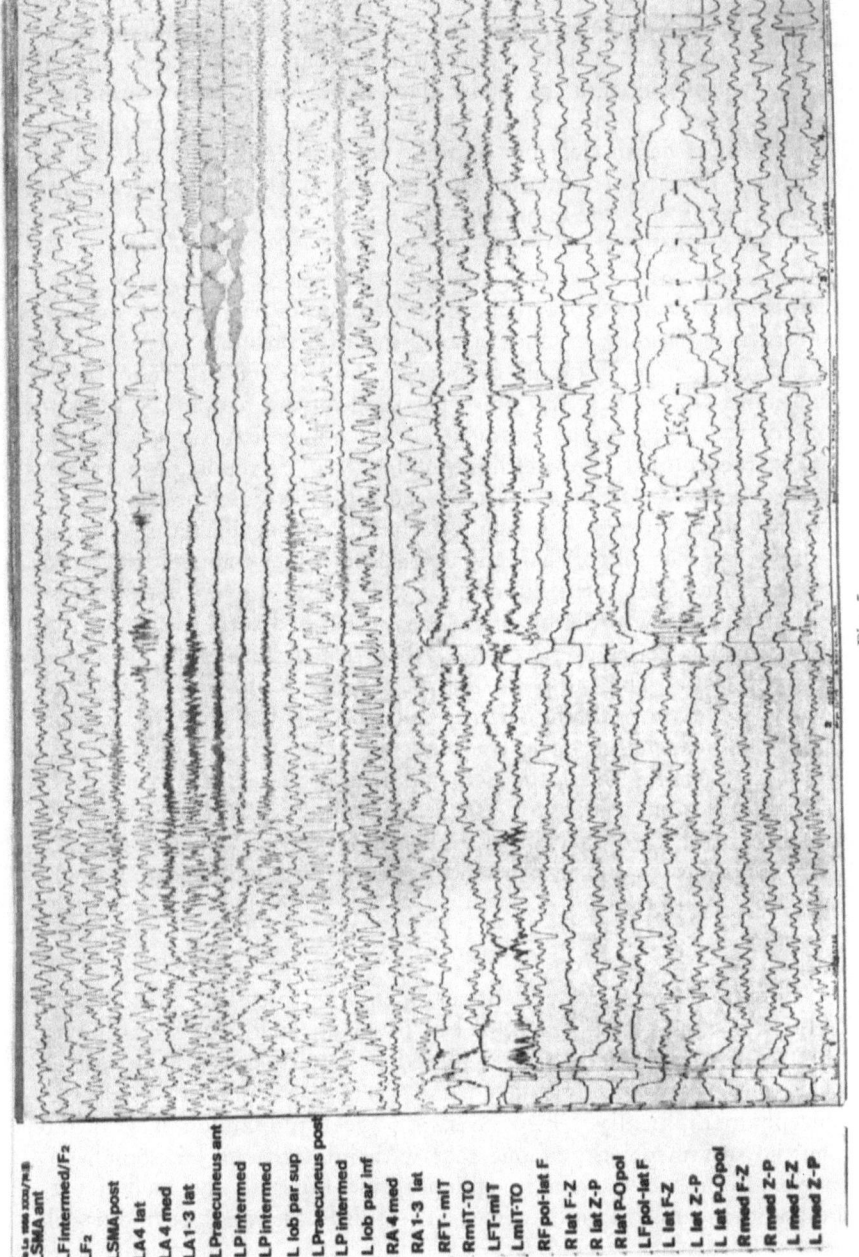

Fig. 5

This study confirms the safety of the method of Talairach and shows that depth electrodes can be used in small children safely. We are also able to prove that epilepsia partialis continua in children, which can not be controlled with drugs and which have no convincing neuroradiological signs, can be improved surgically only if depth electrode exploration has been attempted and has shown a demarcated focus. The removal of the epileptogenic area can be therefore made minimal.

The problem of cortical, subcortical or corticosubcortical origin of epilepsia partialis continua is still a matter of controversy. Juul-Jensen and Denny-Brown [4] had stressed the importance of multiple subcortical lesions in the occurrence of continous clonic jerks. Kristiansen et al. [5] are in favour of the subcortical origin of the continous seizure activity which persisted during temporary blocking of cortical function by craniocerebral cooling (to 15 °C) through an extracorporeal carotid shunt. Botez et al. [3], reporting a case of well-delineated subcortical astrocytoma of the right precentral and central area, are of the opinion that epilepsia partialis continua usually signifies subcortical lesions that sometimes compress the motor cortex. Reviewing the literature extensively, Löhler and Peters [6] found 76 cases with lesion of the cortex verified surgically or pathologically in a series of 78 cases. Subcortical lesions were mentioned only in 19%. This supports the view of Bancaud et al. [1] in 1970, who stated that both the seizures and the isolated jerks result from a Rolandic discharge. The study of our 3 cases confirms Bancaud's opinion. In all 3 cases, the extirpation of a delineated focus of the Rolandic region could stop the jerks and the seizures. In case 2, absences and rare facial jerks persisted postoperatively, which is probably due to an insufficient cortex excision, but can now be controlled with drugs.

Summary

Somatomotor status epilepticus in infants consisting of continous repetitive clonic jerks as a sequel of involvement of the sensorimotor area cortex has rarely been explored by multiple depth electrodes. The authors report 3 cases, which were examined stereo-electroencephalographically. Two girls, a 5 year old and a 3 year old showed sustained jerks of one foot with intermittent Jacksonian seizures. Both had a primary epileptogenic focus in the medial prerolandic and postrolandic cortex. The third case, an 8 year old girl, was a borderline case of Koževnikov epilepsy. All 3 patients were operated on following the stereo-electroencephalographic exploration and the focus was removed. The study shows that it is possible to explore children with depth electrodes and that this exploration is the safest way to localize a focus and, consequently to cure the patient by surgery.

References

1. Bancaud, J., Bonis, A., Talairach, J., Bordas-Ferrer, M., Buser, P. (1970), Syndrome de Kojewnikow et accès somato-moteurs (Étude clinique, EEG, EMG et SEEG). Encéphale 59, 391—493.
2. Bancaud, J., Talairach, J., Bonis, A. (1967), Physiopathogénie du syndrome de Kojewnikoff (Interprétation des données électrographiques). Rev. Neurol. 117, 507.
3. Botez, M. I., Brossard, L. (1974), Epilepsia partialis continua with well-delimited subcortical frontal tumor. Epilepsia 15, 39—43.
4. Juul-Jensen, P., Denny-Brown, D. (1966), Epilepsia partialis continua. Arch. Neurol. 6, 23—39.
5. Kristiansen, K., Kaada, B. R., Henriksen, G. F. (1971), Epilepsia partialis continua. Epilepsia 12, 263—267.
6. Löhler, J., Peters, U. H. (1974), Epilepsia partialis continua (Koževnikov-Epilepsie). Fortschr. Neurol. Psychiatr. 42, 165—212.
7. Talairach, J., Bancaud, J., Szikla, G., Bonis, A., Geier, S., Vedrenne, C. (1974), Approche nouvelle de la neurochirurgie de l'épilepsie. Méthodologie stéréotaxique et résultats thérapeutiques. Neuro-Chirurgie 20, suppl. 1, 1—240.

Authors' address: Professor Dr. J. Siegfried and Dr. C. Bernoulli, Department of Neurological Surgery, University of Zürich, Kantonsspital, CH-8091 Zürich, Switzerland.

Acta Neurochirurgica, Suppl. 23, 193—199 (1976)
© by Springer-Verlag 1976

Neurosurgical Clinic of the Freie Universität Berlin, Klinikum Steglitz
(Direktor: Prof. Dr. W. Umbach)

Basic Targets and the Different Epilepsies

G. Bouchard

With 3 Figures

Introduction

About two thirds of all epileptics are successfully treated by anti-convulsant medication [12, 18]. Traditional neurosurgical methods since 1920 provide a resectable focus. However, the selection of suitable focal cases leaves most of the therapeutically poor patients without a chance of improvement. Walker [19] noted in 1974: "The percentage of patients who are offered surgery may be no more than 5%. The concept of the epileptic focus has changed as experience has accumulated." Talairach and Bancaud [14] noted in 1973 an 2/5 increase of resections with increasing reliability of their intricate stereotactic investigation method. In the foreseeable future we believe no more than 10% of epileptics would be suitable for the excision or resection methods.

The stereotaxic operations since 1950 were at first based on the same concept, an identificable eleptogenic focus. We believe it useful in cases not appropriate to resection methods to disregard a focus and preferably to search for the structures involved in the various types of seizures. Interruption of their activating and reverberating circuits obviously can raise their threshold.

Own Material

Three diagrams summarise our stereotaxic operations performed on 49 epileptic patients since 1967 (Figs. 1–3). Columns are drawn without, with three grades of shading or black. It means in the time respectively: states free of seizures, occasional seizures, few seizures without interfering with the individual's life, reduced seizures of only theoretical significance without patient improvement, and black columns denoting unsuccessful events. Exacerbations of seizures never occured.

It is hardly possible to give an exact classification in the primary or secondary temporal lobe epilepsies, primary or secondary centrencephalic or generalized forms with one or more focal signs. About half have predominating traits of temporal lobe epilepsies, the other half of centrencephalic or multifocal characteristics. All patients had

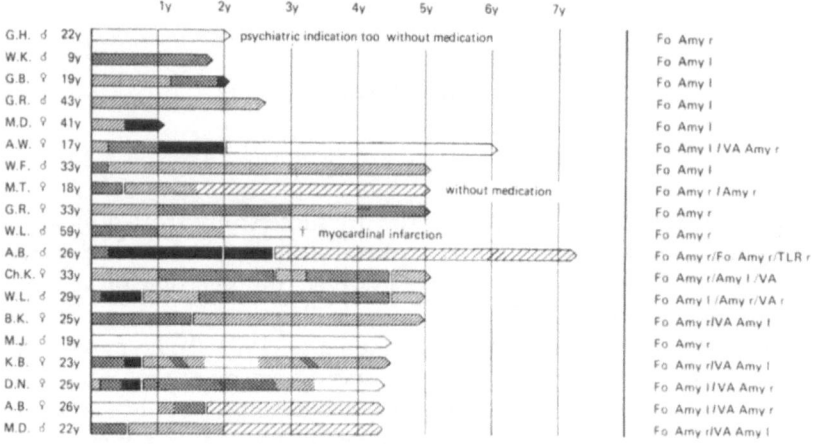

Fig. 1. Diagram of follow up and operations in 19 patients

GM—unconsciousness, bilateral motor phenomena or loss of static control— and minor forms of attacks. Interruptions in the columns indicate 2nd or 3rd stage operations. As a rule several GM, 10 psychomotor seizures or commonly more minor fits occurred per month inspite of medication. In extreme cases daily attacks of GM, of psychomotor seizures or up to 100 short tonic attacks were reported. 23 patients had histories since childhood, 17 since adolescence and 9 after the 20th year of life. At the time of the first operation, a 9 years old child was an exceptional case, 6 patients were between 17 and 19, the majority over 20 years, the oldest were 59 and 51 years respectively. 9 patients suffered from one or several severe epileptic status. 4 survived serious suicidal poisonings. Three had undergone trepanations because of focal epilepsy and one radiation therapy because tumour was suspected.

Three patients had only infrequent seizures, but suffered from chronic psychoses or severe personality disorder resistant to any

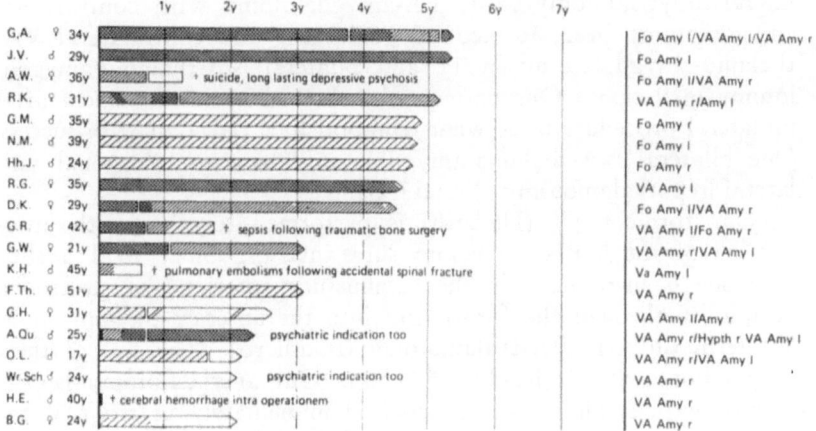

Fig. 2. Diagram of follow up and operations in the subsequent 19 patients

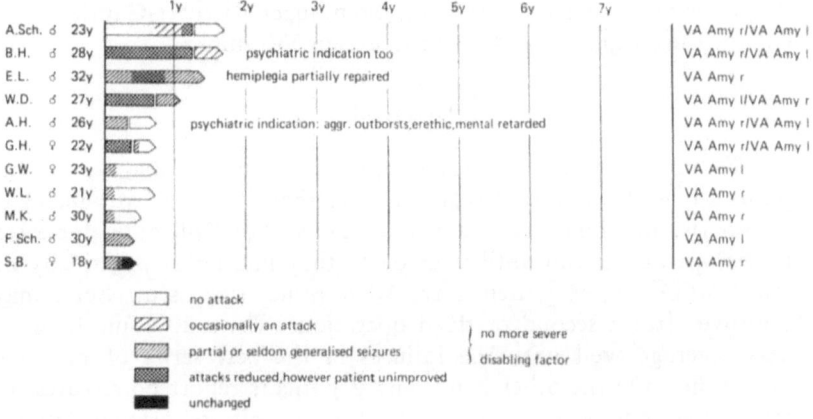

Fig. 3. Diagram of follow up and operations in the last 11 patients

therapeutic procedure. They improved. Psychiatric problems must be reserved for another paper.

No patient has been excluded because of severe organic brain syndrome, low I.Q., excessive number of seizures, hereditary factors or poor somatic condition.

The 49 patients underwent 79 stereotactic operations, 26 unilateral as fornico-amygdalotomy in 14 and VA-thalamo-amygdalotomy in 12 cases. Bilateral and occasional three stage operations were performed in 23 patients, fornico-amygdalotomy with contra-

13*

lateral amygdalotomy in 1, VA-amygdalotomy with contralateral amygdalotomy in 2, fornico-amygdalotomy and contralateral VA-thalamo-amygdalatomy in 11 and bilateral VA-thalamo-amygdalotomy in 9 cases. One patient who showed no improvement after unilateral procedure underwent temporal lobe resection with success. One bilateral VA-thalamo-amygdalotomy had an additional unilateral hypothalamotomy (Jinnai [7], Sano [13]).

Our fornicotomy (Umbach) is performed together with interruption of the bordering commissura anterior. Since 1971 a slide electrode is introduced in the commissura anterior and protruded occipitally through the fornix and into the anterior thalamic pole. We term this our VA-thalamotomy (Bouchard). The size of these coagulations exceeds hardly 150 cmm. Our amygdalotomy is performed with a slide electrode centred immediately in front of the tip of the temporal horn and 20 mm lateral from the midline. The slide electrode is protruded medially, medio-occipitally, laterally and laterooccipitally. The slide electrode is afterwards changed for a thermo-controlled stab electrode (Mundinger-Riechert-Gabriel [10]) to enlarge the coagulation size not more than 350 cmm.

Discussion

We now sum up the results presented in the diagrams: One patient died from intracerebral haemorrhage, thereby producing a 0.75% risk in all our stereotaxic operations. 4 died of causes unrelated to the operations and until their death they had no or practically no seizures. Of the 44 patient alive 10 were not successful. Some may improve after a second or third operation. These 20% unsuccessful cases average well with the failures in the best series of resection operations. On the other hand only 7 patients report no seizures for more than one year. Another 10 report only occasional attacks, giving rise to 36% patients free or almost free of seizures. The remaining 44% demonstrate absence-like fits, short or occasional longer lasting psychomotor seizures or occasional nocturnal GM, all not seriously interfering with daily living. All patient need anticonvulsant medication despite surgical improvement. One tends not to be sceptical of its value. All patients are susceptible to emotional tension due to difficulties in family life and of work. Notwithstanding, 80% of our patients showed valuable improvement, which could not be attained by any other therapeutic procedure.

W. Umbach, one of the pioneers, who has been applying the stereotactic method in epilepsy for over 20 years ago, prefers stereotaxic operations as the first step in surgical therapy [2], traditional methods only where tumor is suspected, in vascular malformations and gross sclerotic areas. D. Jinnai, another pioneer, also engaged in traditional methods, in research of the seizure mechanisms and modern pharmacological potentialities, noted in 1973 [7]: "The stereotactic approach can be fully expected to develop as one of the most reliable surgical procedures. Instead of single lesions it is expected that combined double or triple lesions will produce better results."

In former reports [1, 4, 15, 17] we gave follow ups, quoted the patients who were improved or percentages of abolished seizures summarized from the patients reported. GM were more often abolished than minor partial fits. A tendency to revert to minor forms is also noted. However, in some patients these forms occur more frequently than the greater forms before the operation. As a rule improvement does not occur immediately after surgical management. Seizures in the days or weeks subsequent to stereotactic operation in no way influence the final outcome.

Amydalotomy was first performed by Narabayashi [11]. In the world-wide accepted modification of partial mediodorsal amygdalotomy it is usefully completed by basolateral amygdalotomy in patients with complex psychic performances of psychomotor seizures (Kim 1970 [8]).

Stimulated by Mullan [9] the author modified Umbach's fornicotomy to VA-thalamotomy preferable in patients with centrencephalic traits, however with increasing experience in temporal lobe epilepsies it is given an ever widening range of application. Intraoperative VA-stimulations evoked bilateral cortical afterdischarges and more pronounced activity in medial than in lateral parts of the homolateral amygdala. Some patients show postoperatively homolateral accentuated reduction of spike-wave paroxysms; most of the patients lost these patterns after bilateral operations.

According to the mirror focus research and the kindling mechanisms in limbic structures (Goddard and McIntyre [6]) most of the patients have to await bilateral operations. Some improved unexpectedly after unilateral operation and confirm our efforts in preoperatively selecting the most suitable hemisphere e.g. in secondary centrencephalic epilepsy. In the future we plan our technique to avoid more than two operations, one in each hemisphere at an adequate interval. Until now threestage operations were performed because of fear of producing unwanted side effects. None of our patients however retained vegetative dysregulations as obesity and disturbance of sexual life as long as about three months postoperatively. No changes in the preoperative personalities or organic brain syndromes persisted.

Summary

The follow up of 49 stereotactically operated epileptics is graphically demonstrated and the 79 operations in basic targets within the amygdala and the area of the anterior pole of the thalamus are described. The patients had valuable gaining in 80%. The continued development of stereotactic methods in the future is urgent, so long as 30% of the epileptics respond poorly to drug therapy and only 5–10% are suitable to the traditional resection methods.

Acknowledgements

This paper is dedicated to Prof. Dr. W. Umbach, on the occasion of his 60th birthday.

The author wishes to thank Dr. Bridgewater for his assistance with the translation.

References

1. Bouchard, G. (1970), Long-term results of stereotaxic fornicotomy and amygdalo-fornicotomy in patients with temporal lobe epilepsy showing behavior disturbances. In: Special topics in stereotaxis, pp. 53—64 (W. Umbach, ed.). Stuttgart: Hippokrates.

2. — Umbach, W. (1972), Indication for the open and stereotactic brain surgery in epilepsy. In: Present limits of neurosurgery, pp. 403—406 (I. Fusek, Z. Kunc, eds.). Prague: Avicenum Czechoslovak medical press.

3. — — (1973), Langzeitergebnisse der stereotaktischen Therapie bei psychomotorischer Epilepsie. In: Limbisches System und Epilepsie, pp. 90—93 (F. Heppner, ed.). Bern: H. Huber.

4. — (1974), Stereotactic operations in generalized forms of epilepsy. Acta Neurochir. Suppl. 21, pp. 15—24 (F. J. Gillingham, E. R. Hitchcock, J. W. Turner). Wien-New York: Springer.

5. — Kim, Y. K., Umbach, W. (1975), Stereotaxic methods in different forms of epilepsy. Confin. neurol. 37, 232—238.

6. Goddard, G. V., McIntyre, D. C. (1973), Some properties of lasting epileptogenic trace kindled by repeated electrical stimulation of the amygdala in mammals. In: Surgical approaches in psychiatry, pp. 109—115 (L. V. Laitinen, K. E. Livingston, eds.). Lancaster: Medical and Technical Publishing.

7. Jinnai, D., Mukawa, J. (1973), Surgery for epilepsy. In: Progress in neurological surgery, vol. 5, pp. 267—271, 275 (H. Krayenbühl, P. E. Maspes, W. H. Sweet, eds.). Basel: S. Karger.

8. Kim, Y. K. (1970), Effects of basolateral amygdalotomy. In: Special topics in stereotaxis, pp. 69—78 (W. Umbach, ed.). Stuttgart: Hippokrates.

9. Mullan, S., Vailati, G., Karasick, J., Mailis, M. (1967), Thalamic lesions for the control of epilepsy. Arch. neurol. 16, 277—285.

10. Mundinger, F., Riechert, T., Gabriel, E. (1960), Untersuchungen zu den physikalischen und technischen Voraussetzungen einer dosierten Hochfrequenzkoagulation bei stereotaktischen Hirnoperationen. Zbl. für Chirurgie 85, 1051—1063.

11. Narabayashi, H., Shima, F. (1973), Which is better amygdala target, the medial or lateral nuclei? In: Surgical approaches in psychiatry, pp. 129—134 (L. V. Laitinen, K. E. Livingston, eds.). Lancaster: Medical and Technical Publishing.
12. McNaughton, F. (1954), Observations on diagnosis and medical treatment. In: Epilepsy and the functional anatomy of the human brain. London: J. and A. Churchill.
13. Sano, K., Mayanagy, J., Sekino, H., Ogashiwa, M., Ishijima, M. (1970), Results of stimulation and destruction of the posterior hypothalamus in man. J. neurosurg. *33*, 689—707.
14. Talairach, J., Bancaud, J. (1973), Stereotaxic approach to epilepsy. In: Progress in neurological surgery, vol. 5, p. 350 (H. Krayenbühl, P. E. Maspes, W. H. Sweet, eds.). Basel: S. Karger.
15. Umbach, W. (1954), Die Fornikotomie, ein vorläufiger Versuch zur Behandlung der temporalen Epilepsie. Internat. Symposion Neurochir. Freiburg.
16. — Riechert, T. (1964), Elektrophysiologische und klinische Ergebnisse stereotaktischer Eingriffe im limbischen System bei temporaler Epilepsie. Nervenarzt *35*, 482—488.
17. — (1966), Elektrophysiologische und vegetative Phänomene bei stereotaktischen Hirnoperationen, pp. 117—121. Berlin-Heidelberg-New York: Springer.
18. Walker, A. E. (1972), Surgical treatment of epilepsy. In: Comprehensive management of epilepsy in infancy, childhood and adolescence, p. 410 (S. Livingston, ed.). Springfield, Ill.: Ch.C Thomas.
19. — (1974), Surgery for epilepsy. In: Handbook of clinical neurology, vol. 15, The epilepsies, pp. 740, 744 (P. J. Vinken, G. W. Bruyn, eds.). Amsterdam: North Holland Publishing Company.

Author's address: Dr. G. Bouchard, Klinikum Steglitz, Neurochirurgische Klinik, Hindenburgdamm 30, D-1000 Berlin 45.

Acta Neurochirurgica, Suppl. 23, 201—204 (1976)
© by Springer-Verlag 1976

II. Neurologic Clinic and Neurosurgical Clinic, Comenius University,
Bratislava, ČSSR

Effects of Stereotactic Operations in the Treatment of Epilepsies—Neurological Aspects

L. Cigánek, M. Šramka, P. Nádvorník, and G. Fritz

Summary

In 81 patients with intractable epileptic seizures 121 stereo-electroencephalographic (SEEG) examinations and 91 operations with stereoencephalotomy (SET) were carried out. SEEG and SET targets were chosen in 22 different subcortical structures and in the medial frontal cortex. In 6 of 18 temporal epilepsy cases SET was followed by classical hippocampectomy. With the exception of temporal lobe cases all others were unsuitable for classical neurosurgery. Of 61 controlled patients 24.5⁰/o were cured or greatly improved cured, 39.5⁰/o improved and 36⁰/o unimproved. Correlations among the clinical, EEG and SEEG findings, SET and therapeutic effects are discussed together with the role of stereotactic procedures.

In our experience (Cigánek 1962) among patients unsuccessfully treated by conservative methods over 60⁰/o are unsuitable for classical procedures based on the criteria of the Montreal neurosurgical school, because of the absence of leading epileptogenic area or because they represent cases with completely or almost completely generalized seizures. In these cases stereotaxy offers prospects diagnostic refinement and treatment.

Material and Methods

The referred group consists of 81 patients with intractable epileptic seizures. With the exception of the temporal lobe cases all were unsuitable for the classical procedures. We performed 121 stereoelectroencephalographic (SEEG) examinations, in 28 cases repeated, maximally four times in one patient. One or two rigid electrodes with nine contacts were used and in 14 cases also flexible steel electrodes implanted for one week. Most patients (54) suffered from multiform types of seizures which were often generalized. Some more or less defined subgroups could be distinguished in these patients: those with a prominent epileptogenic area on the medial frontal surface (detected by the SEEG) often with epileptic EEG activity projecting to the frontal convexity and the hippocampi;

cases with combined temporal and frontal symptomatology; patients with extensive general disorder or conversely poor electrographic localization; 18 patients had typical temporal lobe epilepsy, 6 were of progressive myoclonic epilepsy type, 2 had Jacksonian seizures and one case was classified as primarily grand mal type. The SEEG targets—in later stages of our work selected in four standard trajectories—were: 12 different thalamic nuclei, amygdala, hippocampus, hypothalamus, n. ruber, putamen, pallidum, n. caudatus, anterior commissure, Forel's H field, fornix and different points of the medial frontal cortex. In all cases targets for the SEEG were chosen after pathophysiological analysis of seizures and according to the neurological and EEG findings. 91 of the operations stereoencephalotomy (SET) was performed by means of electrocoagulation in one or more of the epileptically active structures (estimated by SEEG). 17 patients had more than one (maximally three) operations with SET. In six patients with temporal epilepsy SET was later followed by direct removal of the hippocampus.

Results

In different cases all structures examined by means of SEEG were occasionally found to be the site of specific epileptic electrographic, intercritic or critic discharges.

The effect of the operation was observed in 61 patients over a period ranging from 6 months to 6 years postoperatively. Fifteen patients (24.5%) were seizure free or had not more than two seizures annually. 24 (39.5%) were substantially improved and 22 (36%) were unimproved.

The treatment of temporal lobe epilepsy was most successful. In two cases of Jacksonian seizures improvement occurred with lesions in the ventro-oral anterior nucleus of the thalamus. In other types of epilepsies the effects of the treatment were less satisfactory. In spite of the large number of structures operated upon these were divided among a great number of patients with different types of seizures and were made in different combinations. Also in this group the improvement appeared to correlate mainly with SET of the amygdala and hippocampus, further in the anterior commissure, reticulatum thalami (mainly in its anterior part) n. caudatus and Forel's H field. Forel's H field lesions seems to suppress contralateral adversive seizures. Lesions in the medial thalamic lamina were found mostly in unimproved cases. On the other hand in the improved patients we made—simultaneously or successively—on average nearly twice as many SET lesions in different subcortical structures as in the unimproved cases.

Discussion

In temporal lobe epilepsy the SEEG very often provides more information than that obtained from clinical and EEG examination. SET of the amygdalo-hippocampal system is less risky though also less complete and radical than the classical operation. In case of failure, classical hippocampectomy or temporal lobectomy can be done.

The operations described in Jacksonian seizures were made with the aim of suppressing the epileptogenic threshold in the central region by reducing afferent impulses to this part of the cortex.

According to Schaltenbrand et al. (1966 a, b) and Romodanov (1972) multiple lesions in different localisations may be more effective. As formulated by Nádvorník et al. (1975) the aim of this type of operation is to separate a complex and effective epileptogenic system into a number of less effective components. This concept also justifies operation upon structures which do not represent the so called primary epileptogenic area (probably the majority if not all subcortical gray structures), as well as upon neural pathways.

Our results raise the following possibilities:

1. In the three dimensional space of the brain the SEEG can detect structures with epileptic activity and perhaps also primary epileptogenic areas in the classical sense which are inaccessible and indetectable by other methods and which can be removed by means of SET.

2. SEEG completes our knowledges about the type of spread of epileptic discharges from known epileptogenic areas as well as their generalization.

3. The problem whether the subcortical gray matter can play the primary role in the mechanisms of at least some types of epileptic seizures can now be solved.

4. Stereotactic operations lead to a new concept of a dynamic epileptogenic system in the three dimensional brain, which is represented by knots of gray matter, connected by edges of the neuronal pathways to a grid-like system with different connections and dependencies (Šramka et al. 1972). In this concept the aim of treatment by combined, simultaneous and successive lesions is to separate such an epileptogenic system into isolated and less effective or even ineffective components.

5. Stereotactic operations have a therapeutic effect not only in cases insuitable for classical surgery, but also in other cases with the advantage of being less risky and less mutilating.

The benefits of stereotactic operations in epilepsy will probably increase as we learn more about seizure mechanisms during stereotactic operations.

References

Cigánek, L. (1962), The possibilities of the surgical treatment of focal epilepsies (in Slovak). Bratislava: The Publishing House of the Slovak Academy of Sciences.

Nádvorník, P., Šramka, M., Gajdošová, D. (1975), A critical view on stereotactic treatment of epilepsy (in Slovak). Čs. Neurol. Neurochir. *38*, 15—18.

Romodanov, A. P. (1972), Combined surgical interventions on the brain for epilepsy. In: Present limits of neurosurgery (I. Fusek, Z. Kunc, eds.). Prague: Avicenum.

Schaltenbrand, G., Spuler, H., Nadjimi, M., Hopf, H., Waren, W. (1966 a), Die stereotaktische Behandlung der Epilepsien. Confin. neurol. (Basel) *27*, 111—113.

— — — — — (1966 b), Die stereotaktische Behandlung der symptomatischen Epilepsien. Münch. med. Wschr. *108*, 1707—1712.

Šramka, M., Nádvorník, P., Lojka, J., Cigánek, L. (1972), Relations of the anterior thalamic reticulum to epilepsy. In: Present limits of neurosurgery (I. Fusek, Z. Kunc, eds.). Prague: Avicenum.

Authors' addresses: Dr. L. Cigánek, II. Neurologic Clinic, Comenius University, Limbová 17, 809 46 Bratislava, ČSSR, Dr. P. Nádvorník, Dr. M. Šramka, Dr. G. Fritz, Neurosurgical Clinic, Comenius University, Limbová 17, 809 46 Bratislava, ČSSR.

Acta Neurochirurgica, Suppl. 23, 205—209 (1976)
© by Springer-Verlag 1976

Neurosurgical Department of the Clinic of Neurology and Psychiatry University Medical School, Debrecen, Hungary

Effects of Stereotactic Lesions in Intractable Epilepsy

J. Hullay, R. Gombi, and Gy. Velok

With 2 Figures

Two periods of surgical treatment of epilepsy can be distinguished before the stereotactic era. In the first period the preliminary data, the symptoms, and the careful seizure-observation constituted the basis of the focus-determination, the PEG confirmed, and the electric cortical-stimulations identified the surgical focus. In the second period the role of the scalp-EEG and electrocorticography (ECoG) came to the foreground. If the EEG focus coincided with the lesions determined by classical methods, then surgery needed to be considered even in cases of epilepsy controlled by anticonvulsants. In the case of psychomotor epilepsy associated with severe personality and behavioural disorders or predisposition to psychosis, we very often relied only on scalp-EEG. The stereo-EEG meant a further improvement of EEG as well as revising the localization value of scalp-EEG and our conception of epilepsy. An account of our observations concerning the stereo-EEG and the present significance of electrostimulation (ES) is reported in another paper (by Dr. Gombi and collab.). In this paper we shall deal only with the operative attempts.

Material

From 1951 to 1975 102 epileptics were operated upon. The first 15 years may be called the period of temporal epilepsy, since until 1965 54 temporal epileptic patients had received operations. In 39 merely the scalp-EEG served as the basis for exposure, and only 15 had radiologically objective lesions of localizational value. The operative and histological finding verified the scalp-EEG in 38 cases (in 8 cases atrophy and microgyria were found, in 8 cases angiomatous abnormalities or angioma, in 7 cases leptomeningeal thickening, adhesion or cyst, in 1 case cortical heterotopy, and in 1 case bone spicule. Histology of the removed pole or lobe in 5 patients revealed

Table 1

The left side shows the site of the lesions, the right side the result and in the middle the numbered circles signify the cases

Site of stereotactic lesions	Cases	Results
I. STRUCTURES, WHERE SEIZURE WAS ELICITES BY ES		
Supplementary motor area · · · · ·	(14)°(1)(15)° · ·	2 improved 1° unchanged
Supplementary sensory area · · · · ·	(2) · · ·	improved
Rostral cingulum · · · · · · · · · · (simultaneously thalamus-subthalamus)	(3)(4)(5) · ·	2 improved 1 unchanged
Septal region · · · · · · · · · · · (previously z. innominata)	(6)* · ·	unchanged
Hippocampus · · · · · · · · · · · ·	(7)* · ·	SEIZUREFREE
Hippocampus, Amygdala · · · · · · ·	(8)(9)° · · ·	2 improved
II. DIFFERENT TARGET STRUCTURES		
Fornix · · · · · · · · · · · · · · ·	(10)* · · ·	unchanged
Thalamus (Ce, V. im. i.) · · · · · · · ·	(11) · · ·	improved
Thalamus (V.o.), Subthalamus · · · · (Z. i., Ra. prl.)	(5)(12)(4)(3) · ·	2 improved 2 unchanged
Subthalamus (Forel field, n. ruber) ·	(16)(13) · · ·	2 improved

○* Patients with sever psychotic manifestations

° after conventional resection became seizurefree

Ammon's horn sclerosis, and in a further 3 macroscopically intact lobes there were incisural sclerosis and leptomeningeal or cortical lesion). In these cases the ECoG as well as the ES was generally corroborative. After the operation, which (except for 2 cases with exploration only) consisted of pole or lobe resection involving the amygdala and the hippocampus in most 26 patients (50%) became seizure-free (20 out of the cases with temporal lobe lesions).

Results were similar in 21 cases as non-temporal epilepsy, although the EEG-focus was identifiable in most of cases. Of these, two successful hemispherectomies deserve mention. Considering the 50% seizure-free result, this period could not be termed bad.

The introduction of the Talairach-Bancaud stereo-EEG took place in 1967, though we had been carrying out deep-electrode EEG

investigations and ES during temporal epilepsy since 1952 and stereotactic operations since 1961. The new method with multi-electrodes
triggered off more exact focus-searching and localizing attempts. The
long and not entirely harmless investigation, which many would consider an intervention, we felt was justified—only in those cases where
there was nothing to be lost, *i.e.* with such patients who were not
only intractable epileptics but also severely retarded or deteriorated

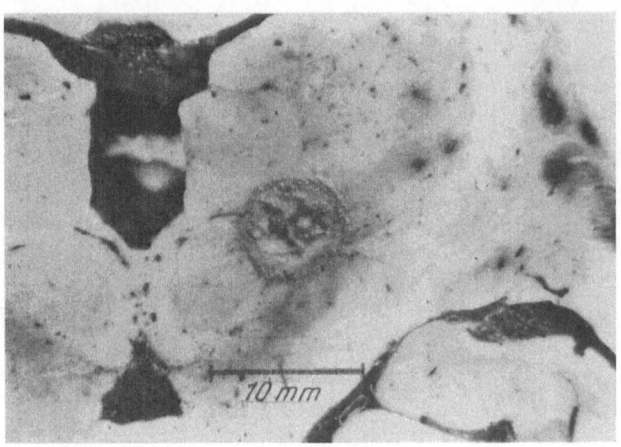

Fig. 1. Size of the thermo-lesion performed by Vitatron apparatus (in a case of
m. Wilson)

and who had behaviour disorders. This means that on the basis of
more than 30, partly repeated investigations, all in all only 15 patients (5 temporal and 10 non-temporal epilepsy cases) had appropriate operative exposure with complete procedures in only half of
the cases. Of these, 7 patients became seizure-free, while the number
of attacks of the remainder decreased.

Stereotactic procedures were carried out on 16 patients (Tab. 1).
Lesions with thermo-coagulation about 6 mm diameter (Fig. 1) were
performed with a Vitatron apparatus. In 11 cases, in the site of the
seizures elicited by means of ES during stereo-EEG, in 4 of these
previously or simultaneously in other structures too, in 5 cases in the
fornix and thalamus, and/or in the subthalamus (Fig. 2). In a few
cases (* on the Table) the procedure was mainly intended to improve
behaviour disorder.

Postoperatively 1 patient became seizure-free and 10 improved.
Five remained unchanged but three of them after conventional focus

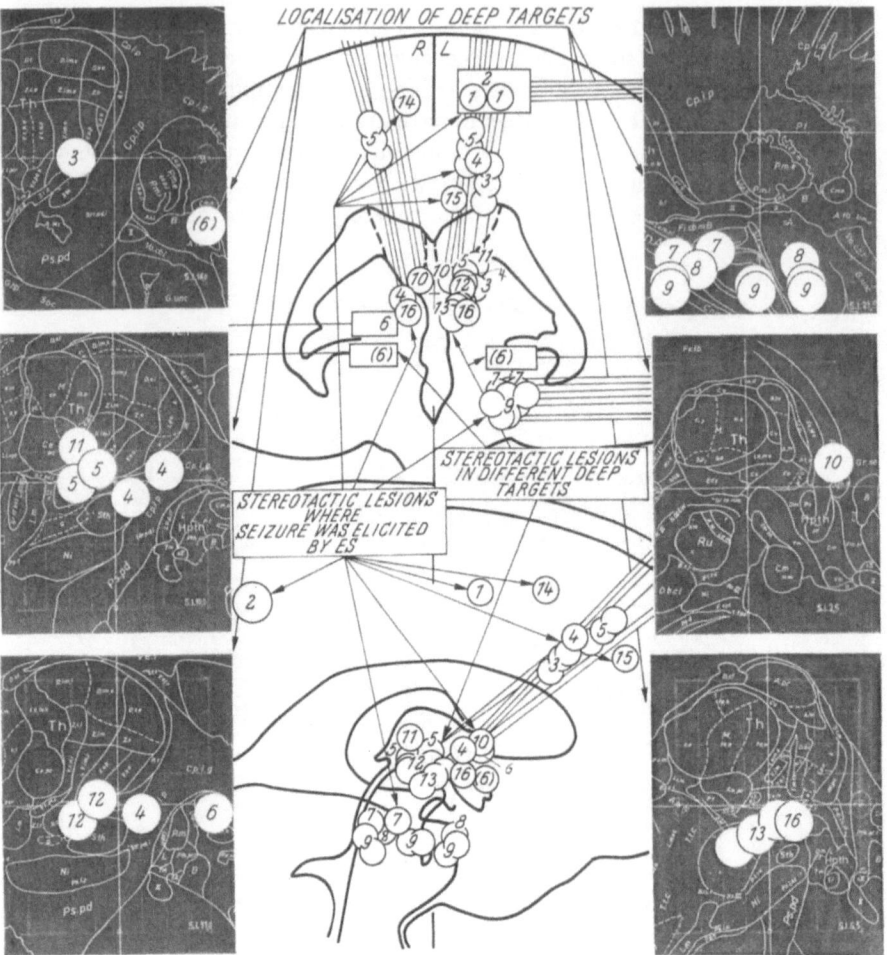

Fig. 2. In the middle, in a–p and lateral projection, can be seen the summation of the lesions corresponding to the case marked by its ordinal number. The horizontal electrodes mean the lesions performed by the Talairach apparatus, the others are those performed by the Riechert apparatus. In both sides of the picture the sites of the deep-cerebral lesions are shown by the S.l. 2.5–21,5 mm figures outlining the structures of the Schaltenbrand atlas

resection became seizure-free. Generally the improvement meant a decrease of seizure frequency and diminution of epileptiform anomalies in EEG activity. The improvement of the psychic picture was noteworthy only in the case of the seizure-free patient and favourably modified in one improved case.

Discussion and Conclusion

This material does not seem to be suitable for comparison with the operations carried out before the stereo-era because of different indications. Moreover, the number of stereo-interventions is small and the follow-up time is short.

In our experience stereo-EEG focus-determination is more exact, but more time consuming complicated and risky. The lesion produced in the site of the seizure elicited by ES during the stereo-EEG may be effective chiefly in the amygdala and hippocampus, a nonspecific lesion however decreases the number of seizures at the most.

Therefore we believe that

1. an adequate operative solution in the future can only be an appropriate exposure and removal of the identified lesion, and focus determined by ECoG and ES,

2. stereotactic intervention blindly carried out in the site of the elicited seizure can not be expected to destroy precisely an area sufficient to stop the seizure, so that an effective lesion by this method occurs by chance rather than design.

3. Nonspecific stereo-interventions are ineffective at the present time probably because the target-structures have not determining role. The effective target can only be in a structure which selectively activates the coded seizure-pattern. Its determination would mean an important advance in our field.

Summary

The eras of surgical treatment of epilepsy are described and experience with the epilepsy operations, especially those obtained in the course of temporal epilepsy operations, and stereotactic attempts based on multielectrode EEG investigations, and ES. Classical, exposure and resection still seems adequate whilst stereotaxy develops in the selective elimination of the structure activating the coded seizure-pattern.

Authors' address: Prof. Dr. J. Hullay, Neurosurgical Department of the University Medical School, H-4012 Debrecen, Hungary.

Acta Neurochirurgica, Suppl. 23, 211—214 (1976)

Department of Functional Neurosurgery and Clinical Neurophysiology,
Neurosurgical Clinic, University of Wien, Austria

New Possibilities of Stereotactic Treatment of Temporal Lobe Epilepsy (TLE)

J. A. Ganglberger

With 1 Figure

Quite frequently limbic seizures are combined with mostly nocturnal major seizures of the grand mal type. While the major seizures are more easily controlled by anticonvulsive drugs it is a well known fact that clearly defined limbic seizures, especially the psychomotor attacks, are often highly resistant to pharmacological treatment.

Open major surgery (resection of one or both temporal poles and of the amygdala etc.) produced a variety of undesirable long-lasting effects or even irreparable side effects so that a growing animosity against such operations was created. A more promising surgical treatment with no risks or lasting side effects, the combined unilateral stereotactic fornico- and anterior commissurotomy has been inaugurated in Freiburg in Breisgau in 1954 (Umbach, 1954, 1966). The concept was to interrupt the majority of the pathways leading away from the epileptogenic focus within the hippocampal-amygdaloid complex. But the initial expectations were not fully realized by this operation. After an initial marked improvement seizures recurred and increased in frequency again after some months or years in a number of cases. This was the reason why after 1961 stereofornico- and anterior commissurotomy has been combined in one or in a second session with ipsilateral medial amygdalotomy (Narabayashi, 1961; Watanabe et al., 1961). Even better results were claimed to be achieved by Kim (1971) by placing the lesion in the baso-lateral amygdala.

Until recently it has been commonly but erroneously believed that the break-through of limbic seizures to other structures of the brain takes place within the so-called limbic cortex. When Ganglberger et al. (1971) found that distant extinction (a period of lowered ex-

14*

citability following an initial single response to high frequency stimulation—originally described as a local phenomenon only by Dusser de Barenne and McCulloch, 1937) could be elicited over prefrontal areas on stimulation of the ipsilateral amygdala, the latency of

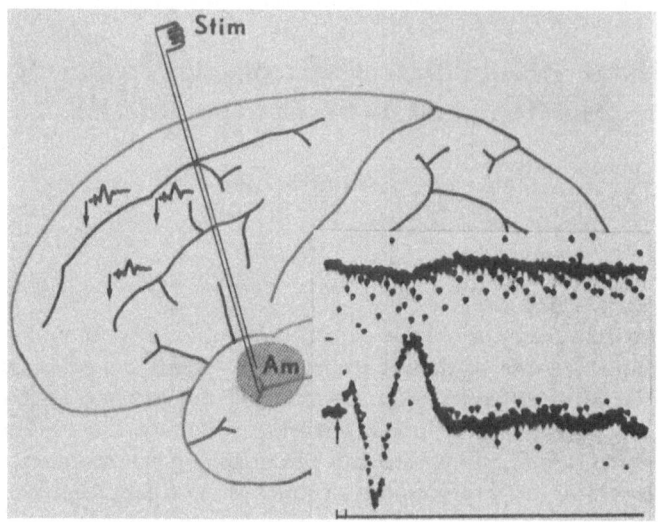

Fig. 1. Distant extinction over prefrontal areas evoked by 50 per second stimulation of ipsilateral amygdaloid nucleus in a 19 years old female temporal lobe epileptic (A. G.). Arrows in frontal region mark site of subdural AgAgCl-electrodes introduced through stereotactic trephine hole. 30 trains of 50 per second rectangular stimuli of 0.05 milliseconds duration were averaged (DISA-Multistim, LABEN-Correlatron 4096). Channel 1 of original inset is from vertex to mastoid recorded, channel 2 from one of the cortical electrodes.
Arrow markes onset of stimulus train, straight black line shows train duration, the two initial vertical bars give the time mark of 20 msec corresponding to the pulse interval. Channel 2 shows clearly a positive-negative-positive response to the initial pulse of the train followed by extinction. The points off the main trace of channel 1 are not „lost" analysis points but stimulus artifacts

20 milliseconds suggested a multisynaptic pathway with a detour via the medial thalamus, the main projector to the prefrontal regions (Fig. 1).

A study of the literature revealed the existence of pathways from the baso-lateral amygdala to the medial (or dorso-medial) nucleus of the thalamus, described by Fox (1949). Still more important were the anatomical studies carried out on human brains by Klingler and Gloor (1960) who proved the existence of a fibre tract passing from the amygdala and from the anterior temporal cortex via the ansa peduncularis and the pedunculus thalami extracapsularis to the medial thalamic nucleus. (Interested readers are refered to the excellent figures in the original publication of Klingler and Gloor.) But the most important fact was brought to our attention by Brazier at a Vienna Symposium on Synchronization of EEG Activity in Epilepsies, September 1971 (1972). Based on experiences with more than 50 cases of temporal lobe epilepsy with continuous recording from indwelling multi-electrodes Brazier could prove beyond any doubt that the break-through of limbic seizures to other brain structures invariably takes place in the medial thalamic nucleus and certainly not in the so-called limbic cortex as had been commonly believed.

A few weeks after Brazier revealed the important fact of the thalamic break-through of limbic seizures the first stereotactic operation was carried out in order to interrupt the above mentioned pathway on the rostro-ventral margin of the medial thalamic nucleus. The male subject (G. W.) had previously undergone a stereofornico- and anterior commissurotomy in 1967 at the age of 17 years. Prior to the first intervention the basically intelligent patient had been unable to finish his school education and unable to work because of his frequent major seizures of the grand mal type and still more frequent psychomotor attacks. As a result of the first operation the psychomotor attacks were considerably reduced in frequency, severity and duration, while the major seizures of the grand mal type were completely stopped. After the second stereotactic operation with the new target point in 1971 the patient is completely free of seizures. In the meantime he has successfully completed his school education while working, participated successfully a training course in massage, and is now occupied as an orderly in the operation theatre of a major surgical department.

All in all only six patients were operated in this target point until the end of last year, all of them had previously undergone stereofornico- and anterior commissurotomy, one female subject also an additional medial stereoamygdalotomy. Three out of these six patients are now completely free of seizures, two have still minor seizures, but less frequently and of shorter duration. The one female patient with two previous interventions before the last one seems to be a failure. This patient suffers additionally from a slight hemiathetosis combined with a slight hemiatrophy of the right side of the body and of the left cerebral hemisphere due to a birth injury.

We still have some reservations regarding this operation, but we think it can be done in one session, combined with stereofornico-

and anterior commissurotomy by using the lateral drive-out or stylet-electrode. This conclusion may be drawn from a careful study of the operation protocols of our most successful cases of stereofornico- and anterior commissurotomy. Some of those patients are already morethan 10 years free of seizures. It became evident that in these cases bigger lesions were made in the latero-posterior direction as necessary for the interruption of the fornix alone. And the pedunculus thalami extracapsularis lies at some point slightly behind and slightly lateral to the pars tecta columnae fornicis. It could be that thus this pathway could have been interrupted ensuring the excellent effect in these cases.

References

Brazier, M. A. B. (1972), Interactions of deep structures during seizures in man, pp. 409—424, H. Petsche and M. A. B. Brazier (Eds.): Synchronization of EEG activity in epilepsies. Wien-New York: Springer.

Dusser de Barenne, J. G., McCulloch, W. S. (1937), Local stimulatory inactivation within the cerebral cortex, the factor for extinction. Am. J. Physiol. *118*, 510—524.

Fox, C. A. (1949), Amygdalo-thalamic connections in Macaca mulatta. Anat. Rec. *103*, 537.

Ganglberger, J. A., Groll-Knapp, E., Haider, M. (1971), Computer analysis of electrophysiological phenomena during stereotactic fornico- and amygdalo-tomy, pp. 149—155, W. Umbach (Ed.): Special topics in stereotaxis. Stuttgart: Hippokrates-Verlag.

Kim, Y. K. (1972), Effects of basolateral amygdalotomy, pp. 69—78, W. Umbach (Ed.): Special topics in stereotaxis. Stuttgart: Hippokrates-Verlag.

Klingler, J., Gloor, P. (1960), The connections of the amygdala and of the anterior temporal cortex in the human brain. J. Comp. Neurol. *115*, 3, 333—369.

Narabayashi, H. (1961), Stereotaktische Amygdalektomie zur Behandlung von abartigem Verhalten mit oder ohne Anomalien des Elektroencephalogramms. Excerpta med. Int. Congr. Ser. *36*, 140.

Umbach, W. (1954), Die „Fornikotomie", ein vorläufiger Versuch zur Behandlung der temporalen Epilepsie. Int. Sympos. Neurochir., Freiburg im Breisgau.

Umbach, W. (1966), Elektrophysiologische und vegetative Phänomene bei stereotaktischen Hirnoperationen. Berlin-Heidelberg-New York: Springer.

Watanabe, S., Miwa, K., Takeuch, Y. (1961), Studien über die Amygdalektomie zur Behandlung der subcorticalen Epilepsie. Excerpta med. Int. Congr. Ser. *36*, 178.

Author's address: Prof. Dr. med. J. A. Ganglberger, Department of Functional Neurosurgery and Clinical Neurophysiology, Neurosurgical Clinic, University of Wien, Alser Straße 4, A-1090 Wien, Austria.

Acta Neurochirurgica, Suppl. 23, 215—219 (1976)

Dr. Hans Berger Kliniek, Breda,
Department of Neurosurgery, University Groningen,
Leyenburg Ziekenhuis, Den Haag, The Netherlands

Results of Amygdalotomy and Fornicotomy in Temporal Lobe Epilepsy and Behaviour Disorders

A. E. H. Sonnen, J. v. Manen, and B. van Dijk

Introduction

Amygdalotomy is an accepted therapeutic tool for drug resistant temporal lobe epilepsy, especially in combination with aggressive behaviour. Because of the danger that in these difficult patients the decision to operate is taken too easily a national committee to which all these cases for operation are presented was formed in Holland, consisting of neurosurgeons, neurologists, psychiatrists, electrophysiologists and epileptologists. The cautious procedure of this independent comittee explains the small series we present to-day.

Material

The series consists of 2 female and 6 male patients of 12–16 years and 1 patient of 26, all suffering from psychomotor epilepsy, sometimes in the past combined with generalized tonic clonic seizures and isolated myoclonic jerks for more than 6 years and clinically treated for 2½–7 years. The range of I.Q. was 30–80, of seizure frequency 0.06–2.3 : a day. The main indication for operation was only twice the seizure frequency and 6 times the behaviour disturbance, consisting of impulsive aggressiveness with dangerous outburst of rage, in 1 case with an attempt at homicide and suicide. 3 Patients were nearly constantly separated from others. Some were hyperkinetic, and others slow and uninterested. One patient was psychotic. All usual anti-epileptic drugs had been given in various combinations including in several cases complete withdrawal of the medication. Psychoactive drugs and conditioning strategies produced only limited success.

Methods

3 Patients underwent bilateral amygdalotomy and ipsilateral fornicotomy in 3 stages with an interval of 3 months. 3 Patients underwent only a bilateral amygdalotomy, in 1 patient an ipsilateral amygdalotomy was sufficient and in 1 case contralateral amygdalotomy followed an ipsilateral temporal lobectomy. The stereotactic

device of van Hoytema and van Manen was used. The lesion in the fornix was about spherical with a diameter of 5–6 mm and located just lateral to the median plane of the brain at a level just above the anterior commissure.

The amygdaloid nucleus was localized just in front of the temporal horn and 5 mm above the lowest point of the horn on this line. On the AP radiograph the lateral border of the nucleus was supposed to be at the medial border of the lateral cleft of the temporal horn, as indicated by Spiegel and Wycis.

In our material this meant 30 mm (27–33) lateral from the median plane. The width of the nucleus was estimated 13–17 mm, the mean centre of the lesions was 23 mm (21.5–28.5) lateral from the middle of the brain.

The first few patients were given neurolept anaesthesia but because most patients were too uncooperative all later operations were performed under full anaesthesia.

The location of the tip of the electrode was controlled by X-ray, EEG recording and stimulation with ether and electric current. The EEG during the operation and the reactivity of the patient was however greatly influenced by the anaesthesia. Stimuli were administered with a constant current stimulator with pulses of 1 msec, $1/2$–4 mA and 1–100 c/s, during 5—20 seconds.

Unipolar and bipolar lesions were made by a series of temperature controlled high frequency coagulations resp. 70, 80, 90 and 90° C during 60 seconds on a range of 12 mm along the trajectory above the targetpoint. The lesions were approximately 17 mm in length along the trajectory, of 4–6 and 8–10 mm thick resp. on the deepest and the highest point in the AP direction and 8 and 12 mm wide in the frontal plane.

On the lateral radiograph the position in relation to the commissura anterior was 3.5 mm behind and 19 mm below.

We supposed the lesion to be in the centre of the nucleus. The patients were discharged from the clinic after 1–5 months and followed for 1–3 years. To rate the behaviour we used an observation scale and additionally the daily notes of the staff members. The medication remained constant during the observation period.

Results

1. Operation

a) EEG recordings: although all patients but 1 had spikes in the EEG before operation, in only 9 out of 15 operations these spikes were seen in the surface recording. During operation surface and depth recording were positive in 6 cases, negative in 3 cases, only the surface positive in 3 cases and only the depth recording positive in 3 cases. The depth recording was just as often positive on the contralateral as on the ipsilateral side. Reaction to stimulation of the amygdala consisted of swallowing, chewing, licking, eye movements, looking amazed, feeling of uneasiness, nausea, sometimes combined with flattening of the EEG but mostly without any change. Reactions were seen in 6 out of 7 cases of ipsilateral and in 5 out of 7 cases of contralateral amygdala stimulation and in 2 out of 3 cases of ipsilateral fornix stimulation.

An after discharge in the area of stimulation during 10–180 seconds was mostly accompanied by widening of the pupils, eye movements, slowing of the pulse rate and respiratory arrest. These effects were seen with a current of 3–4 mA and 30–60 pulses/second. Coagulation of the amygdala produced in some cases change in respiration, mouth movements and mumbling. Coagulation of the fornix produced short tachycardia and once a widening of the pupils, mouth and eye movement and looking amazed.

Although all patients were stimulated with ether inhalation we never saw the spikes that were described by Narabayashi.

b) complications: 4 patients showed a sudden rise in temperature to 40° C, once caused by a pneumonia, in the other cases unexplained. Once the blood pressure rose to 240/150 on the first day. In 1 patient there was a slight contralateral hemiparesis of a few hours' duration, in 1 patient a contralateral hemiparesis lasted for 1 month.

2. Seizure Control

In 4 patients there was no change at all, in 1 patient the seizure frequency increased, especially after the fornicotomy and in 1 patient the nature of the seizure changed from psychomotor attacks with automatisms to vague feelings of fear, probably more frequent than the attacks before. In one case there are fewer seizures but the frequency varied also considerably before the operation and finally 1 patient is nearly seizure-free but the improvement did not appear before his transfer to another institute. Summing up there is no definite improvement that is unquestionably the result of the operation.

3. EEG Recording

The amount of spikes and spike waves discharges remained the same. In 2 patients the focus of maximal activity shifted to the other side.

4. Behaviour

In 4 patients the behaviour was as bad as before, in 1 case worse and in 3 cases definitely better, two immediately and once after a delay of two months after the operation. Additionally 2 more patients improved, 1 after transfer to another institute and 1 after a considerable decrease in medication.

5. Psychological Tests

There was no definite change in verbal or performance tests of I.Q., concentration, accuracy, speed or perceptomotor ability.

Discussion

Amygdalotomy and fornicotomy were chosen, because there is now considerable experience, the danger is small and the reported results are good. Our results are not very encouraging for epileptologists. It may be argued that the lesion was too small as Adams found in consecutive temporal lobectomy after the failure of the amygdalotomy to produce satisfactory results. Maybe the location of the lesion was not right or the case material was different. Our target was more lateral, than that of Mundinger and Narabayashi and it seems that the intelligence was lower. It may be that since we have treated the patients ourselves for years and the patients are observed by the same staff and in the same surroundings as before that we are more aware of the so-called spontaneous fluctuations in behaviour and in seizure frequency. These may be caused perhaps by the arrival of a new patient in the group, the expectation of the patient's family or the doctor of the result of the operation, the transfer to another institute etc. It is moreover difficult to measure the degree of epilepsy by counting attacks, what is an attack and who observes the patient. For many attacks the cooperation of the patient in reporting his feelings is necessary. Maybe the patients do not want to disappoint the doctor. Maybe the fact that we both are of a rather sceptical nature has spoiled our results. Double blind operations are still difficult to perform.

Summary

8 patients with drug-resistant epilepsy underwent amygdalotomy in some cases followed by fornicotomy. There was no definite improvement in seizure frequency. The behaviour improved in 3 cases.

References

1. Adams, J. E., Rutkin, B. B. (1969), Treatment of temporal lobe epilepsy by stereotactic surgery. Confin. Neurol. *31*, 80—85.
2. van Manen, J., (1967), Stereotactic methods and their applications in disorders of the motor system. Holland: v. Gorcum ed.
3. Narabayashi, H. (1972), Stereotaxic amygdalotomy in: The neurobiology of the amygdala, p. 459—483. New York: Plenum Press.
4. Spiegel, E. A., Wycis, H. T. (1952, 1962), Stereoencephalotomy, Part I and II. New York: Grune and Stratton.
5. Umbach, W. (1966), Elektrophysiologische und vegetative Phänomene bei stereotaktischen Hirnoperationen. Berlin-Heidelberg-New York: Springer.
6. Valenstein, E. (1973), Brain control. New York: J. Wiley.

Authors' addresses: Dr. A. E. H. Sonnen, Dr. Hans Berger Kliniek, Breda, The Netherlands, Dr. J. v. Manen, Department of Neurosurgery, University Groningen, Groningen, The Netherlands, Dr. B. v. Dijk, Leyenburg Ziekenhuis, Den Haag, The Netherlands.

Acta Neurochirurgica, Suppl. 23, 221—223 (1976)

Department of Neurosurgery, Medical Research Centre
Polish Academy of Sciences, Warsaw, Poland

Stereotactic Amygdalotomy in the Light of Neuropsychological Investigations

E. Łuczywek and E. Mempel

The aim of this paper is to describe on the basis of comparative psychological studies the effect of partial amygdalectomy on the behaviour and cognitive processes of patients with acute forms of epilepsy whose long-term pharmacological treatment, and in some cases also conventional surgical treatment, had been unsuccessful.

Method

A number of clinical examinations were made, including EEG, stereo-EEG and contrast studies, and neurological and psychiatric examinations.

The psychological tests were made before the operation, in the near post-operative period, 6 months after the operation, and then every year. The following techniques were employed: clinical history with the patient's family, history and conversation with the patient, observation of the patient's behaviour in the clinic, in difficult and conflicting situations, intelligence tests, neuropsychological tests, inventory of complaints, Eysenk's presonality inventory, Taylor's personality scale of manifest anxiety, the thematic aperception test of Bandura and Walters, Goodenough's human figure drawings, questionnaires, description of behaviour and its alterations given in writing by the patients themselves.

It should be stressed that during the pre-operative period it was possible to make all of the planned examinations in only 50% of the patients due to frequent difficulties in making contact with the patients, large differences in age and intelligence.

Material

The study was performed in the years 1967–1974 on 46 patients (17 female and 29 male). The age of the patients at the time of surgery ranged from 6 to 42 years. The most numerous group were school-age patients from 7 to 18 years old (28 persons). The duration of the disease ranged from 1 to 18 years. 26 patients had been suffering from the disease for 6–15 years. In 30 patients epileptic fits occurred a number of times per day. A great majority of the patients had several types of fits such as: petit mal (absence), tonic-clonic fits, tonic fits, adversive fits, flexion fits, "salaam" fits, temporal absence, psychomotor automatisms, and dysthymic fits. The latter occurred in 37 patients, and in 8 patients such fits were the only symptom of the disease, also reflected by disturbed bioelectrical activity of an epileptic character in the temporal region.

31 patients had been hospitalized in psychiatric clinics or neurological departments more than once.

The post-operative observation period in this group amounted to 1–6 years (of which 33 patients were observed for 3–6 years).

In accordance with the suggestion put forward by Mempel [1], selective stereotactic lesions were made in the dorsal and medial part of the amygdala; the lateral and ventral parts being spared, as they affect the behaviour of essential systemic reactions.

In 36 cases, bilateral amygdalotomy was performed, and in 7 cases the lesion also covered the rostral part of the hippocampus.

With pathologically changed nervous processes, mental retardation, severe inhibition of mental development or even debility, and also unfavourable environmental conditions, one can hardly expect the patient to formulate a proper picture of the environment and himself, his basic tasks and vital needs, and the general foundations for fulfilling his needs and for determining his behaviour in relation to other people, objects and situations.

Before surgery the patients' mental state ranged from I.Q. = 38 to I.Q. = 124. 28 patients had an I.Q. below 90, of which 23 persons were below 80. As regards age of onset, it was established that in a group of 20 patients in whom the first fit took place between 1 to 5 years of age, 13 had on I.Q. above 70 and 6 between 70 and 89.

Analysis of cognitive processes showed that, beside specific defects in the form of disturbed visual and spatial analysis and synthesis, dyscalculia, there were also disturbances in thinking and, above all, memory.

Results

After the operation 17 patients had an improved intelligence quotient, gradual extension of the direct memory range, and improvement of understanding and learning.

As regards formal patterns of behaviour, we observed very clear neurodynamic changes in 37 patients. During the post-operative period we observed, among other things, a distinct decrease in emotional tension in 18 out of 22 patients, improvement in control of reactions in 30 patients, decrease in excessive activity in all patients showing this pattern of behaviour before the operation.

Disturbances in the patients' needs and motives for action usually manifested themselves by constant emotional excitation (26 patients) and by the need to relieve excessive psychic tension, aggressive attitude (24 patients). Disturbances in the patients' attitudes and reactions in difficult situations manifested themselves in the form of a fixed aggressive attitude (24 patients), particularly towards the family and, above all, towards the mother. A whole range of different behaviour patterns was observed, from simple problems of child to periodic bouts of antisocial behaviour (15 patients). In the period before the operation, 27 patients exhibited disturbances in social development.

In all the patients studied, surgery resulted in a distinct decrease in constant psychic overtension and this, in turn, resulted in a considerable improvement as regards aggressiveness and aggressive attitudes in difficult situations.

It is worth stressing that out of a total of 18 patients with an I.Q. above 90, 15 persons showed improvement; however out of 28 patients with an I.Q. below 90, only 15 showed improvement.

By eliminating or decreasing the frequency of epileptic fits, amygdalotomy improves the disturbed functions of the central nervous system and enables the patient to return to life in society. It should be stressed that in retarded patients, a stereotaxic operation gives only the foundations for the future development and shaping of the patient's emotional and social maturity.

Of great importance to the degree of improvement and its permanency is the type of environment the patient is subjected to.

14 patients were able to return to school, three of whom passed their final matriculation examinations. The rest finished specialized job-training schools, or were still studying in such schools at the time of writing. Two patients with clinical improvement were sent to psychiatric-care establishments because of bad care at home. 16 patients were engaged in various jobs, half of them being in special employment for mentally disabled persons.

References

1. Mempel, E. (1972), The influence of partial (dorso-medial) amygdalectomy on emotional disturbances and epileptic fits in humanes. In: Present Limits of Neurosurgery. Prague: Avicenum.

Authors' address: Dr. Elżbieta Łuczywek and E. Mempel, Department of Neurosurgery, Medical Research Centre, Polish Academy of Sciences, Warsaw, Poland.

Acta Neurochirurgica, Suppl. 23, 225—234 (1976)
© by Springer-Verlag 1976

Institute of Neurology of Madras, India

Stereotactic Surgery of the Limbic System in Epilepsy

V. Balasubramaniam and T. S. Kanaka*

With 2 Figures

Introduction

This paper analyses the various targets in the limbic system, the elimination of which has a beneficial effect on epilepsy. We prefer to include the amygdala, certain nuclei in the hypothalamus and the internal medullary lamina in this "so-called limbic system". The reasons for inclusion of these under one title of behavioural brain have been published in our earlier papers [2, 4]. Under the broad term epilepsy we propose to discuss many varieties of paroxysmal disorders. These will be detailed in the course of our analysis. It has to be pointed out at this stage that practically all the targets were eliminated only with one main idea and that was to control the various behavioural phenomena. These behavioural phenomena were either continuous or (only in some cases) episodic—the latter conforming to a grouping under temporal lobe or psychomotor seizure. The patients were brought in for the behavioural disorders and the surgery was performed only for this. These cases were operated upon from 1964 and are being followed up regularly to date, *i.e.* 1975.

During our follow up we found that many of them had a welcome relief from the convulsions. The relief was one of many kinds. Patients who had uncontrollable seizures even with maximum tolerable anticonvulsant medication found their seizures now manageable, or there was a reduction in intensity and/or frequency.

In the routine follow up some cases had EEG performed in the post-operative phase and this was found to have "improved" con-

* We thank Prof. B. Ramamurthi, Director, Institute of Neurology, Madras, and the Superintendent, Government General Hospital, Madras, for giving permission to present this paper. We thank the Neurologists Prof. G. Arjundas, Prof. K. Jagannathan, and Dr. C. U. Velmurugendran who read and reported on the EEG.

siderably. At about this time Narabayashi [9] published his observations on stereotaxic amygdalotomy.

We have now analysed all our cases to find out what effect surgery directed at the limbic system has on seizures.

Materials and Method

260 patients had stereotaxic amygdalotomy and 54 had stereotaxic hypothalamotomy. In addition 5 cases had stereotaxic ablation of the internal medullary lamina. 5 cases had elimination of the centrum medianum bilaterally to control salaam seizures.

Except in the group of salaam seizures, as indicated earlier, all of these patients were cases with behavioural aberration. The aetiology of behavioural disorders in patients with seizures varied and they are given in Table 1. In most of the cases the behavioural disorders were due to uncontrolled seizure or an attack of "encephalitis". In some there were other causes like cerebral agenesis, schizophrenia, meningitis, trauma etc.

For purposes of our analysis only cases who had fits are considered. Usually the patients had seizures which were not temporally connected with the behaviour disorder. In some, however, the behavioural disorders and the seizure maintained a see-saw realtionship. The types of fits met with in this analysis are given in Table 2.

These patients were treated by producing lesions in the amygdala, hypothalamus and internal medullary lamina. Some had centromedianum thalamotomy bilaterally. All the operations were done stereotactically. Our technique of stereotaxy has been described earlier [1-3]. The machine used was the Leksell's machine. The lesions were made either by diathermy or by injection of oil-wax prepared according to the formula of Narabayashi. The operations performed and the analysis of seizures are correlated in Table 3.

One word of explanation is necessary at this stage. Our own policy in the management of behavioural disorders is to do bilateral amygdalotomy at one stage initially. If amygdalotomy fails then hypothalamotomy is done. Usually it is necessary to do hypothalamotomy for these patients on only one side. This has been called secondary hypothalamotomy. In a few cases where the patients were severely retarded and for the sake of comparison hypothalamotomy was done straight away—bilateral but staged. This is referred to as primary hypothalamotomy. The details of this and the comparison of amygdalotomy and hypothalamotomy have been given in a previous paper [5].

The diagnosis of seizures and their nature was made in many

Table 1. *Aetiology of Behavioural Disorder*

Post epileptic	50
Post "encephalitic"	34
Miscellaneous	23

Table 2. *Types of Fits*

Grandmal	85
Focal—General	15
T. L. E.	5
Absence attacks	1
Myoclonus	1
Total	107

Table 3. *Behavioural Abnormalities ± Fits and Surgery Done*

Relationship of fits to behavioural abnormality	Amygdalotomy	Hytothalamotomy		Thalamolaminotomy
		Prim.	Sec.	
No fits	82	6	19	0
No relation to fits	96	3	8	5
Fits only in infancy	42	5	6	0
Fits—behaviour (see-saw)	2	0	1	0
Pre Ictal	1	0	0	0
Post Ictal	1	0	0	0
Fits controlled Behaviour problems	35	0	5	0
Others	1	0	1	0
Total	260	54		5

cases only by the history and clinical examination. EEG was not done in all cases.

The follow-up was done using a proforma mainly intended for the effect on behaviour. Where the patient had fits, more details were obtained by directing questions to the patient (when possible) or to the relatives.

Results

The cases analyzed here were those operated upon up to December '74. Thus the shortest follow-up is for 4 months and the longest is over 10 years. A few cases could not be followed for beyond 2 or 3 years.

From an overall point of view, out of 107 cases 76 had a welcome relief from seizures, *i.e.* 71% did well. This is given in detail in Table 4.

In 36 cases the seizures were completely abolished as seen in prolonged follow-up. These patients were on anticonvulsant medication preoperatively and were having fits at varying frequency. Following the operation there were no fits at all; however, the anti-

Table 4. *Relief from Seizure*

Number of patients with seizure	107
Totally abolished	36
Nearly abolished	30
Well controlled	10
Relief from seizure—Total	76

Table 5. *Analysis of Quality of Relief—Type of Seizures*

Quality of Relief	Overall Result	T.L.E.	Myclonus	Absence	General—Focal-seizures
Fits totally abolished	36	3	1	1	31
Fits nearly abolished	30	1	0	0	29
Fits well controlled	10	0	0	0	10

convulsant medication could not be stopped straight away for ethical considerations. The dosage, however, was reduced. In 30 cases out of 107 there were some fits rarely, once in a while, after the operation. These are labelled as nearly abolished. In 10 cases post-operatively the fits were much less in intensity and/or frequency. These are referred to as well controlled.

On further analysis of these 76 cases the fits were totally abolished in 3 out of the 5 patients with temporal lobe epilepsy. In 1 they were nearly abolished. Only 1 patient did not do so well.

One patient who had "absence" at least 2–3 times daily was seizure-free for more than 6 months. Now he gets an attack, once in a while. He had bilateral amygdalotomy for behaviour disorder, consisting of low rage threshold.

One patient with myoclonus and behavioural problems had total relief following amygdalotomy and unilateral hypothalamotomy.

The break-up of our cases is shown in Table 5.

We found that 70 patients who had general or focal seizures became generally improved. Of these, 4 had total abolition of fits following thalamolaminotomy.

This group also includes 15 cases of infantile hemiplegia with

Table 6. *Grading of Results*

A	Where there is no need of any drug. Patient is able to mingle easily with others
B	Very docile and given to occasional outbursts only
C	Manageable when given drugs though not leading a useful life
D	Transient improvement but relapsed
E	No change
F	Died

Table 7. *Relief from Behavioural Problems—Follow Up Study of 1 to 10 Years*

Total	107
Grade A	4
Grade B	45
Grade C	43
Grade D	9
Grade E	0
Grade F	6

behavioural problems and focal or general seizures. In all these patients unilateral amygdalotomy (of the damaged hemisphere) has totally abolished the seizures. There has been a welcome change in behaviour also. These were once candidates for hemispherectomy.

To reiterate, we find that 76 out of 107 did well from the point of view of seizures.

Of these 107 patients the relief from behavioural disorders is also given. Our grading is given in Table 6.

The results given in Table 7 show that nearly 86% had good relief. One patient died of acute Pulmonary oedema in the post-operative period, the other five in the course of 10 years due to various unrelated conditions.

Secondary Hypothalamotomy and Fits

10 cases had hypothalamotomy following amygdalotomy because their behavioural problems were not controlled. Following amygda-

lotomy the fits were controlled in 5 of them, though behavioural problem were not. After hypothalamotomy the fits were controlled in 3 cases out of 5 who still had fits. The behavioural problems were controlled in 7 of them.

Cases of Special Interest

Patient "K" aged 6 years was a regular visitor to the Neurosurgical Department (from the age of 6/12) where he was treated for bilateral subdural empyema. At the age of 4 he showed signs of aggressive behaviour associated with minor motor seizures. These were not controlled by medication. Bilateral amygdaloid lesions controlled the seizures as well as the aggression.

Patient A, male, aged 18 years, was admitted with a history of severe generalized seizures and aggressive behaviour of 8 years' duration. He was on maximum doses of Hydantinates, Phenobarbitone and Primidone. He was very much retarded. His IQ was 60. Bilateral staged hypothalamotomy was done in July 1973. His improvement with regard to behaviour is very good. He is now very docile. More than this, his seizures have stopped almost completely. He had for the first time a seizure-free interval of one year. He had one seizure almost daily pre-operatively, each attack lasting for ½ hour. After hypothalamotomy he had only two attacks in a period of twenty months. His pre-operative EEG report was "Active epileptic seizure dysfunction involving both hemispheres synchronously with no localization or lateralization of activity—Idiopathic genetically linked seizure". His EEG eight months after the operation was reported as follows. "5-6 theta activity seen equally. Paroxysmal frontally predominant synchronous activity at 3-4 c/s of 50-100 micro volts. No seizure activity dysfunction both hemisphere."

Discussion

It was pointed out as early as 1967 [1] that stereotaxic amygdalotomy can be considered as an alternative to temporal lobectomy in patients with temporal lobe epilepsy. Subsequently a paper recording the experiences in 8 cases was published by Ramamurthi and Balasubramaniam [11]. This was followed by another from our Institute, presented at The Hans Berger Centenary Symposium by Ramamurthi *et al.* Our experiences leave no doubt that stereotaxic amygdalotomy must be considered as the procedure of choice in temporal lobe epilepsy.

Stereotaxic elimination of the amygdala or hypothalamus has a definite ameliorating effect on generalized seizure in at least 71⁰/₀ of cases. There has been a reduction either in the intensity and/or frequency of seizures. This had been referred to by Narabayashi [9], and Sano [12] also. Of these patients nearly 86⁰/₀ had reduction in behavioural problems also.

The reduction of seizure following surgery of limbic system must mean that this system forms an important link in the circuit responsible for the initiation or propagation of the seizure.

It is very likely that the limbic circuits not only form an important link but possibly the main link in the abnormal circuit. Operations at the limbic level are unlike the operations at the capsular level (Kalyanaraman and Ramamurthi [6]) which only "tend" to block the "physical manifestation" of the seizure.

It is quite probable that the medial temporal lobe structures, when damaged, produce the epileptic discharge which enters the centrencephalon and produce generalized seizure. This was what

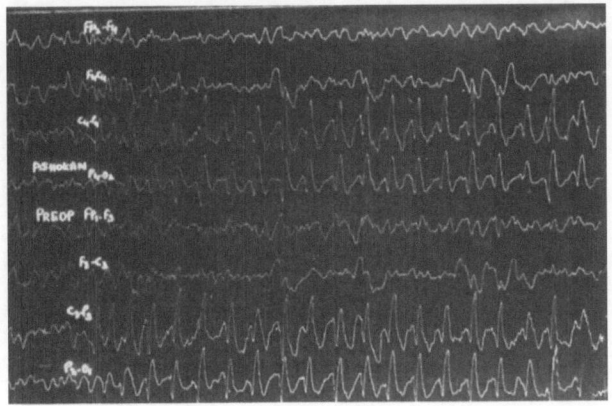

Fig. 1

was postulated by Penfield [10]. The proof for this comes from two levels:

(i) The amelioration of seizure in a patient with infantile hemiplegia who has focal or focal cum general seizure. These are the patients who once benefitted from hemispherectomy and who now have relief following amygdalotomy. Our 15 cases have proved this point.

(ii) The other proof that the limbic structures are not only concerned in the maintenance but probably in the causation of seizures is evidenced by the effect on the EEG following amygdalotomy. Seizure activity recorded from the amygdala in some patients further confirmed this. Because of certain limitations EEG could not be done on all patients but those on whom it has been carried out have shown striking improvement (Fig. 1 and 2) and in some cases there has been a return to a near-normal condition. Proof has also come [1] from the experimental level.

Experiments by Walker and Mayanagi [14] have shown that amygdala lesions produce epileptic discharges which are easily transmitted to the opposite side and also along cortical and transcortical preferential pathways.

The relationship between fits and behavioural problems is a reciprocal one. Many patients who have prolonged and uncontrolled seizures have developed behavioural problems, possibly because of the secondary hypoxic damage to the structures of the limbic or behavioural brain. Many conditions like encephalitis which damage

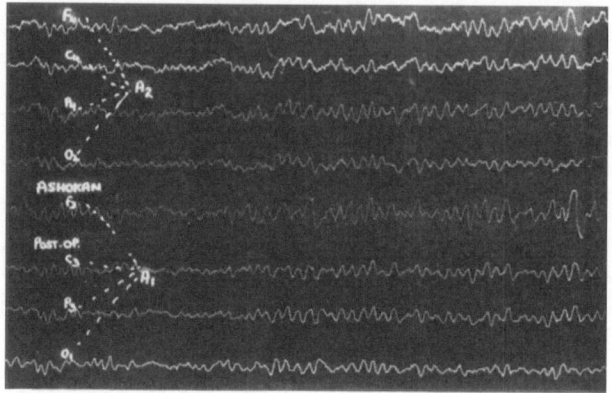

Fig. 2

the behavioural brain also damage structures like the hippocampus. Further, (at least in our minds) the structures responsible for the fits and the behavioural brain overlap to a great extent.

Generally speaking, post-epileptic cases show better relief from behavioural problems than post-encephalitic cases or cases with marked cerebral retardation. There is at present a detectable relationship between amelioration of fits and amelioration of behavioural problems, though some cases who have had no relief from behavioural problems have had relief from seizures, and vice versa.

The question has been asked—which is more effective, amygdalotomy or hypothalamotomy? This is difficult to answer. In our series there have been more cases of amygdalotomy as we usually do hypothalamotomy only when amygdalotomy fails.

The control of seizures by operation like thalamolaminotomy confirms that these areas are pathways in the abnormal circuit of epileptic discharge and that they also form part of the limbic system.

There has been relief of salaam seizure by CM thalamotomy in 4 out of 5 cases.

In cases of petit mal it is accepted that the site of origin is in the thalamus (Meyers et al.[7], Spiegel et al.[13], and Williams[15]. Williams[15], hypothesized that the clinical state of petit mal epilepsy is due to a disturbance in the thalamus which causes a rhythmic discharge throughout the cortex. The effect of this is a failure in afferent integration, resulting in secondary akinesis, flaccidity and amnesia which form the basis of the disability in petit mal attack.

Mullan[8] suggested that symptoms of epilepsy improve because a properly placed lesion in the thalamus blocks the discharge pathway or destroys "dispensable" volume of excitable neurone. Unilateral VA thalamic lesions were made by Mullan[8] in cases of epilepsy with good improvement. It is quite likely that the same mechanism works in akinetic seizures also.

Summary

During the routine follow-up of results of stereotaxic surgery in the patients treated for behaviour disorders, it was found that some of them had a bonus relief from seizures. Out of 260 amygdalotomies, 54 hypothalamotomies and 5 thalamolaminotomies performed for behavioural problems, 107 patients suffered from associated seizure disorder. 76 of them (71%) showed considerable relief from seizures following surgery. This is detailed.

It is hypothesized that probably these nuclei of the "limbic system" either initiate and/or propagate seizure activity. This view is supported by the "improvement" in EEG in addition to the clinical improvement seen in these patients.

References

1. Balasubramaniam, V., Ramamurthi, B., Jagannathan, K., Kalyanaraman, S. (1967), Stereotaxic amygdalotomy. Neurology (India) 15, 3, 119—121.
2. — Kanaka, T. S., Ramanujam, P. B., Ramamurthi, B. (1969), Sedative neuro-surgery—A contribution of the behavioural sciences. J. Ind. Med. Assoc. 53, 8, 377—381.
3. — (1969), Stereotaxic amygdaloid lesions in behaviour disorders. Ph.D. Thesis, University of Madras.
4. — Kanaka, T. S., Ramanujam, P. B., Ramamurthi, B. (1970), Sedative neuro-surgery. Neurol. (India) 18, Suppl. 1, 46—52.
5. — — (1973), Amygdalotomy and hypothalamotomy—a comparative study. Proc. Inst. Neurol. Madras. 3, No. 2, 67—74.
6. Kalyanaraman, S., Ramamurthi, B. (1970), Stereotaxic surgery for generalized epilepsy. Neurol. (India) 18, Suppl. 1, 34—41.
7. Meyers, R., Knott, J. R., Hayne, R. A., Sweeney, D. B. (1950), The surgery of epilepsy. J. Neurosurg. 7, 337—346.
8. Mullan, S., Vailati, G., Karasick, J., Mailis, M. (1967), Thalamic lesions for the control of epilepsy; a study of nine cases. Arch. Neurol. 16, 277—285.

9. Narabayashi, H., Mizutani, T. (1970), Epileptic seizures and the stereotaxic amygdalotomy. Confin. Neurol. *32*, 289—297.
10. Penfield, W., Jasper, H. (1954), Epilepsy and the functional anatomy of the human brain. Boston: Little, Brown and Co.
11. Ramamurthi, B., Balasubramanian, V., Kalyanaraman, S., Arjun das, G., Jagannathan, K. (1970), Stereotaxic ablation of the irritable focus in temporal lobe epilepsy. 4th Symp. Soc. Res. Stereoencephalotomy, New York, 1969. Confin. Neurol. *32*, No. 2-5, 316—319.
12. Sano, K. (1966), Sedative stereoencephalotomy: fornicotomy, upper mes-encephalic reticulotomy and postero-medial hypothalamotomy. In: Progress in brain Research, Vol. 21-B, p. 350—372 (Tokizane, T., Schade, J., eds.). Amsterdam: Elsevier Publ. Co.
13. Spiegel, E. A., Wycis, H. T., Baird, H. W. (1962), Subcortical mechanism in convulsive disorders. In: Stereoencephalotomy, p. 447—452 (Spiegel, E. A., Wycis, H. T., eds.), Part II. New York: Grune and Stratton.
14. Walker, A. E., Mayanagi, Y. (1974), Mechanism of temporal lobe epilepsy in the monkey. Proc. of the Hans Berger Centenary Symposium, p. 48—52 (Philips Hans, Clifford Mawdsley, eds.). Edinburgh-London-New York: Churchill Livingstone.
15. Williams, D. (1953), A study of thalamic and cortical rhythms in petit mal. Brain *76*, 59—69.

Authors' address: Dr. V. Balasubramaniam and Dr. T. S. Kanaka, Institute of Neurology of Madras, Madras, India.

Acta Neurochirurgica, Suppl. 23, 235—239 (1976)

University of Arkansas Medical Center, Little Rock, Arkansas, and
Duke University Medical Center, Durham, North Carolina, U.S.A.

Stereotactic Lesions of the Amygdala and Hippocampus in Epilepsy

H. F. Flanigin and B. S. Nashold

With 2 Figures

Introduction

Although temporal lobectomy has become well established in the treatment of unilateral epileptogenic lesions (Penfield and Jasper [13], Falconer [6], Crandall [5]. Patients with bitemporal epilepsy and with unverified temporal lobe foci have not had the option of surgical treatment available to patients with clearly unilateral temporal lobe seizure discharges.

In 1949 Wycis, Lee and Spiegel [18], using stereotactic techniques implanted depth electrodes in man and recorded from the thalamus and in 1950 Spiegel and Wycis [15] reported thalamic seizure activity. These authors [14] in 1958 proposed pallidotomy and pallido-amygdalotomy for seizures. Talairach and associates [16, 17] created therapeutic lesions in the amygdalae and hippocampi using radioactive yttrium.

Crandall, Walter and Rand [5] and Fisher-Williams and Cooper [7] reported the use of stereotactically implanted electrodes for recording seizure discharges from the temporal lobe followed by open craniotomy for surgical ablation. More recently Narabayashi [11], Heimburger [8], Adams [1], Mark [9], Balasubramaniam and Kanaka [3], Andy [2], Umbach and associates [4], Nadvornik [10], and Nashold and Flanigin [12], have reported stereotactic therapeutic lesions of temporal lobe structures in treatment of seizure disorders.

Own Material

Our experience is based on collaborative studies performed by the authors at Duke University Medical Center and University of Arkansas Medical Center in the investigation and treatment of intractable epileptics using stereotactic techniques. Using the Bertrand and Todd-Wells stereotactic units, multiple contact, teflon insulated, stainless steel wire electrodes with six contacts, 5–10 mm apart are inserted stereotactically through frontal burr holes, or through hollow screws in a technique developed by Crandall and his associates [5]. Beginning 24 to 48 hours following the introduction of electrodes recording of spontaneous activity is begun using Grass Model VI, EEG machines with magnetic tape recording where appropriate. Activation procedures include sleep, both natural and induced and Metrazol.

Table 1. *Electrode Implantation Studies*

Number of patients	27
Stereotactic lesioning	16 (two were lesioned and later resected)
Craniotomy with resection	10 (including the 2 above)
Rejected for intervention	3

Bipolar stimulation has been carried out using Grass S 44 and S 5 stimulators at frequencis ranging from 3 to 200 hertz and voltages from 3 to 20 volts with duration of waves from 1 to 2 milliseconds. Trains of stimuli have ranged from 3 to 8 seconds. In all cases there were recorded slow waves, spikes, spike and waves or repetitive spikes in the amygdalae and hippocampi. A few spontaneous and Metrazol activated seizures were recorded, usually without, but at times with a clear focus of onset. When simultaneous scalp and nasopharyngeal electrodes were used only rarely did spike or sharp wave activity occur in these electrodes to a diagnostic degree although persistent and repetitive abnormal discharges were being recorded from subcortical structures. When surface and nasopharyngeal activity was observed it was frequently not synchronous with the recorded subcortical activity and was observed to be contralateral at times.

Stimulation produced after discharges in both the amygdalae and hippocampi, at times associated with clinical phenomena related to the seizure pattern, and at other times unrelated. These were obtained from the side opposite the presumed primary focus as well as on the side of the presumed focus and usually revealed no accompaning scalp or nasopharyngeal electrode activity.

Of the 27 patients studied by stereotactic electrode implantation in this series three were considered to be unsuitable for recommendation of surgery either by stereotactic lesioning or by open craniotomy. Stereotactic lesioning was performed on 16 patients (Table 1). The procedures included unilateral hippocampal or amygdaloid lesions, unilateral combined amygdaloid and hippocampal lesions and

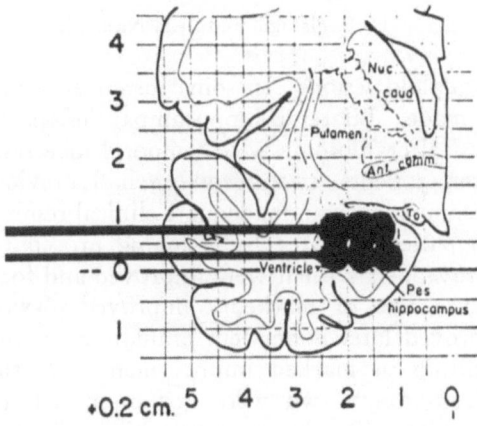

Fig. 1. Location and extent of typical multiple lesions in the amygdala

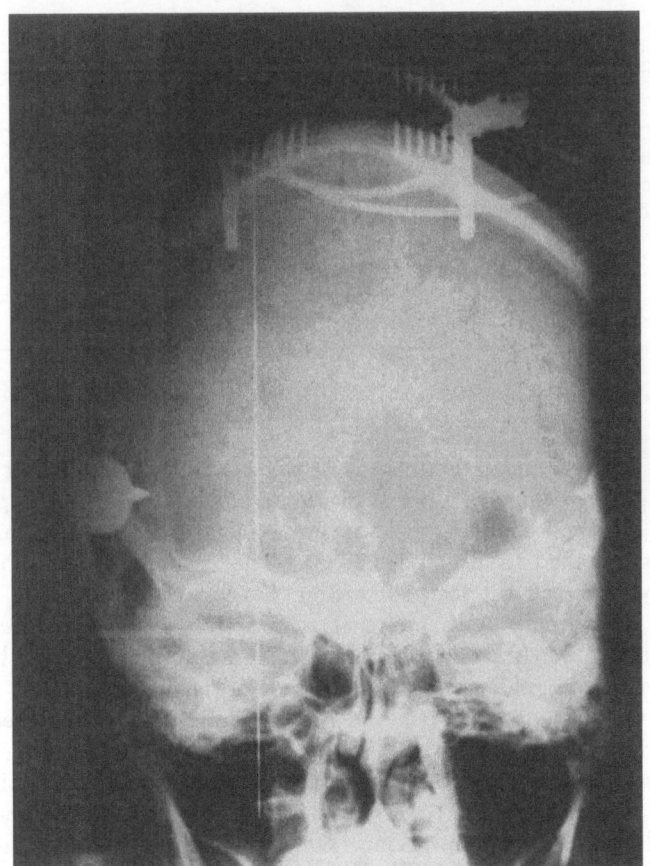

Fig. 2. X-ray showing lesioning electrode introduced by lateral approach while recording electrodes introduced from vertex remain in place

bilateral amygdaloid lesions. In some instances additional thalamic lesions were made. Bilateral hippocampal lesions were of course avoided. Classical craniotomy with temporal lobe resection was carried out in ten patients, two of whom had previously undergone stereotactic lesioning with an inadequate clinical result.

In the 16 patients treated by lesioning procedures, six patients were not improved, six patient were improved and four patients were rendered seizure free or markedly improved. Two patients who were not improved later underwent craniotomy with temporal lobe resection resulting in marked improvement. Of the ten patients undergoing craniotomy, two were not improved, three were improved, and five including the previously lesioned patients were either seizure free or markedly improved (Table 2).

Table 2. *Procedure Results*

	Lesioning	Resection	Total
Seizure free or markely improved	4		9
Improved	6	5	9
Not improved	6 (2 later resected)	3 2	8 (2 later resected)
	16 (2 later resected)	10	26 (including 2 dual procedures)

Discussion

As greater understanding of brain physiology evolves it is increasingly evident that more accurate determination of patho-physiological sites and connections becomes necessary before instituting procedures designed to alter physiology. The sampling of physiological activity obtained by scalp recording has proved inadequate, particularly in patients with bilateral temporal lobe abnormalities. We have found stereotactic implantation of depth electrodes to be free from demonstrable complications and of significant value in the preoperative study of patients to be considered for either stereotactic lesioning or open operative intervention. Stereotactic lesioning by radiofrequency electrodes presents an intermediate therapeutic procedure which may render the more formidable craniotomy and temporal lobe resection unnecessary but does not in any way inferfere with proceeding with this classical procedure if unsatisfactory results are obtained. It should not be overlooked, however, that radiofrequency lesioning does not provide for tissue study and should be considered with caution where the possibility of neoplasm is considered.

References

1. Adams, J. R., Rutkins, B. B. (1969), Treatment of temporal lobe epilepsy by stereotactic surgery. Confin. Neurol. *21*, 80—85.
2. Andy, O. J., Jurko, M. F. (1973), The amygdala in relation to olfaction. VI. Symposium of the International Society for Research in Stereoencephalotomy. Japan.
3. Balasubramanian, V., Kanaka, T. S. (1973), Amygdalotomy and hypothalamotomy—a comparative study. VI. Symposium of the International Society for Research in Stereoencephalotomy. Japan.
4. Bouchard, G., Kim, Y. K., Umbach, W. (1973), Stereotaxic methods in different epilepsies. VI. Symposium of the International Society for Research in Stereoencephalotomy. Japan.
5. Crandall, W. P., Richard, D., Rand, R. W. (1963), Clinical application of studies in stereotactically implanted electrodes in temporal lobe epilepsy. J. Neurosurg. *20*, 827—840.
6. Falconer, M. S. (1973), The place of surgery in temporal lobe epilepsy in childhood and adolescence. VI. Symposium of the International Society for Research in Stereoencephalotomy. Japan.
7. Fischer-Williams, M., Cooper, R. A. (1963), Depth recording from the human brain in epilepsy. Electroenceph. Clin. Neurophysiol. *15*, 568—587.
8. Heimburger, R. F., Whitlock, C. C., Kalsbeck, J. E. (1966), Stereotaxic amygdalotomy for epilepsy with aggressive behavior. JAMA *198*, 165—169.
9. Mark, V. H., Ervin, F. R. (1970), Violence and the brain. Harper and Row.
10. Nádvorník, P., Šramka, N., Gajdosova, D., Kokavec, M. (1973), A new stereotactic approach to the gyrus hippocampi. VI. Symposium of the International Society for Research in Stereoencephalotomy. Japan.
11. Narabayashi, H., Mizutani, T. (1970), Epileptic seizures and the stereotaxic amygdalotomy. Confin. Neurol. *32*, 289—297.
12. Nashold, B., Flanigin, H. (1973), Stereotactic evaluation of bitemporal epilepsy with electrodes and lesions. Confin. Neurol. *35*, 94—100.
13. Penfield, W., Jasper, H. H. (1954), Epilepsy and the functional anatomy of the human brain. Boston: Little, Brown.
14. Spiegel, L. A., Wycis, H. T., Baird, H. W., III. (1958), Pallidotomy and pallidoamygdalotomy in certain types of convulsive disorders. Arch. Neurol. Psych. *80*, 714—728.
15. Spiegel, E. A., Wycis, H. T. (1950), Thalamic recordings in man with special reference to seizures discharges. Electroenceph. Clin. Neurophysiol. *2*, 23.
16. Talairach, J., Bancand, J. (1973), Stereotactic approach to epilepsy. Progr. Neurol. Surg. vol. 5, pp. 297—354. Basel: Karger.
17. — David, M., Tournoux, P. (1958), L'exploration chirurgicale stereotaxique du lobe temporale dans l'épilepsie temporale. Paris: Masson et Cie.
18. Wycis, H. T., Lee, A. J., Spiegel, A. E. (1949), Simultaneous records of thalamic and cortical potentials in schizophrenics and epileptics. Confin. Neurol. *9*, 264—272.

Authors' address: H. F. Flanigin, M.D., University of Arkansas Medical Center, Little Rock, Arkansas, and B. S. Nashold, M.D., Duke University Medical Center, Durham, North Carolina, U.S.A.

Acta Neurochirurgica, Suppl. 23, 241—245 (1976)
© by Springer-Verlag 1976

Juntendo University Hospital, Tokyo, Japan

Lessons from Amygdaloid Surgery in Long-Term Observation

H. Narabayashi

In my first paper on amygdaloid surgery in 1963 [5], it was clearly stated that the idea of the procedure was to minimize the surgical lesion to one certain structure in the depth of the temporal lobe in order to achieve relief of emotional and behavioural disturbances in epileptic patients *in a wide sense,* as well as of seizure problems. This thought might have followed, at least partially, the wide experiences of the Montreal school on temporal lobe epilepsy. For selection of cases for surgery, the first category was of those patients with severely disturbed behavior and with clinical epileptic seizures, either of the grand mal or temporal lobe type, and the second category were those with no clear clinical fits, but with a definite epileptic EEG. The third were those with neither clinical seizures nor epileptic EEG, but presenting various grades of non-progressive feeblemindedness, which suggested non-progressive organic brain-damage in those cases. Most of the cases in the latter had a history of encephalitic convulsions in early childhood. Non-epileptic patients with normal intellectual ability, and behaviour problems only, and those with major psychosis were excluded from my series.

The surgical technique using stereotaxic instrumentation for siting the amygdaloid nucleus has been described elsewhere and will not be repeated here again. The nucleus is radiologically detectable without much difficulty, as lying on the antero-dorsal wall of the temporal horn tip. However it is more important to differentiate the different subnuclei within this big nuclear mass and this becomes possible by applying several physiological devices, such as analysis of difference of olfactorily evoked potentials from its medial and lateral subnuclei. It is much larger and active in the medial nuclei than in the lateral. High frequency electrical stimulation of the medial nuclei and of the area of stria terminalis produces

16

remarkable autonomic changes, such as pupillar dilatation and arrest of respiration at the inspiratory phase, even in the slightly anaesthetized state. Similar stimulation of the lateral nuclei produces much fewer changes. Also unitary recording from the nucleus through the microelectrode can identify the border of the nucleus.

From our observations, medially located lesions and especially lesions in the intermediate zone between the medial and the lateral nuclei have been found to be most effective, and it is presumed that the fibers of the stria terminalis converge in this area. However, since no postmortem study of the operated brain has yet been available, the final interpretation should be postponed for future study. As reported previously by us, the effect of surgery is observed and summarized in three different aspects [6, 7, 8, 9]. These are in relieving the emotional hypertension, in reducing the severity of epileptic clinical seizures, as well as improvement of EEG paroxysm, and in lowering the threshold of barbiturate to induce sleep.

Clinical Studies

I (Case 127). A twenty-five year old girl suffered from frequent akinetic seizures, followed by prolonged postictal aggression, during which she attacked those around her and sometimes hurt herself. Because of this, she was refused admission to mental hospitals and was kept at home in a specially designed cell. After bilateral amygdaloid surgery, all seizures and postictal phenomena described above completely disappeared and the benefit has been maintained for three years. In preoperative EEG studies repetitive bilateral anterior temporal spikes were present and were completely abolished after the procedure.

II (Case 97). An 8 year old boy was diagnosed as suffering from tuberous sclerosis. He was considered to have a mental age of two years, though he was very difficult to examine. There was marked hyperactivity with almost no concentration and little verbal communication. To keep him quiet for ten seconds was impossible and taking him into crowds, streets or shopping areas always caused trouble. He was not toilet-trained. Multiple intracranial calcification and butterfly-shaped facial adenoma classical manifestations of the disease. Frequent grand-mal attacks were very difficult to control with medication. He was considered as uneducable and refused even classes for the mentally-retarded.

Surgery was carried out bilaterally on the amygdaloid nuclei on August 17th, 1968. Postoperatively, epileptic attacks did not return, even though medication was completely stopped six months postoperatively. The few diffuse spikes which existed preoperatively, totally disappeared, but basic slowing did not change. His behaviour makadly improved, becoming educable and he started to visit special classes for the mentally retarded one year later. The boy also became more sociable, manageable and cooperative towards his family, school teachers and classmates. He became toilet trained only one month postoperatively.

He started his first words of speech three weeks after surgery, and his vocabulary then advanced to about 200 in about a year.

Discussions and Comments

The main concern of those considering the operation is the possibility of side effects from surgery, namely intellectual, memory, speech, emotional and behavioural defects and autonomic or hormonal dysfunction, either in immediate postoperative or in long-term follow up period. I was relatively reluctant to begin bilateral amygdaloid procedures, except in a few cases in the early stages of our research, which was done earlier in some other centres abroad. Routine bilateral surgery at the same sitting started late with us, *i.e.* in 1970.

It is now quite clear that relatively small bilateral lesions within the medial part of the nucleus produces no adverse side-effects, *e.g.*

1. Symptoms resembling the Kluver-Bucy Syndrome or so-called temporal lobe symptoms were not observed in our series, except in one instance and this was very slight and temporary, and subsided within two months. Slight increase of appetite was seen in about one-third of patients transiently for several weeks postoperatively with minimum increase of body weight. Changes in olfaction and taste were not experienced.

2. Calming effect on hyperactive behaviour or on easily excitable explosiveness and aggression in these patients is definite, resulting in a return to normal emotional activity. Our fear that patients would become apathetic, unemotional or poorly reactive after surgery proved to be groundless. They were observed to be almost normal in the cases described, and were able to adjust to a milieu, for their particular intellectual level. The school boy re-joins his class, playing and studying like his classmates. Of course, most of them could attend only special classes for the feebleminded. The young adult with normal or subnormal intelligence takes up again or begins a job in a factory, business company, or in farming or family business. Further developments in social activities naturally depend on their intelligence. Some of the young ladies began lessons in the teaceremony or of flower-arrangements which suggest a return of sensitivity. They can and do become excited or angry, when they are badly teased by schoolmate or co-workers. They are not emotionless. Rohrschach tests showed only minimum change, *i.e.*, very slight increase of total responses in a few cases.

It should be emphasized, that patients with epilepsy either with clinical manifestations or EEG changes which were subjected to surgery, all had an acquired etiology.

3. The sexual behaviour of patients seems also to be unaffected by surgery. Postoperatively, menstruation is normal or starts at the normal time. Two patients have married with an almost normal

sexual life and one patient is pregnant! There was only one instance of postoperative hypersexuality and that was slight and transient.

4. Memory loss was not detectable at all to clinical testing or to psychometric estimations but not all patients could be studied pre-operatively because of hyperactivity. Penfield *et al.* recently confirmed that the amygdaloid nuclei have no role in memory function [10].

5. Speech function in adults in our series is not changed. However interesting observations were made on patients of early school age. Basic changes are similar to those in adults, but since the expression of epileptic emotional disturbance in a child is usually not the same as in the adult, it is very often manifested as poor and short-lived concentration, motor-restlessness or hyperactive and minor destructive behaviour. After the procedure, the period of concentration is prolonged almost to the subnormal pattern, enabling the child to attend the classroom or to learn by television. Drs. Nagahata and Sumino established an objective measurement of behaviour and particularly for hyperactivity and short concentration span [4, 8]. As a result, they became educable and their I.Q. was very often observed to be elevated. This may be a secondary improvement of intellectual performance due to improvement in attitude and concentration. We believe *the most important aim of the procedure for such children of schoolage, is to make them educable in order to give them the most basic and primary education at the right time.*

Another important change is in patients diagnosed as idiots with no speech. In twelve epileptic children aged between 5 to 10, none could speak before surgery, though some manual expression for hunger or toiletting did just exist. More than two thirds of these started to have their first word, at the most, within three to four weeks postoperatively, and usually not later than that. Vocabulary then increases slowly. Most of these patients showed spikes in the EEG which disappeared almost completely after surgery. This might suggest that some overflow of hyperactive discharges from the nucleus might have inhibited the further development of cortical functions such as language which were still preserved but latent.

These situations are quite similar to our observations of pallido-tomy or thalamotomy in parkinsonism and some of the severely disabled dystonic cerebral palsy. Following operation muscle tone is lowered and returned to normal, but without hypotonia, followed by marked improvement in facility of movement in parkinsonism. In patients with cerebral palsy improvement in motor performance was slower and depended on intensive postoperative rehabilitation.

Finally, it is well known that destruction of the medial nuclei of the amygdala is effective and useful for improving several epileptic traits, if the symptoms are strongly drug resistant. However, it should not be the treatment of choice for abnormal emotional conditions due to other unknown etiology. At the present stage of my knowledge, the procedure is considered not applicable to the emotional behavioural problems of the major psychosis, psychoneurotic states or violence based on complex psychopathology [2, 3].

References

1. Heimburger, R. F., Whitlock, C. C., Kalsbeck, J. E. (1966), Stereotaxic amygdalotomy for epilepsy with aggressive behavior. J. Amer. med. Ass. *198*, 741.
2. Hitchcock, E., Cairns, Valerie (1973), Amygdalotomy. Postgraduate Medical Journal *49*, 894—904.
3. Kiloh, L. G., Gye, R. S., Rushworth, G. R., Bell, D. S., White, R. T. (1974), Stereotactic amygdaloidotomy for aggressive behaviour. J. Neurol., Neurosurg., Psych. *37*, 437—444.
4. Nagahata, M. (1968), Behavior disorder and minor brain damage. Shonika Shinryo *31*, 1193. (In Japanese.)
5. Narabayashi, H., Nagao, T., Saito, Y., Yoshida, M., Nagahata, M. (1963), Stereotaxic amygdalotomy for behavior disorders. Arch. Neurol. *9*, 1—16.
6. — Mizutani, T. (1970), Epileptic seizures and the stereotaxic amygdalotomy. Confin. neurol. *32*, 289—297.
7. — (1971), Stereotaxic amygdalotomy for behavioral disorders of epileptic etiology. Excerpta Medica International Congress Series No. 274. Psychiatry (Part I), pp. 175—184.
8. — (1972), Stereotaxic amygdalotomy. In: The neurobiology of the amygdala (Eleftheriou, Basil E., ed.), pp. 459—483. New York-London: Plenum Press.
9. — Shima, F. (1973), Which is the better amygdala target, the medial or lateral nuclei? (For behaviour problems and paroxysm in epileptics.) Surgical Approaches in Psychiatry, Medical and Technical Publishing Co., Ltd., edited by Laitinen, L., and Livingston, K., pp. 129.
10. Penfield, W., Mathieson, G. (1974), Memory. Arch. Neurol. *31*, 145—154.

Author's address: Professor Dr. H. Narabayashi, Juntendo University Hospital, Tokyo, Japan.

Acta Neurochirurgica, Suppl. 23, 247—250 (1976)

District Mental Hospital, Pezinok, ČSSR

Evaluation of Psychopathological Changes in Epileptic Personality after Stereotactic Treatment

J. Pogády and Ľ. Kočiš

The basic requirement for collection and sorting of materials relating to the indication and evaluation of the therapeutic effect of stereotactic treatment consists in a thorough anamnestic investigation and a precise psychopathological analysis at the plane of symptom, syndrome, nosologic or nosographic entity. The information obtained by means of these methods from the patient help to decide to which neurophysiological structures the intervention should be directed and which cluster of symptoms or syndromes should be affected by this intervention. Only a thorough knowledge of the patient's personality in its cross-section justifies considerations on indications of a stereotactic treatment.

However, besides the clinical, further evaluations are to be made at other planes, primarily at those of a psychological and neuropsychological diagnosis. A self-evident condition for the intervention is a complex check-up of the patient's inner environment, whose changes must be known and evaluated as well as the psychopathological ones.

Therefore, at the present time psychopathological changes can be registered and evaluated and sorted out at the clinical, psychological and neuropsychological plane. The latter fills the gap between neurophysiology and the theory of higher nervous activity on the one hand, and general, or developmental psychology and psychopathology on the other.

Only such a complex process of making the complicated phenomenon more exact with the aid of the above methods will enable us to apply the general rules of a stereotactic intervention. We speak of formalization by which we understand in the broadest sense of the term a precise adjustment of the investigated objects, associated with a construing of their content which permits one to operate with them in accordance with the rules of formal logic with an exclusion of their firm "substance" in constantly moving, changing objects. This exclusion is realized by abstraction, idealization, schematization and other processes and achieves its peak at the level of neurocybernetics.

In studying psychopathological changes we start from the personality structure. This constitutes the primary phenomenon. The remaining phenomena ensue through a qualitative reduction of disposing properties of the various elements forming the given psychopathological phenomenon. We are supported by principles which seem to us to be adequately verified.

Two circumstances are to be considered first and foremost: what is the relationship of an objective manifestation of personality hence of behaviour to a subjective manner of its experiencing in the consciousness and in what measure is assigment of psychopathological changes conditioned by neurophysiological concepts. The latter circumstance is of course of interest to us mainly in relation to stereotactic treatment.

Contrary to the behavioural conception of personality, we understand the relationship between the objective and the subjective in terms of the theory of reflection. We realize that in a description of the psychopathological phenomenon the subjective and objective constituent of the phenomenon cannot be exactly differentiated. If we do it, it is solely in order to take into account both the aspects of the phenomenon. In one case this may involve an invisible objective substrate, in another a subjective reflection.

In order to be able correctly to evaluate clinically a chronic symptom or group of symptoms, we must start from a certain working hypothesis, eventually from what we have termed an integrating theory of symptom and syndrome and its resistance. A pathological symptom is a process phenomenon which, because of its complexity, requires to be analyzed at various levels or planes (psychological, psychopathological, neurophysiological, neurochemical, psychosocial, etc.). At the present time, however, we do not possess a sufficient quantity of facts whose synthesis would enable us thoroughly to explain and understand the symptom. In our view, the integrating theory of symptom and syndrome and their resistance will permit us to avoid all forms of reductionism and to understand psychopathological phenomena as related to — the psychosocial or biological-structural aspect of personality, in the present case of cerebral structures.

Symptom resistance in dependence on personality structure will from the clinical or psychopathological aspect be the greater, the more centrally the phenomenon is localized, the smaller are the compensatory possibilities of other structures, the more complex is the structure of the phenomenon, and the more highly differentiated are the controlling structures.

The more highly organized structural entities then put up a greater resistance in disintegration than do the structurally poorer, lower entities. Consequently, also the resistance of the higher and lower structural psychopathological manifestations will be different. At the same time, resistance of these structures will be all the higher, the more centrally they are localized in the personality structure, and it will be all the lower, the more peripherally they are.

The pathological manifestations of epilepsy in our material relate to epileptic paroxysms and concomitant psychopathological changes of personality that cannot be influenced by current therapeutic methods. It is only natural that the primary task of therapeutic interventions in epilepsy ought to be to depress the frequency of paroxysms. This, however, is more in the neuropathologists's competence. We are interested primarily in the personality changes referred to here, where we encounter among other manifestations, affective outbursts, dysphorias, assaultive behaviour, periodic rage reactions and other kinds of uncontrollable aggressive behaviour.

We have already spoken on another occasion of our attitude towards the so-called epileptic personality and changes of its character. We do not subscribe to the view of a univocal, unambiguous organic determination of the singularities of epileptic's personality. Everyday practice, informs us and this is supported by considerable literature on the subject, that the major part of the psychopathological picture of an epileptic personality is of a psychoreactive origin. Insofar as we confine outselves to the aggressive syndrome, or more generally speaking to the hyperreactive syndrome, we presume that part of these disorders is reactively motivated. In such a case, the phylogenetically younger cerebral structures are principally involved in setting up the structure of this syndrome.

However, one part of these disorders may also be inferred from a deliberated automatic behaviour anchored and controlled mainly by phylogenetically older structures, whether these disorders are met with at the level of equivalents of epileptic paroxysms, or as the so-called ictal or episodic disorders of behaviour without any simultaneous disorders of consciousness.

These phenomena have been evaluated by means of the above procedures. However, the available batteries of psychometric methods have not permitted us to differentiate between the various components or types of the hyperreactive syndrome. Therefore, in the evaluation, emphasis was laid on an exact anamnestic investigation and psychopathological analysis.

We referred the patients for Prof. Nádvorník's team who carried them out at the stereotactic department of our District Mental Hospital, Pezinok. Since 1971, eleven patients with serious behavioural disorders within the basic diagnosis of epilepsy, have been operated upon.

The first case involved a patient with an increasing frequency of epileptic fits, with onset of traits of impulsivity, unadaptability and aggressiveness. Concomitant alcoholism made treatment of epilepsy practically impossible. After an intervention into the left amygdalo-hipocampal complex, there was a radical withdrawal of the aggressive behaviour, frequency of fits decreased while impulsiveness was only partly affected.

In the second case, stereotactic treatment was indicated because of affects of anger resonant moods, hostility, persecution and querulant delusions. The intervention was again directed to the left amygdalohippocampal complex, but in addition, a bilateral posterior hypothalamotomy was also performed. This resulted in an improvement in the resonant moods and affects of anger and a restructuralization of the delusions. Aggressiveness, hostility and impulsivity were affected only partially.

In two further cases with a dominance of the aggressivity syndrome, a radical bilateral hypothalamotomy or intervention into the amygdalohippocampal complex resulted also in only a partial reduction of aggressive behaviour. Similar results were obtained in our fifth patient in whom a bilateral posterior hypothalamotomy was combined with an intervention into the left amygdalohippocampal complex.

In the remaining patients, stereotactic intervention was indicated because of an aggressive or hyperreactive syndrome. Posterior hypothalamotomy was performed in all the patients. The results proved to be practically uniform—a moderation or total disappearance of aggressive manifestations.

Secondary symptoms noted in the patients were sporadic insomnia and disorders of memory which perhaps may be related to a lesion to the mammillothalamic tract. However, these side symptoms tended spontaneously to recede.

The follow-up did not show any reduction of intellectual or clinical neurological status in a single patient.

Author's address: Ass. Prof. J. Pogády and Dr. Ľ. Kočiš, District Mental Hospital, Pezinok, ČSSR.

Acta Neurochirurgica, Suppl. 23, 251—255 (1976)
© by Springer-Verlag 1976

Mental Hospital Jankomir, Zagreb, Yugoslavia

Centrencephalic Epilepsy and Suboccipital Derivations

B. Faber and F. Hajnšek

With 2 Figures

Introduction

There is a special group of epilepsies whose primary source lies within so called "centrencephalic" regions and are commonly characterized by loss or impairment of consciousness during the attack and by a characteristic EEG pattern which shows bilaterally synchronous discharges of the spikes and wave complex of various frequency (Penfield-Jasper). Frequently, however, these specific discharges are often overlooked in standard recording performed from the scalp where merely slow activity or biphasic slow waves can be detected. Apart from this, the occurrence of these "centrencephalic" discharges is not always bilaterally synchronous from the very beginning, as was believed earlier (Rovit *et al.*, Hajnšek *et al.*) (Fig. 1). These facts led us to use suboccipital EEG recordings for epilepsy where the primary source appeared to lie within centrencephalic regions. This approach was used in order to record activities originating in the suboccipital area in the regions termed "centrencephalic". The technique of needle-electrode application is as follows: The needle is introduced and placed extracranially starting from the back part of the mastoid process of the temporal bone half a centimetre upwards from its crest. The needle is then led vertically to the sagittal plane of the skull and lightly slant-wise upwards terminating at the atlanto-occippal joint (Fig. 2). If the needle is introduced at the right point there is no danger of lesion of any structures in these regions.

Material

This method of detection has been applied for the last four years in cases with infratentorial symptomatology (posterior cranial groove) and in patients suffering from various forms of epilepsy, and particularly in those with so-called primary generalized attacks. The

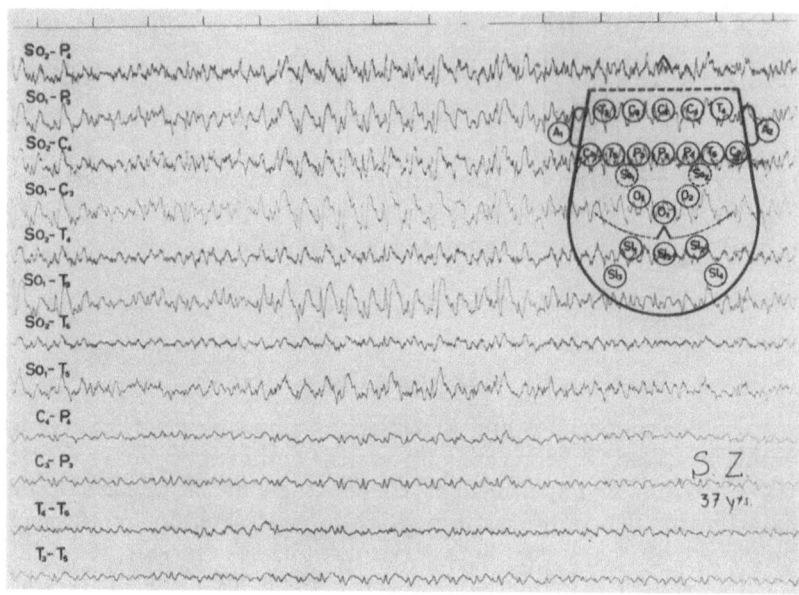

Fig. 1

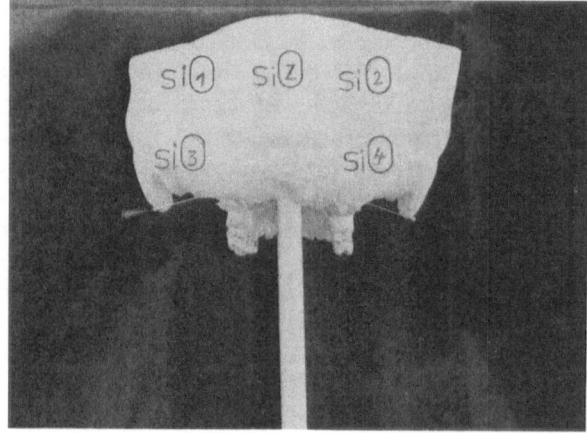

Fig. 2

recordings performed were either standard or combined with chemical activations by Megimid or Epontol (Faber *et al.* 1973). Thus we could make an exact diagnosis of space occupying lesions and other "macrofactors" in 18 out of 25 cases studied, and in 10 patients with "forced normalization" according to Landolt, the application of suboccipital derivations with Epontol activation detected epileptogenic activity in the phase of "hypernormal" EEG and the productive

Table 1

EEG	F + C	Csv	Cmv	Cfv	C 3/s	F	Dpd	Dd	B	N	Σ
Dpd	1			4							5
Dd	5		2	4	1			8			20
B				1		1		2	3		7
Total	6		2	9	1	1		10	3		32

Legend: F + C = Primary subcortical focus with secondary bilateral discharges of the centrencephalic type. Csv = Centrencephalic discharges—slow variant (2–2½ seconds). Cmv = Centrencephalic discharges—mixed variant (2–5 c/seconds). Cfv = Centrencephalic discharges—fast variant (3½–5 c/seconds). C 3/sec = Centrencephalic discharges—3 c/seconds spike and wave complex. Dd = Diffuse "dysrhythmic" discharges (slower than alfa, as a rule). B = Border case finding. N = Normal finding.

psychosis in all the cases. Out of 74 epileptic patients studied, 32 showed centrencephalic changes in EEG, 24 suffered from symptomatic epilepsy (clinically diagnosed as grand mal attacks) and in 12 cases major attacks (grand mal) were combined with psychomotor crises.

The group of patients with centrencephalic type of epilepsy [32] were treated separately. In this group the EEG tracing recorded by standard scalp derivations differed greatly from the records obtained by suboccipital electrodes in a relatively large number of cases (Table 1).

Discussion

In a relatively large number of cases with primary generalized epilepsy the attacks are often hard to differentiate on the basis of case history only. The standard EEG scalp tracing often reveals non-specific slower waves or non-specific changes only. When sub-occipital recordings were applied in such cases, we detected highly specific epileptic elements in the EEG tracing as spike and wave complexes of various frequencies with or without a primary subcortical focus. Many successive recordings by standard scalp electrodes do not always reveal the real nature of the disease although the clinical data are persistently indicative of the epilepsy of the centrencephalic type. In such cases the application of sub-occipital electrodes is the method of choice for electrographic veri-fication of a specific form of epilepsy. In order to provide early detection of probable primary focus we have applied a combined recording by suboccipital electrodes and with Epontol or Megimide. This technique enabled the detection of the primary focus in 6 cases.

According to Table 1 in our group of 32 patients with previous data indicative of epileptic attacks corresponding to those of "centr-encephalic" type, there was not a single case with centrencephalic changes in EEG when the standard recording method was carried out. The application of suboccipital electrodes detected such changes in 18 patients. The only "variant" not detected and recorded was the slow variant, which is quite understandable since this form occurs mainly in younger patients and usually accompanies more wevere forms of epilepsy. Also, only one case of pure spike and wave complex of 3 c/sec. was detected. In 10 case the changes remained marked as "diffuse dysrhythmic" although clinically speaking there were elements indicative of primary generalized epilepsy. Only three patients continued to show non-specific changes and were classed as borderline cases. In the last two groups Epontol activation was applied and consequently a further 5 centrencephalic tracing samples were obtained. It is interesting to observe that paroxysmal discharges change and are clearly differentiated as centrencephalic ones. This fact calls for a more precise differentiation of paroxysms, which is particularly important in determining the optimal therapy. When simultaneous recording using both suboccipital and scalp electrodes is performed, a stereo-technique is obtained in the simplest way possible.

Summary

1. The application of suboccipital electrodes provides earlier and safer detection of pathological activities within deep infratentorial structures than the standard recording techniques.

2. Spike and wave complexes are better differentiated with regard to frequency, duration and possible primary focus, which is of basic importance in determining the optimal therapy.

3. The combination with chemical activation methods increases the number of positive findings and thus contributes to a better diagnosis.

4. The technical procedure is not complicated or dangerous for the patient. It causes less pain and inconvenience than the application of the needle in sphenoidal electrodes.

5. Suboccipital electrodes applied alone or in combination with the scalp and sometimes with sphenoidal electrodes represent the simplest technique of recording and detecting deeply located focal centres as well as electrographic changes originating in deep infratentorial structures, without demaging the meninges.

References

Faber, B., Hajnšek, F. (1973), Propanidid (Epontol)—A new activation method in EEG. Epilepsia (Amst.) *14*, 3, 357—362.

Hajnšek et al. (1969), Frequency analysis of EEG in centrencephalic epilepsy using Petersen's analyser and photic stimulation. Neuropsihijat. *17*, 3—4, 21—27.

Hajnšek, F., Faber, B. (1974), A new derivation with suboccipital placement of electrodes. A preliminary report. Acta med. iug. *28*, 135—142.

Landolt, H., Lorentz de Hass, A. M. (1958), Lectures on epilepsy. Amsterdam-London-New York-Princeton: Elsevier.

Penfield, W., Jasper, H. H. (1954), Epilepsy and functional anatomy of the brain. Boston: Little, Brown and Co.

Rovit, R. L., et al. (1961), Sphenoidal electrodes in the electrographic study of patients with temporal lobe epilepsy, an evaluation. J. Neurosurg. *18*, 151.

Authors' address: Dr. B. Faber and Dr. F. Hajnšek, Mental Hospital Jankomir, Zagreb, Jugoslavia.

Acta Neurochirurgica, Suppl. 23, 257—262 (1976)
© by Springer-Verlag 1976

Research Laboratory of Clinical Stereotaxy at Neurosurgical Department,
Comenius University, Bratislava, ČSSR

Some Observations in Treatment Stimulation
of Epilepsy

M. Šramka, G. Fritz, M. Galanda, and P. Nádvorník

With 1 Figure

Introduction

In recent years, surgeons dealing with epilepsy appear to be abandoning ablative procedures on large anatomical brain structures endeavouring now to change function with minimal injury.

These procedures were heralded by the Baldwin method [1] of local brain cooling under simultaneous administration of a single high dose of antiepileptic medication. The low temperature of the brain was supposed to increase the permeability of the haematoencephalic barrier and to bring about, under the effect of chemical compounds, quite a favourable change of nervous system function. A different, though similarly orientated method, was that of stimulation of nervous structures which is supposed to have originated from acupuncture, as well as the application of impulse technique of nervous structures stimulation which might well imitate the acupunctures. Favourable results obtained in stimulating the dorsal surface of the spinal cord in the process of pain according to Shealy [6] led to the stimulation being applied in epilepsy therapy as well. The first steps here were made by Cooper [3] who stimulated the cerebellar cortex, *i.e.*, Purkynje cell in cerebellar cortex which were assumed to have an attenuating effect on both the tonic and phasic motions.

The stereotactic method provided the opportunity of direct stimulation even in deep brain structures and, therefore, experiments are now being made to extend the method to the treatment of epilepsy. For a programme of stimulation the dentate nucleus and the caudate nucleus particularly the head of the caudate are considered the most useful areas.

Material

In the Research Laboratory of Clinical Stereotaxy at Neuro-surgical Department, Medical School of Comenius University, in Bratislava experience with a group of 10 patients suffering from epilepsy in whom therapeutic stimulation was performed three times in nucleus dentatus and five times in nucleus caudatus (one patient was stimulated in both structures simultaneously). In seven patients generalized form of grand mal type, in two patient partial temporal form and in one myoclonic epilepsies were found (Table 1).

Structure stimulations were made by means of chronic electrodes. Simultaneously, by means of other electrodes introduced most frequently into gyrus hippocampi and the nonspecific thalamus system, stimulation—provoked changes were followed. The registration from subcortical structures was, moreover, compared to that taken on the head surface. The stimulation itself was programmed and arranged so that the appropriate structures were stimulated once a day by electric impulses, with the frequency of 10 and 100 Hz of one milli-second duration and, the voltage of 10 V, for as long as three minutes. The stimulation would be performed during 1–8 days.

Stimulating nucleus dentatus, when chronical electrodes had been introduced from the occipital approach, increased actively of only nucleus dentatus was registered under simultaneous late depression of the activity of gyrus hippocampi of the other side. In one of the patients the changes were not quite convincing and, since the epi-leptical activity of gyrus hippocampi proved to be a marked one and of the focal type, it was decided to apply stereotactic longitu-nal hippocampectomy. Caput nuclei caudati was stimulated using the same technique but with electrodes introduced from the coronal approach. Stimulation was performed only once by means of a pace-maker and once by normal rhythm from the hypothalamus of the same patient recorded on magnetic tape.

Following stimulation, the spontaneous activity of caput nuclei caudati increases under simultaneous decrease of mediobasal struc-tures of temporal lobe and even of non-specific thalamic structures (Fig. 1).

In one of the patients, who wa ssubjected, two years ago, to stereotactic surgery in the anterior thalamic reticulum, chronic elec-trodes were introduced into the amygdalo-hippocampal complex and non-specific thalamus and functioned by mechanical irritation of these structure. The epileptic activities both within and on the head surface completely disappeared after three days.

Table 1

Patient	Surgery	Diagnosis	Structures	Stimulation	Days of treatment	Result
U. M., f. 45 years	15. 2. 1974	ep. P	Dt bilat.	10 and 100 Hz 1 ms, 10 V, 3 min	1	temporary improved
M. M., m. 34 years	1. 3. 1974	ep. P	Dt bilat.	10 and 100 Hz 1 ms, 10 V, 3 min	1	temporary improved
O. J., m. 16 years	18. 7. 1974	ep. GM	Dt bilat. Cd sin	10 and 100 Hz 1 ms, 10 V, 3 min	4	improved
M. J., m. 19 years	3. 9. 1974	ep. GM	Cd bilat.	10 and 100 Hz 1 ms, 10 V, 3 min	4	improved
D. A., f. 23 years	17. 9. 1974	ep. GM	Cd bilat.	10 and 200 Hz 1 ms, 10 V, 3 min	6	without seizures
M. Š., f. 33 years	23. 10. 1974	ep. GM (p)	Cd bilat.	10 Hz 1 ms, 10 V, 3 min	6	without seizures
Č. V., m. 21 years	25. 1. 1975	ep. GM	Cd bilat.	10 and 100 Hz 1 ms, 10 V, 3 min	8	improved
B. M., f. 34 years	29. 1. 1975	ep. GM (p)	Cd bilat.	permanent stimulation by pace marker	10	temporary improved
O. J., m. 28 years	13. 2. 1975	ep. myoclonica	Dt sin cortex cerebelli	10 and 100 Hz 1 ms, 10 V, 3 min	8	temporary improved
K. J., m. 31 years	30. 10. 1972	ep. GM (p)	A-G. hp bilat. La. m bilat.	mechanical stimulation	3	without seizures

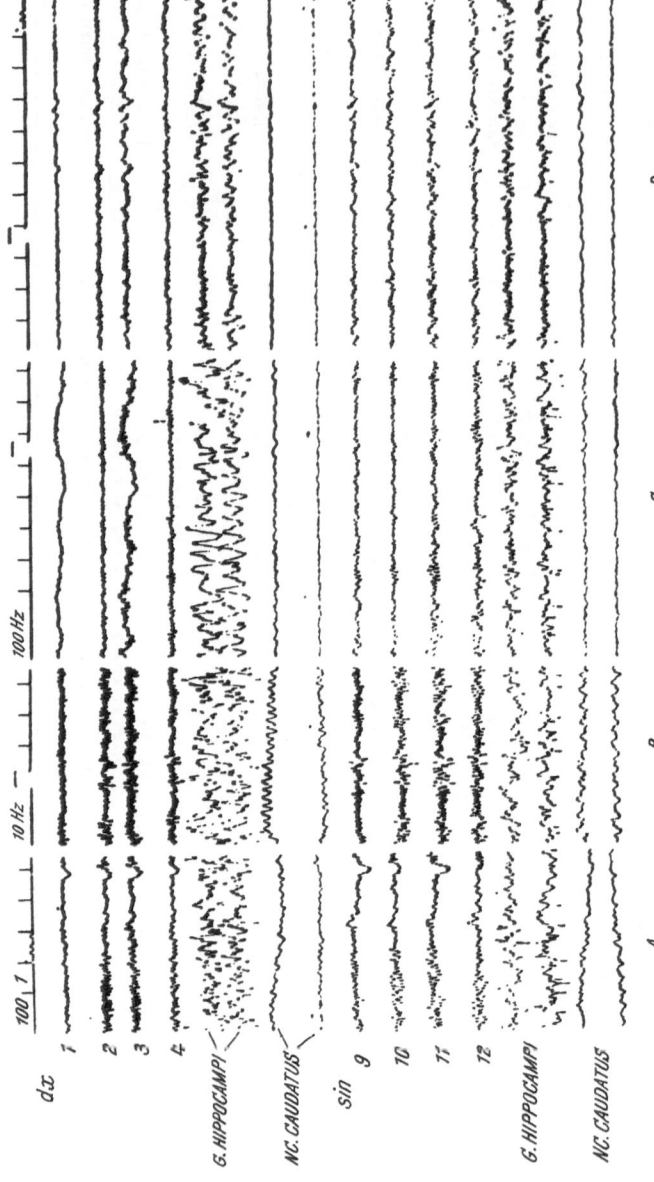

Fig. 1. Stimulation of caput nc. caudati bilat. A Before stimulation, B after stimulation, C after stimulation 1st day, C after stimulation 2nd day, D after stimulation 5th day. *1* F-P cortex dx, *2* P-O cortex dx, *3* F-T cortex dx, *4* T-O cortex dx, *5–6* g. hippocampi dx, *7–8* nc. caudatus dx, *9* F-P cortex sin, *10* P-O cortex sin, *11* F-T cortex sin, *12* T-O cortex sin, *13–14* g. hippocampi sin, *15–16* nc. caudatus sin (*1–16* EEGrecords)

Discussion

Stimulation of nervous structures in epilepsy appears to be a new approach in the treatment of attack-like diseases which has so far not been sufficiently elucidated. Our knowledge in this field might only be widened by the active work of Cooper [2, 3] and Nashold [5].

Apart from the favourable results expected we should also take account of some serious complications. We have met with them in one female patient, stimulated in the posterior sensitive thalamic structures on account of pain. In this patient, 3 weeks stimulation resulted in iatrogenic epilepsy. This complication is quite similar to the phenomenon known from experiments on animals. By stimulating the amygdalo-hippocampal complex and septal structures of these animals, epilepsy may be provoked easily and permanently. This experience was described by Goddard [4] as "kindling phenomenon". The stimulation to remove epilepsy is the antikindling phenomenon and may well be considered as the transformation of the function of nervous structure, i.e., a special case of brain function transplantation.

Summary

In a group of 10 patients suffering from epilepsy therapeutic stimulation was applied by means of chronic electrodes and a technical stimulator three times in nucleus dentatus, five times in nucleus caudatus, once in both structures simultaneously. Once chronic electrodes were introduced into the amygdalo-hippocampal complex and non-specific thalamic system bilaterally. One patient was stimulated by means of a pacemaker and once by normal rhythm from the hypothalamus of the same patient using magnetic tape. The patients were subjected to stimulations once a day for a period of 1–8 days.

The results obtained are being discussed with respect to Goddard's kindling phenomenon.

References

1. Baldwin, M., Ferrier, R. (1963), Cerebral deposition drugs at low temperatures. J. Neurosurg. 20, 2, 637—646.
2. Cooper, I. S., Amin, I., Gilan, S., Waltz, J. M. (1974), The effect of chronic stimulation of cerebellar cortex on epilepsy in man. In: The cerebellum, epilepsy and behavior (Cooper, I. S., Riklan, M., Snider, R. S., eds.), pp. 113—171. New York: Plenum Press.
3. — Gilman, S. (1973), The effect of chronic cerebellar stimulation upon epilepsy in man. 98th Annual Meeting Amer. Neurol. Assoc., July 11–13, 1973, Montreal.

4. Goddard, V. G. (1967), Developed of epileptic seizures through brain stimulation at low intenzity. Nature *214*, 1020—1021.
5. Nashold, B. S., Wilson, W. P., Fulghum, J. (1975), Cerebellar stimulation and
brain activity. Symposium on stereotactic treatment of epilepsy. Collection
of Abstracts, SLS, Bratislava, 1975, pp. 79—80.
6. Shealy, C. N., Mortimer, J. T., Hagfors, N. R. (1970), Dorsal column electro-
analgesia. J. Neurosurg. *32*, 560—564.

Author's address: M. Šramka, M.D., Neurosurgical Department, Medical
School, Comenius University, Bratislava, ČSSR.

Acta Neurochirurgica, Suppl. 23, 263—269 (1976)

Department of Surgical Neurology, University of Edinburgh, and
The Royal Infirmary and Western General Hospital, Edinburgh, Scotland

Stereotactic Lesions for the Control of Intractable Epilepsy

F. J. Gillingham, W. S. Watson, A. A. Donaldson,
and V. M. Cairns

With 2 Figures

Since 1955 somewhat over a thousand patients with Parkinsonism have been treated by stereotactic central lesions and the incidence of epilepsy has been very low, in fact in only two instances. In one of them it was strictly of a Jacksonian type and related to a cortical scar at the site of the burrhole in the premotor area. This is of interest in view of the observations of Williams (1965)—"Whilst focal attacks are confined to the cortex and subcortex focal attacks leading to a generalised convulsion abnormally activate the thalamic reticular structures which are essential to the development and diffuse spread of the general discharge. The thalamic mechanisms responsible must be intact for this process of activation and propagation for generalised epilepsy to occur." Jinnai et al. (1963) attempted to define the conduction pathways of the focal epileptic convulsion in animal experiments and came to the conclusion that these might be interrupted with benefit at the most strategic point, namely the field of Forel (Fig. 1). He then applied this knowledge to some of his patients who were totally incapacitated and deteriorating because of uncontrolled severe and frequent epileptic attacks. The longterm results were promising and a number lost all major attacks. In these cases the pathways were interrupted by the stereotactic method using electrocoagulation. Our interest in Jinnai's work began because of an observation in 1958 on a patient with postencephalitic Parkinsonism who suffered from attacks of compulsive calculation and disturbed consciousness many times a day so that he became almost inaccessible. The stereotactic lesion was placed more anteriorly than usual because of particular difficulty in abolishing his tremor.

Tremor was abolished but the lesion also reduced the frequency of
the compulsive attacks to one or two a week so that he has been
totally rehabilitated since (Gillingham *et al.* 1960). The important
point about this is that the area of destruction required to relieve his
tremor transected the posterior limb of the internal capsule which
included Jinnai's pathway but at a higher level than his point of
interruption (Fig. 2). It is, of course, realised that this was not a

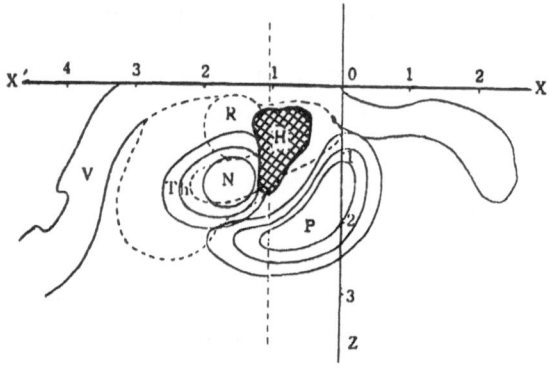

Fig. 1. Stereotactic map of Forel-H fields

case of epilepsy in the true definition but there are some similarities.
During our own stereotactic procedures we have used a technique
based on that of Guiot (Gillingham *et al.* 1960). Accuracy does not
only depend on the precise engineering of the guiding apparatus or
indeed on the precision of radiological techniques but also on the use
of physiological parameters such as stimulation and depth micro-
electrode recording (Guiot, Hardy and Albe Fessard, 1962). The
micro-electrode which is 10 μ at its tip protrudes from the main electrode and as it is passed through the brain it records the various
types of electrical discharge from the different nuclei and the borders
of grey and white matter of the basal ganglia (Gaze *et al.* 1964).

In our work on epilepsy the tendency has been with succeeding
patients to move from the field of Forel to the ventrolateral nucleus
of thalamus (v.o.p. and v.o.q.) and later to the posterior limb of the
internal capsule and finally to the pallidocapsular zone at the genu
of the internal capsule. The field of Forel is a crowded area and
deficits occur more easily in our experience with errors of placement
of lesions, *e.g.*, dysarthria. It is not yet certain which of these sites
is most effective in the diminution of fits in patients with intractable

epilepsy as the numbers are as yet too small and the follow-up not long enough. The results of operations on 10 patients are shown in Table 1.

Pre- and post-operative psychometric studies were carried out in the first eight patients and the results follow.

Intellectual level: In all eight patients function was below average level intellectually, with five falling below normal limits.

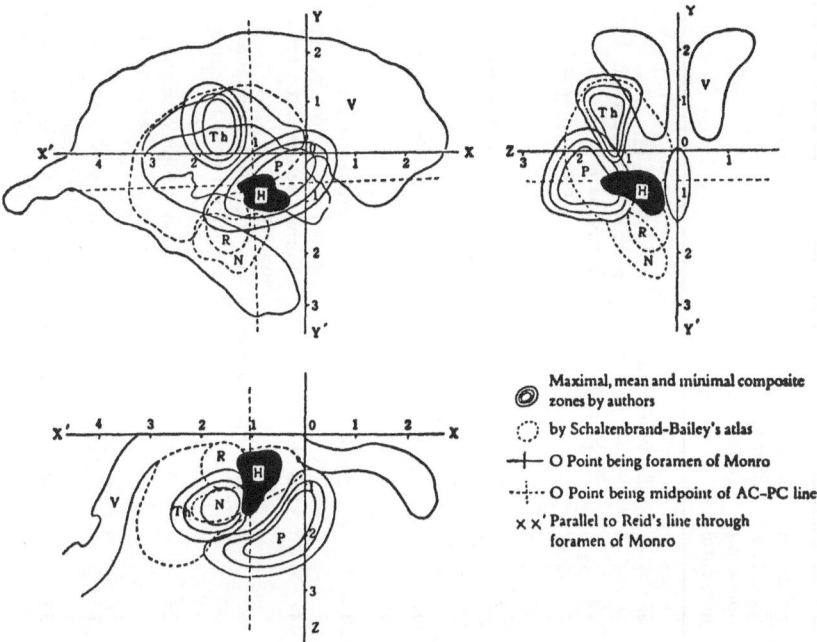

Maximal, mean and minimal composite zones by authors

by Schaltenbrand-Bailey's atlas

O Point being foramen of Monro

O Point being midpoint of AC–PC line

x x' Parallel to Reid's line through foramen of Monro

Fig. 2. Slow voluntary movements of flexion and extension of the left wrist. The tremor in the control record is clearly seen in the velocity force and in the electromyograms. The instability is less marked after the lesion has been placed in the right pulvinar

Changes in cognitive function: Minimal increases in scores on a test of non-verbal reasoning occurred postoperatively in six of the eight cases (in the later cases this was noted on testing as early as one week postoperatively). Minimal decreases in scores on a vocabulary test have been noted, more particularly following bilateral lesions. Learning and memory function show no consistent changes.

Psychomotor speed: This was investigated through studies of

Table 1. *Results of Operations on 10 Patients, Stereotactic Brain Lesions in Intractable Epilepsy*

Patient and age	Lesion side and sites spacing in months	Follow up since last operation in months	Reduction in fit frequency and severity	Neurological state	Personality change since operations
[1] W. M. ♂ 34	[R] F. F./2 months [L] F. F.	87	By two thirds	Mild ataxia [R] after second operation	None, stable invalid living at home
[2] J. D. ♂ 35	[R] V. L. Th/7 months [L] Cap/21 months [R] V. L. Th/9 months [R] Cap	29	By half	Motor paresis [L] limbs before and after operation	Cerebration slowed, stable living in long stay hospital
[3] L. A. ♂ 30	[R] Cap/3 months [R] Cap/8 months [L] V. L. Th	27	By half	Normal before and after operation	Much more stable, working as gardener
[4] M. McC. ♀ 19	[L] Cap/6 months [R] V. L. Th	51	By three quarters	Normal before and after operations	None, stable intellectually more alert dull living at home
[5] A. P. ♂ 44	[R] Cap/3 months [L] Cap	43	By one quarter	Mild dysarthria following second operation	More stable, working in sheltered workshop
[6] D. M. ♂ 13	[R] Pal/Cap/FF/1 month [L] Pal/Cap	34	By half	Normal before and after operations	Dull and backward since birth, much less aggressive
[7] B. R. ♂ 19	[R] Pal/Cap/20 months [L] Pal/Cap	7	By three quarters	Right cerebrum atrophic since birth normal before and after operation	Stable, normal youth
[8] D. P. ♂ 14	[R] Pal/Cap/2 months [L] Pal/Cap	25	By three quarters	Receding right face and limb paresis after second operation	Stable, normal youth
[9] T. C. ♀ 46	[L] FF	24	By half	Temporary mild weakness of the right hand	None, stable person
[10] F. C. ♀ 21	[R] Pal/Cap/V. L. Th	22	By half	Postoperative receding very mild weakness of the left face and arm	None, stable clerkess

reaction time, using a visual stimulus. In individual cases there have been postoperative changes, but no consistent trends emerge for the group of eight as a whole.

Personality and behaviour: Conventional questionnaire methods of assessment of personality have only limited application in patients functioning at lower intellectual levels. These were applied where possible and showed little evidence of post-operative change.

Interpretation of behaviour must also be made in the context of level of intellectual function. Thus while several of these patients appeared immature in behaviour, no specific areas of personality abnormality or behavioural disturbance emerged. Three of the eight patients have been classed as disturbed: in one there was a history of psychotic episodes, in another a personality disturbance and in a third severe behaviour disturbance, with violent destructive behaviour and marked instability. All three of these cases showed improvement in general effectiveness postoperatively. The first case attended an Industrial Therapy Unit, the second was in open employment and the third resides in an epileptic colony and attends special school, but six months postoperatively showed marked improvement in behaviour.

Discussion

1. It can be seen that a significant though variable reduction in fit severity and frequency has been achieved by these operations in the ten patients.

Owing to the well known practical difficulties in calculating and evaluating fits of patients living at home more precise figures would not be reliable.

The results in fit reduction are in practice based on a comparison of the patients' state in the six months leading upt to the first operation, and the period following, the six months, after it. It is necessary to discard the person's epileptic state whilst operations are in progress and for at least six months after the last operation.

2. In each patient the size of lesion was small (5 mm × 5 mm × 7 mm) and it might be argued that larger lesions might have been more effective but the risks of morbidity might well have been higher particularly in bilateral lesions.

3. The variability in fit reduction in the different patients might suggest that either the field of Forel, ventrolateral nucleus of thalamus or posterior limb of internal capsule was the most effective lesion site. No firm deduction can be made from the results in these patients, although it is probable that we are interrupting a conduc-

tion system similar to that already defined in the surgical management of Parkinsonism (Gillingham, 1970) but of course different to some extent in anatomical distribution.

4. The lack of neurological complications in Cases 2, 3, 4, 6 and 7 is encouraging.

5. Various kinds of intellectual deterioration and personality abnormality are, of course, common in severe chronic epileptic patients often on complex drug regimes. Only in patient 2 was there a significant deterioration of personality associated with the operations. There were in this patient many complicating factors such as repeated status epilepticus and concussional head injuries. In this respect bilateral operative lesions, particularly if sited inaccurately, are likely to lead to intellectual slowing for a time.

6. Patients 1, 2 and 4 showed marked E.E.G. changes of a focal and generalised pattern before the operations, and these abnormalities persisted afterwards despite a very considerable reduction in their epileptic fits. It is of interest that patients 3 and 5 have at no time ever showed interseizure E.E.G. changes.

In summary, therefore, experience over 7 years with these patients would suggest that there is a place for stereotactic central lesions in selected epileptic patients, particularly when seizures are severe, frequent drug resistant and likely to be intractable. These operations might more profitably be carried out at a much earlier age and before the epileptic pattern has become so firmly established. In this group the best results showed a 75% elimination of fits which was achieved in patient 4 who was operated on when 17, although on psychometric assessment patients 5, 7 and 10 are regarded as the most effectively treated at present in terms of occupational attainments and personal relationships.

References

Cairns, Valerie, M. (1974), Epilepsy, personality and behaviour. In: Epilepsy; proceedings of Hans Berger Centenary Symposium (Harris, P., and Mawdsley, C., eds.), pp. 256—268. Edinburgh: Churchill Livingstone.

Gaze, R. M., Gillingham, F. J., Kalynaraman, S., Porter, R. W., Donaldson, A. A., Donaldson, I. M. L. (1964), Microelectrode recordings from the human thalamus. Brain *87*, 691—706.

Gillingham, F. J. (1969), Introduction to scientific sessions. In: Third Symposium on Parkinson's Disease (Gillingham, F. J., and Donaldson, I. M. L., eds.), pp. 1—5. Edinburgh: E. & S. Livingstone Ltd.

— Watson, W. S., Donaldson, A. A., Naughton, J. A. L. (1960), The surgical treatment of Parkinsonism. Brit. med. J. *2*, 1395—1402.

Jinnai, D., Nishimoto, A. (1963), Stereotaxic destruction of Forel-H for treatment of epilepsy. Neurochirurgica *6*, 164—176.

Mullan, S., Vailati, G., Karasick, J., Mailis, M. (1967), Thalamic lesions for the control of epilepsy. A study of 9 cases. Arch. Neurol. (Chicago) *16*, 277—285.
Williams, D. (1965), The thalamus and epilepsy. Brain *88*, 539—566.

Authors' addresses: Professor Dr. F. J. Gillingham, Dr. W. S. Watson, Department of Surgical Neurology, University of Edinburgh, Scotland, and Dr. A. A. Donaldson, Dr. V. M. Cairns, The Royal Infirmary and Western General Hospital, Edinburgh, Scotland.

Acta Neurochirurgica, Suppl. 23, 271—281 (1976)
© by Springer-Verlag 1976

University of Southern California, Department of Physiology, Los Angeles,
California, U.S.A.

Experiences with Pharmacological Methods
for the Lateralization of Temporal Epileptic Foci

N. A. Bercel

With 9 Figures

Introduction

Of 96 temporal lobe epileptics treated since 1950, only 55%
responded favorably to medication (before carbamazepine). Of the
rest, 75% had bilateral temporal spikes (independent or synchronous),
23% had unilateral spikes and 2% had a normal record, wake and
sleep. Since the bilateral spike cases respond most poorly to medication, they would need most a new approach, such as surgery, to
rehabilitate them. However, they are not doing as well after temporal lobectomy when compared to those who had unilateral spikes.
Falconer [1] (1963) found the operation successful in only one out
of ten bitemporal cases while two out of three of his unilateral spike
patients did well. He concluded that it is best to exclude from
surgical consideration all cases of bilateral temporal spikes approaching a 50/50 parity. The idea of bitemporal lobectomy including the
hippocampus is generally discarded because of its predictable cata-
strophic effect on recent memory.

Crandall [2] and collaborators found that 30% of their patients
had unilateral temporal spikes and 36% had bilateral ones. They too
had best results with unilateral spikes as did originally Bailey et al. [3]
whose patients were seizure free after surgery in the ratio of only
one out of six when the spikes were bilateral, but one out of three
when they were unilateral.

Considerable effort has gone into the determination of the primary site in bitemporal spike cases in order to introduce more precision in delineating the area that has to be excised. In spite of this,
however, the results continue to favour heavily the unilateral cases.
For the record, one should mention the very elaborate programme

of Crandall and Walter [4] who use bilateral implanted depth electrodes, telemetered recording, observing the patients for one month,
looking for spontaneous psychomotor attacks, reproducing these at
least on three occasions with pentylenetetrazol and studying electri-
cally-induced after-discharges and corresponding seizures. Other
methods used consist of fractionated intracarotid injection of pentylenetetrazol by Gloor [5].

Tedious and hazardous as these methods may be, some vexing
problems remain. Laboratory proof is not incontrovertible that a
well identified pathology is responsible for a seizure. Even when a
depth electrode picks up the earliest manifestation of the attack,
there is no guarantee that the seizure does not originate in some other
part of the brain where no recording electrodes are in place.
Frequently after-discharges cannot be generated on the suspected side.
The excision of the primary focus sometimes increases the spike
activity in the contra-lateral secondary location rather than decreasing it. Penfield always stated that neurosurgeons do not remove
spikes. Spike activity is only a clue and even before EEG, surgery
apparently was performed with good results. In the present state
of the art, it is not surprising to read about Gibbs' [6] speculation
that "conceivably the section of fiber tracts might be more effective
in blocking spread and eliminating clinical seizure than surgery aimed
at the removal of the primary discharging areas".

A careful statistical treatment of the results, however, indicates
that the most complete sampling of spike and seizure will isolate best
the offending focus and Ajmone-Marsan et al. [7] had better results
with the more extensive rather than the limited removal of tissue.

Material and Method

This paper concerns itself with a study partly going back to 1946
when we [8] described a slow, intravenous method of injection of
pentylene tetrazol for the double purpose of activating the threshold
seizure discharge (minimal threshold EEG or MTEEG) and reproducing the focal (or temporal lobe) seizure. This was modified in
1948 by the use of I.V. drip infusion of the convulsant at 30–60 drops
per minute. A few years later sleep activation with barbiturates was
added to the routine. The latter increased the probability of spike
discharges by 100% over the wake tracing but it did not differentiate
the primary from the secondary focus with any degree of reliability.

In the late fifties, we began to substitute chlordiazepoxide
1 mg/kg for the barbiturates and this, combined with pentylene
tetrazol, gave us the best results with regard to lateralization.

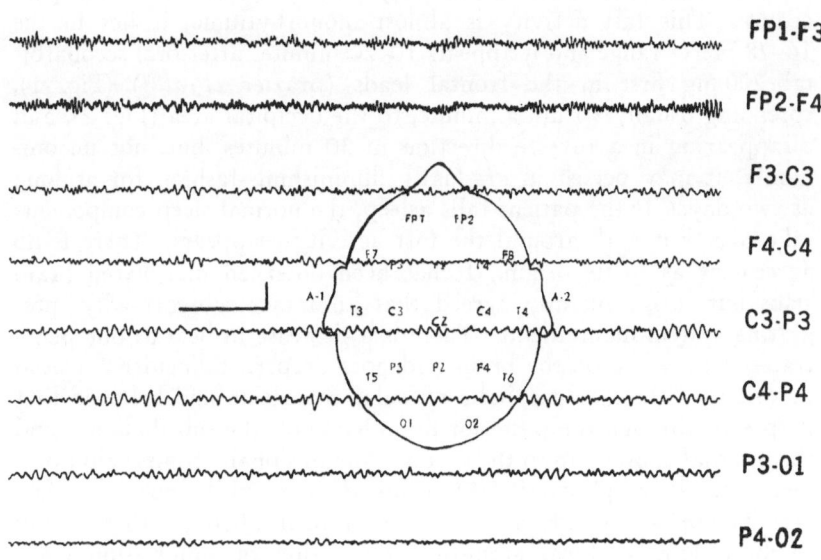

Fig. 1. Sedative-induced fast activity first appearing in the frontal leads

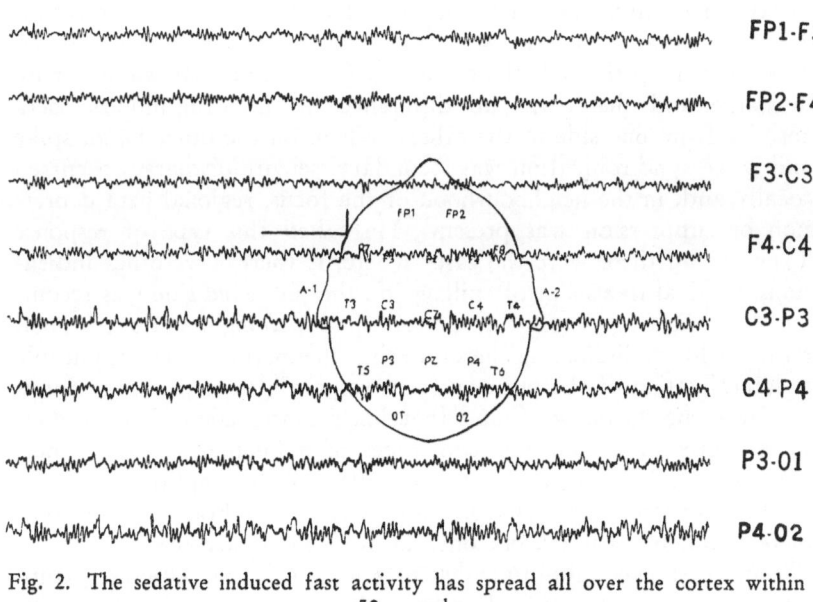

Fig. 2. The sedative induced fast activity has spread all over the cortex within 50 seconds

The sedative-induced fast activity plays a major role in this procedure. This fast activity is almost monorhythmic, it lies in the 16–28 Hertz range and it appears 10–20 minutes after oral secobarbital 200 mg first in the frontal leads (Brazier et al.[9]) (Fig. 1), spreading usually within a minute, to the occipital area (Fig. 2), and disappearing in a reverse direction in 30 minutes, but, not uncommonly, it may persist in gradually diminishing fashion for as long as two days. If the patient falls asleep, the normal sleep components take over but with arousal the fast activity reappears. There is no agreement as to its origin. It has been observed in isolated brain slabs but it is generally agreed that an intact sub-cortically integrating system maintains it. There is a decrease in beta as one penetrates the surface of the brain and goes deeper. Schneider[10] traced its origin to the mesancephalic reticular formation and believed that it spreads through the posterior hypothalamus, the sub-thalamus and the internal capsule up to the cortex. Mesancephalic transsection prevents it. Pampiglione[11] (1952) noted that while normally fast activity appears symmetrically over both hemispheres, if there is any cerebral damage, focal amplitude depression or suppression takes place.

Lombroso[12] (1970) studying bilateral spike and wave bursts, mostly in children, used I.V. thiopental to sleep-activate the record and found that if bilateral spike and wave synchronization was primary, e.g. in petit mal, there was no focal spike and wave seizure discharge and there was no difference in the drug-induced beta activity from one side to the other. When, on the other hand, spike and wave synchronization was secondary, seizure discharges occurred focally and, in the neighbourhood of the focus, regional beta depression or suppression was present. He called this type of response Type II and these were the cases where, if there were other indications, surgical treatment of epilepsy on the suspected side was recommended and, over a followup period of two to eight years, the good results held up, indicating therefore that the methods were applicable to lateralization of the primary focus responsible for partial seizures.

Over the years, we found that barbiturates commonly produce some degree of asymmetry, sometimes of a fluctuating type which, however, rarely amounts to more than 50% of the amplitude.

In 64 controls taking barbiturates who had no brain disease, complete symmetry was present only in 50%. Fast activity was absent 5% and it showed amplitude deficit in 45% (Fig. 3). Discreet pathology was commonly covered up by the very pronounced fast activity produced by I.V. barbiturates at a time when asymmetry in the normal spontaneous sleep spindles did point to the area of the lesion.

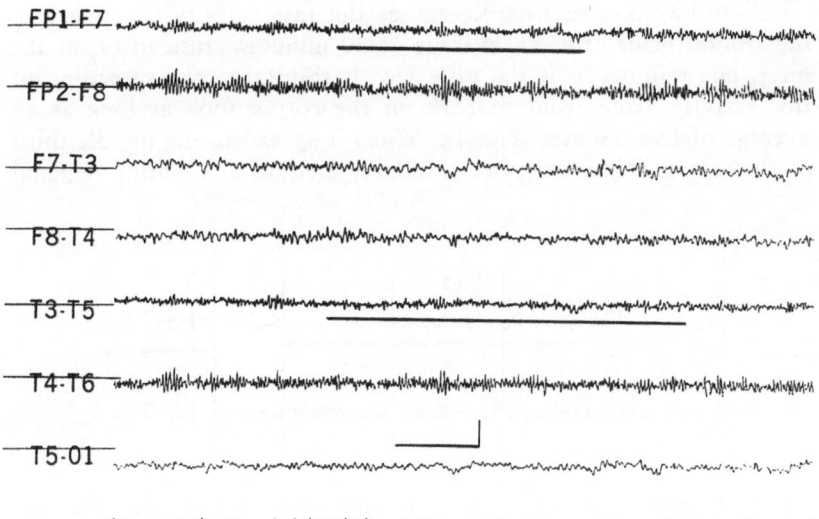

Fig. 3. Amplitude deficit in normal controls given fast acting, injectable barbiturates

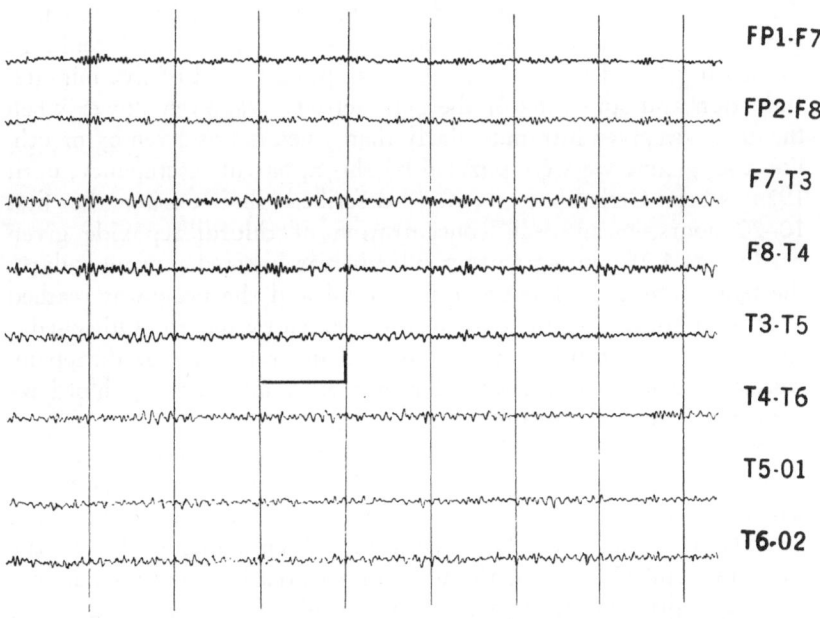

Fig. 4. Slow spreading of fast activity after chlordiazepoxide 1 mg/kg *i.m.*—without obliterating the alpha background

18*

Chlordiazepoxide 1 mg/kg causes the fast activity to appear in
the frontal leads after an average of 30 minutes. Instead of, at the
most, one minute, as is the case with barbiturates, the spreading of
this activity from front to back on the cortex took as long as an
average of five minutes (Fig. 4). When it spread to the middle third
of the cortex, it proved to be a reliable method of isolating regional

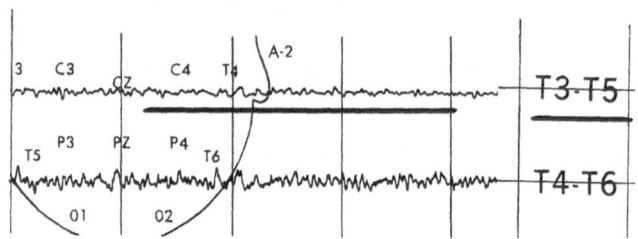

Fig. 5. Regional beta suppression in the left temporal lead after chlordiazepoxide 1 mg/kg *i.m.*

beta depression in that hemisphere which produced the primary spike
in cases of bilateral temporal lobe spikes (synchronous or indepe-
dent) (Fig. 5). The long period of spreading allowed for the emergence of even discreet focal beta depression which then could be
studied in great detail over the long sampling period of five minutes.
Induction and spreading of the beta activity was even slower when
the drug was given intramuscularly than when it was given by mouth.
For a long time we were puzzled by this apparent discrepancy, until
1974 when Greenblatt et al. [13] described that during the first
10–20 hours, mean peak concentration of chlordiazepoxide given
orally was 1.75 microgram per ml whereas injected intramuscularly
the figure was only 1 microgram per ml and the peak was reached
$1^1/_2$–$10^1/_2$ hours later than when it was given by mouth. Other seda-
tives, such as non-barbituric hypnotics, meprobamate or diazepam,
were better than barbiturates but not even approaching chlordiazepoxide in the slow spreading time.

We were especially concerned about bitemporal spikes that were
synchronous or nearly so. In animals, a primary alumina cream
seizure focus easily gives rise to a secondary "mirror" focus. It is
believed that this secondary synchrony in epileptics is due to the
constant bombardment of the uninvolved area by seizure discharges
from the primary focus which then lend the secondary area an
epileptic potentiality (Roger [14]).

Once the regional beta depression was determined by this method, within one hour, pentylenetetrazol 1⁰/o was injected by I.V. drip infusion, 60 drops per minute, in an attempt to confirm the correctness of the lateralization (Fig. 6). The average range was 150–200 mg. Both procedures were repeated a second time, when enough of the convulsant was given to reproduce the patient's habitual seizure short of the onset of automatism, which was all that the patient was able

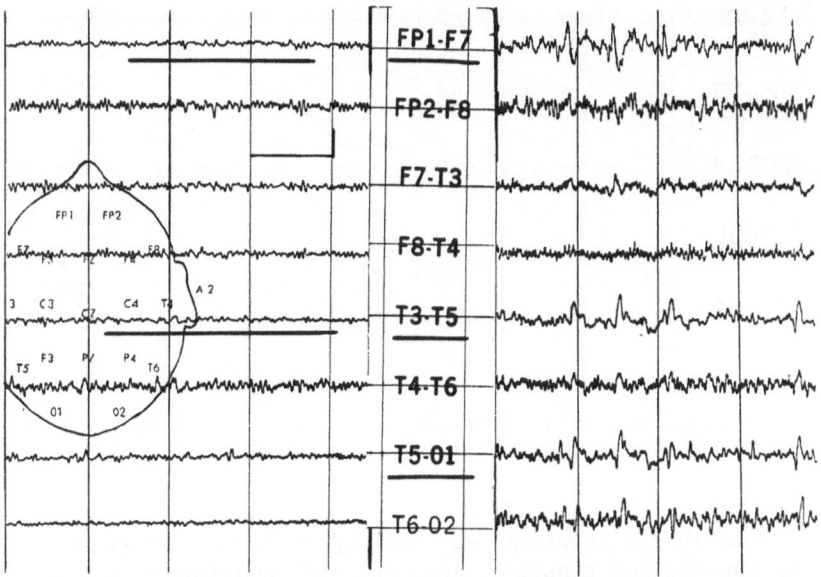

Fig. 6. On the left, left temporal beta suppression brought about by chlordiazepoxide. On the right, one hour later, lateralization to the left is confirmed by the threshold spike activity induced by pentylenetetrazol 1%

to recall. As soon as the threshold seizure discharge occurred (Fig. 7) sodium phenobarbital 130 mg was forcefully injected into the rubber tube above the intravenous needle in order to keep the patient from having a seizure. When it was our intention to have the patient reproduce his seizure, the convulsant was allowed to drip till the onset of automatism when the barbiturate was added to keep the patient from having this time a major convulsion. After the focal discharge (which may have been a fast or a slow single spike, sharp wave or multiple spike) highly synchronized spike flurries or, even more commonly, spike and dome bursts appeared in all the leads attributed to properties of the convulsant, which therefore for our purposes were useless (Fig. 8).

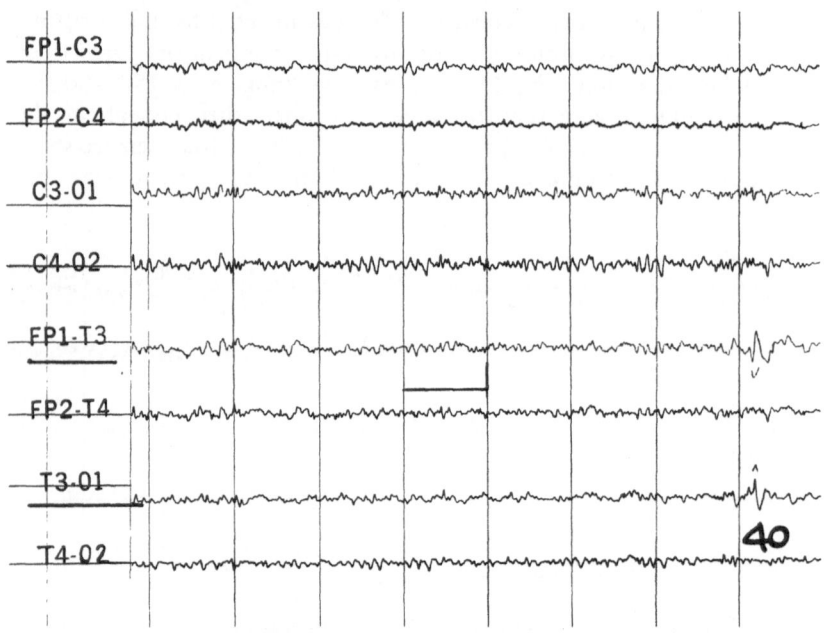

Fig. 7. Left mid-temporal threshold spike after pentylenetetrazol 1%—at the site of regional amplitude depression brought on by chlordiazepoxide 1 mg/kg *i.m.*

The chlordiazepoxide was usually sufficient to counteract the apprehension commonly accompanying pentylenetetrazol injection, and it alerted the patient enough so that within 30–60 minutes he was ambulatory.

Results

All ten patients with bitemporal spikes showed regional beta depression of more than 50% in terms of amplitude deficit or complete focal suppression of the fast activity brought on by chlordiazepoxide. In two of the ten, unilateral temporal spikes appeared, at least briefly, as the patient drifted toward sleep. In all others, the spikes were bilateral in sleep (Fig. 9). This is in contrast with the findings of Lombroso whose patients with secondarily synchronized spike and dome bursts showed the focal appearance of this type of discharge around the focus of regional beta depression with the onset of sleep.

Pentylenetetrazol activation reproduced the patient's seizure, but in one case a grand mal could not be obviated.

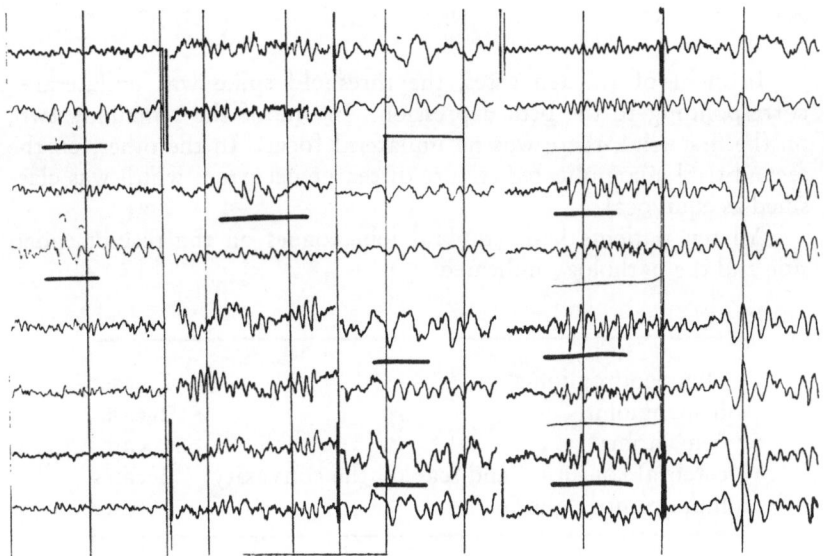

Fig. 8. The first three samples on the left show varieties of the focal temporal threshold spike after pentylenetetrazol activation. The fourth and fifth sample on the right shows the appearance of bilateral sharp wave bursts after threshold as the patient enters a clinical psychomotor attack, but before the onset of automatism

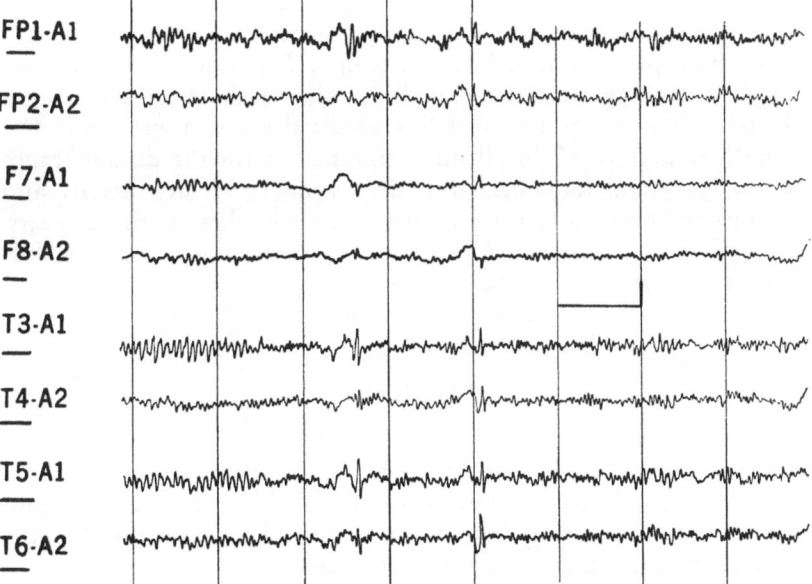

Fig. 9. As the patient drifts toward sleep, bilateral (and fairly synchronous) temporal spikes appear—after chlordiazepoxide 1 mg/kg

In eight of the ten cases, the threshold spike was unilateral— corresponding to the beta depression. In one of the remaining two, on the first trial, there was no unilateral focus. In the other, on the second trial a complicated seizure discharge occurred, which was classified as equivocal.

All ten patients had temporal lobectomies on the recommended side and the pathology indicated

oligodendroglioma	2 cases
hemangioma	2 cases
hemartoma	1 case
cerebral contusion and scar on the convexity	2 cases
hippocampal gliosis	3 cases

In the assessment of post-operative results "good" means no seizures (or no more than a couple a year) after the first year. Eight patients belonged to this category. One patient had no seizure during the first year in spite of the persistence of occasional spiking on the operated side, but then seizures resumed and averaged at the most three a year. Another, who had hippocampal gliosis and whose activated record gave the equivocal lateralization, actually has gotten worse with persistence of bilateral temporal spiking. In the remaining two cases of hippocampal gliosis, the results were good, even though spikes on the operated side persisted for two weeks and five months respectively. In all other instances, with the disappearance of the ipsilateral focal discharge, the secondary seizure activity also disappeared eventually for a follow up time of three to fifteen years. Four of the ten had grand mal seizures during the first month following surgery and all were maintained on medication which was either diphenylhydantoin or phenobarbital for at least one year.

Conclusion

Ten temporal lobe epileptics with bilateral spikes were tested with a simple non-invasive method that combines the chlordiazepoxide-induced beta asymmetry and threshold seizure discharge and seizure reproduction by 1% pentylenetetrazol infusion for the purpose of lateralizing the primary spike focus.

References

1. Falconer, M. A., Serafetidines, E. A. (1963), A follow-up study of surgery in temporal lobe epilepsy. J. Neurol. Neurosurg. Psychiat. *26*, 154—165.
2. Crandall, P. A. (1975), Postoperative management and criteria for evaluation. Advances in Neurology, Vol. 8, pp. 265—279. New York: Raven Press.
3. Bailey, P., Green, J. R., Amador, L., Gibbs, F. A. (1953), Treatment of psychomotor states by anterior temporal lobectomy. (Chapter 29 in "Psychiatric Treatment", 341—346.)
4. Walter, R. D. (1973), Tactical considerations leading to surgical treatment of limbic epilepsy. Epilepsy, its phenomena in man. Academic Press Inc., pp. 99—119.
5. Gloor, P., Rasmussen, T., Garretson, J. A. N. (1964), Fractionized intracarotid metrazol injection. Electroenceph. Clin. Neurophysiol. *17*, 322—327.
6. Gibbs, F. A., Amador, L., Rich, C. (1958), Electroencephalographic findings and therapeutic results in surgical treatment of psychomotor epilepsy. In: Temporal lobe epilepsy (Baldwin, M., and Bailey, P., eds.), p. 364. Springfield, Ill.: Ch. C Thomas.
7. Ajmone-Marsan, C., Baldwin, M. (1958), Electrocorticography. In: Temporal lobe epilepsy (Baldwin, M., and Bailey, P., eds.), pp. 368—395. Springfield, Ill.: Ch. C Thomas.
8. Ziskind, E., Bercel, N. A. (1946), Studies in convulsive thresholds in epileptics and non-epileptics. Tr. Amer. Neurol. Assoc. 1946.
9. Brazier, M. A. B., Finesinger, J. E. (1945), Action of barbiturates on the cerebral cortex. EEG study. Arch. Neurol. Psychiat. (Chicago) *53*, 51—58.
10. Schneider, J., Thomalske, G. (1956), L'éxploration pharmacodynamique cortico-sous-corticale et ses critères électrographiques. Electroenceph. Clin. Neurophysiol. *8*, 353—369.
11. Pampiglione, G. (1952), Induced fast-activity in the EEG as an aid in the location of cerebral lesions. Electroenceph. Clin. Neurophysiol. *4*, 79—82.
12. Lombroso, C., Erba, G. (1970), Primary and secondary bilateral synchrony in epilepsy. Arch. Neurol. *22*, 321—334.
13. Greenblatt, D. J. (1974), Slow absorption of intramuscular chloridiazepoxide. N. Engl. J. Med. *291*, 116—118.
14. Roger, A. R. (1955), Contribution à l'étude expérimentale de l'épilepsie partielle. Thèse de Marseille. Laval, Impr. Barneoud, 60 pp.

Author's address: Dr. N. A. Bercel, 9201 Sunset Boulevard, Los Angeles, CA 90069, U.S.A.